SKOKIE PUBLIC LIBRARY

3 1232 00685 8510

MAR   2013

RESUSCITATE!

D1314765

RESUSCITATE!

How Your Community Can Improve Survival from Sudden Cardiac Arrest

SECOND EDITION

MICKEY S. EISENBERG, M.D.

A SAMUEL AND ALTHEA STROUM BOOK

UNIVERSITY OF WASHINGTON PRESS   SEATTLE AND LONDON

This book is published with the assistance of a grant from the Samuel and Althea Stroum Endowed Book Fund.

All royalties from this book are donated to a cardiac arrest research fund at the University of Washington.

Please visit these Web sites for further information:
www.resuscitationacademy.org; www.learncpr.org; www.learnaed.org

© 2009 and 2013 by Mickey S. Eisenberg
Printed in the United States of America
Second edition, 2013
Design by Ashley Saleeba
17 16 15 14 13   5 4 3 2

All rights reserved. No part of this publication may be reproduced or transmitted in any form or by any means, electronic or mechanical, including photocopy, recording, or any information storage or retrieval system, without permission in writing from the publisher.

University of Washington Press
P.O. Box 50096, Seattle, WA 98145 U.S.A. www.washington.edu/uwpress

Library of Congress Cataloging-in-Publication Data
Resuscitate! : how your community can improve survival from sudden cardiac arrest / Mickey S. Eisenberg. - 2nd ed.
p. ; cm. "A Samuel and Althea Stroum book."
Includes bibliographical references and index.
ISBN 978-0-295-99246-4 (pbk. : alk. paper)
I. Title.
[DNLM: 1. Cardiopulmonary Resuscitation. 2. Heart Arrest—therapy. 3. Community Health Services. 4. Death, Sudden, Cardiac—prevention & control. 5. Emergency Medical Services. WG 205]
616.1'23025—dc23   2012035732

The paper used in this publication is acid-free and meets the minimum requirements of American National Standard for Information Sciences—Permanence of Paper for Printed Library Materials, ANSI Z39.48–1984.∞

Contents

Foreword by Roger D. White, M.D. ix
Preface to the Second Edition xi
Acknowledgments xv
Guide to Terminology xix

ONE   How We Die Suddenly 1
TWO   A History of Resuscitation 19
THREE   Causes of Sudden Cardiac Death 44
FOUR   A Profile of Sudden Cardiac Arrest 58
FIVE   Who Will Live and Who Will Die? 77
SIX   Location, Location, Location: Best Places to Have a Cardiac Arrest 120
SEVEN   What Can Your Community Do? 150
EIGHT   A Completed Life 160
NINE   Putting It All Together 168
TEN   A Plan of Action 175
ELEVEN   A Vision of the Future 209

Addendum: Resuscitation Academy 221

Notes 229
Index 257

To the emergency dispatchers, emergency medical technicians, and paramedics of Seattle and King County. I admire and applaud your professionalism. You are the best.

And to the faculty of the Resuscitation Academy. Thank you for your hard work in providing the knowledge and skills so that other communities throughout the nation and the world can improve survival from cardiac arrest.

Resuscitation Academy

The Resuscitation Academy is offered twice a year in Seattle and is provided tuition free. It is sponsored by Seattle Medic One, King County Emergency Medical Services, and the Medic One Foundation. Support is also provided by the University of Washington, Harborview Medical Center, Seattle Fire Department, Public Health—Seattle and King County, Asmund S. Laerdal Foundation for Acute Medicine, Life Sciences Discovery Fund, and the Medtronic Foundation HeartRescue Program.

The tag line for the Academy is "Improving cardiac arrest survival—one community at a time." Lectures and hands-on workshops provide attendees with the tools to transform cardiac arrest resuscitation in their home communities. *Resuscitate!* serves as the textbook for the Academy. Supplementing the textbook is a comprehensive set of tool kits for establishing a cardiac arrest registry, high-performance CPR, dispatcher-assisted telephone CPR, police defibrillation, community public access defibrillation, end of life issues, and foundation and fund raising. The tool kits provide the details and supporting documentation and material on how to implement the various programs. Copies of all tool kits, as well as information about the Resuscitation Academy and how to register for a future class, may be found at resuscitationacademy.org. The kits and all material on the Web site are available at no charge.

Foreword

Cardiac arrest occurs in people's homes as well as in public places. It can strike anytime. For decades, it has been the leading cause of death among adults. Given the magnitude of this public health problem, you might suppose that the highest priority of emergency medical services (EMS) would be to improve survival rates. It is true that EMS systems in a few communities do manage cardiac arrest reasonably well. Regrettably, however, most do not. In fact, if you were to suffer sudden cardiac arrest while on vacation in some cities, you would be *dozens of times* more likely to die than if you had gone on vacation somewhere else.

What accounts for this amazing variance in rates of survival? In this book, Mickey Eisenberg, an expert EMS medical director, gives you the answers, and he lays out a specific action plan consisting of fifteen steps for EMS systems that are serious about raising survival rates in their communities. The book, intended for Dr. Eisenberg's fellow medical directors and for EMS administrators as well as for elected officials and concerned citizens, outlines what all of us can do to help more people survive sudden cardiac arrest. If you care about sudden cardiac arrest in your community, and about how your community's EMS system is responding to this critical emergency, I can think of no more important book for you to read than this one.

Nor can I think of anyone more qualified to have written it than Mickey Eisenberg. He has been conducting research since 1975 on how communities manage cardiac arrest in King County, Washington, where he established one of the world's first community-level surveillance programs for cardiac arrest. But he didn't stop there. Not content just to measure and chronicle cardiac arrest, Dr. Eisenberg also took what he had learned and used that information to found innovative programs aimed at improving survival rates. In 1980, he and his colleagues began the first program in the world to let emergency medical technicians (not just paramedics) perform defibrillation, and shortly thereafter they started the world's first systematic program for emergency dispatchers to tell callers over the phone how to perform cardiopulmonary resuscitation while waiting for help to arrive. The published research stemming from these two programs alone has had a profound impact on EMS care, and the paradigms for both programs are now universally accepted and endorsed by international organizations. Dr. Eisenberg and his research team have also explored innovative methods of teaching CPR and defibrillation to the public. They continue to push the envelope of resuscitation from sudden cardiac arrest, and as the authors of more than 150 scientific articles on the topic, they are widely recognized as leaders in research and education related to the field.

Dr. Eisenberg names three communities as having high rates of survival for cardiac arrest—the city of Seattle, the greater King County area, and my own community of Rochester, Minnesota. The book describes, in very accessible language, the reasons for these communities' success. Their EMS systems have several things in common— strong medical and administrative leadership, high-quality training and continuing education, continuous quality improvement, high expectations—all of which add up to an uncompromising culture of excellence, one in which the question on everyone's lips is always "How can we do better?" If you take this book to heart, so to speak, I guarantee that you will improve survival rates in your community, too.

ROGER D. WHITE M.D., F.A.C.C., MAYO CLINIC
Department of Anesthesiology and Division of Cardiovascular Diseases,
Department of Internal Medicine
Medical Director, City of Rochester and Olmsted County Early Defibrillation Program
Co-Medical Director, Gold Cross Ambulance Service, Rochester, Minnesota

Preface to the Second Edition

In my line of work there is nothing more gratifying than speaking with a survivor of sudden cardiac arrest. Survivors are, needless to say, extremely grateful to their rescuers. The most common question they ask is how they can thank the people who saved their life. The rescuers are the people who are part of the EMS system and respond to the emergency—the dispatchers who help with telephone CPR instructions, the EMTs who perform CPR and deliver defibrillatory shocks, and the paramedics who provide airway control and medications. It is unfortunate that among those who have cardiac arrest, survivors comprise the minority—and in most communities throughout the nation a very, very small minority. When the patient dies we should ask why? Was death inevitable? Did the system fail? Was there something we could have done better? How can we improve? That's what this book is all about—to provide the knowledge and tools to improve.

Perhaps only 1 percent of all calls to 911 involve attempted resuscitation from sudden cardiac arrest, but this 1 percent brings into play everything that is good and everything that is not so good about a community's EMS system. The elements of care needed to resuscitate a victim of cardiac arrest are the same ones needed to help the victim of a car crash, a child with severe asthma, or people with other medical and traumatic emergencies. Every improvement in the treatment of sudden cardiac arrest benefits everyone who will ever need emergency care. And that's why an EMS system's management of cardiac arrest serves as a surrogate for the system itself. In short, survival from cardiac arrest is the metric upon which an entire EMS system's quality may be judged.

The book is for the people—medical and administrative directors, fire chiefs, dispatch directors, and program supervisors—who direct and run EMS systems all across the country. But it will also have value for paramedics, EMTs, training officers, dispatchers, nurses, doctors, and other EMS professionals, as well as for elected officials, health services researchers, healthcare administrators, and ordinary concerned citizens. Because not every chapter will be equally relevant to every reader, those familiar with emergency medical services and resuscitation can skim or skip chapters 1–3. Those really pressed for time should read chapters 7, 9, and 10.

Chapter 1, "How We Die Suddenly," describes sudden cardiac arrest and laments its generally low survival rates and its diversity in survival throughout the United States.

Chapter 2, "A History of Resuscitation," gives a brief account of resuscitation starting with Biblical times and ending with how modern emergency medical services came to pass.

Chapter 3, "The Causes of Sudden Cardiac Arrest," describes the common and uncommon causes of this event.

Chapter 4, "A Profile of Sudden Cardiac Arrest," provides demographics and elements of successful resuscitation and goes into some detail characterizing the time elements involved in providing care for cardiac arrest patients.

Chapter 5, "Who Will Live and Who Will Die," identifies fifty factors associated with the likelihood of surviving or not surviving cardiac arrest. They are grouped into patient, event, system, and therapy factors and do much to explain why communities succeed or fail in the management of cardiac arrest.

Chapter 6, "Location, Location, Location: Best Places to Have a Cardiac Arrest," gives details on the EMS systems in Seattle and King County, WA, and Rochester, MN, and profiles leaders in these EMS programs.

Chapter 7, "What Can Your Community Do?" challenges a community to assess its own performance with a Community Report Card.

Chapter 8, "A Completed Life," poses the difficult question of who should be resuscitated, on the assumption that not everyone in cardiac arrest should be brought back to life.

Chapter 9, "Putting It All Together," provides a framework for successful programs.

Chapter 10, "An Action Plan," provides a specific path with 15 concrete steps toward improvement. and lays out 4 immediate steps a community can take to improve survival. The first edition of *Resuscitate!* included 25 steps, but from listening to EMS administrators and medical directors, I have pared down and refocused the list to 15 steps. The national steps remain the most challenging to accomplish; they are included because I think attention must continue to be focused on the need for these changes, however difficult they may be.

Chapter 11, "A Vision of the Future," describes both a short-term and a long-term vision. Currently, the national survival rate from cardiac arrest is abysmally low, yet it can be raised considerably higher. Though I may be constitutionally optimistic, I hope my vision is solidly based in reality. Time will tell.

Shortly after the publication of the first edition of *Resuscitate!* in 2009, my colleagues and I had the opportunity to put its lessons and principles to the test. We started the Resuscitation Academy. The Academy is a partnership between King County EMS, Seattle Medic One, and the Medic One Foundation and is held in Seattle (more information about the Academy is found in the addendum and at resuscitationacademy.org). We offer two academies a year and, though the length varies slightly, the typical academy is two days. Each class has about 30–40 attendees—primarily EMS managers, medical directors, QI officers, and EMS training officers. They have come from throughout the United States and from nine other nations, representing the spectrum of EMS systems from large urban programs to tiny rural volunteer EMS organizations. We are pleased to see the concept spreading with state and regional Resuscitation Academies springing up.

It is always a question as to whether change best starts from the top or from the bottom. Though both probably happen, I think lasting change occurs mostly from the bottom up—the seeds of change have to germinate on soil tended by local leaders and local residents. The Resuscitation Academy attendees have taught me much, not only about the diversity of EMS systems but also about real world challenges EMS managers face—realities compounded by increasing demand and falling resources. The real joy of teaching at the Academy is twofold: first, I get to mount my soapbox and orate about the elements of successful resuscitation and, second, I get to learn about the barriers to implementation. Every attendee at the academy wants to improve survival in his or her own community, but it is painfully apparent, as I learn from the alumni who report back on their efforts, that change is hard. Yet improvements are happening and slowly more and more lives are being snatched from the jaws of death. As my colleague Tom Rea, MD, makes clear at each Academy, change happens only gradually. Don't expect to transform your system overnight. Realize that improvement occurs tiny step by tiny step. It is humbling but true.

So I thank the attendees for all they have taught me. With this second edition of *Resuscitate!* I have included lessons learned from the Resuscitation Academy, as well as my own evolving thoughts on how to improve survival from sudden cardiac arrest, one community at a time. This edition contains entirely new material in chapters 9, 10, and 11 and includes an extensive Addendum on the Resuscitation Academy. I hope you will attend a future Academy and we can meet in person.

MICKEY S. EISENBERG, M.D., PH.D.
Seattle, Washington

Acknowledgments

Let me begin by expressing my appreciation to the people who make it all possible—the hundreds of emergency dispatchers, the thousands of EMTs, and the hundreds of paramedics in Seattle and King County. Special thanks also to the dispatch directors, fire chiefs, and training officers. We have a wonderful EMS system, and it is all because of you. I am so proud of the great work you do.

I am indebted to dozens of colleagues and research staff whom I have had the pleasure of knowing and working with over the past thirty-six years. They include Alan Abe, Mary Alice Allenbach, Dan Anderson, Elena Andresen, Felisa Azpitarte, Lance Becker, Deborah Berger, Larry Bergner, the late Marilyn Bergner, Jennifer Blackwood, Barbara Blake, Megan Bloomingdale, Jim Boehl, Bosaiya (who provided many of the figures that appear in this book), Cynthia Bradshaw, Allan Braslow, Margaret Brownell, Dean Brooke, Byron Byrne, Tony Cagle, David Carlbom, Bill Carter, Douglas Chamberlain, Fred Chapman, Helen Chatalas, Al Church, Jill Clark, Don Cloyd, Linda Culley, Richard Cummins, Cip Dacanay, Marlys Davis, Paul Davison, Susan Damon, Gregory Dean, Paula Diehr, Leah Doctorello, Eric Dulberg, Jim Duren, Daniel Eisenberg, David Eisenberg, Devora Eisenberg, Tom Evans, Carol Fahrenbruch, Sylvia Feder, David Fleming, Rob Galbraith, Gayle Garson, Laurie Gold, Tom Gudmestad, Wendy Guirl, Al Hallstrom, Valerie Harris, Blake Harrison, Jerris Hedges, Dan Henwood, John Herbert, Mary Ho, Cynthia Horton, Betty Hurtado, Brooke Ike, John Jerin, Dave Jones, Dawn Jorgensen, Noa Kay, Art Kellerman, Rudy Koster, Paula Lank, Mary Pat Larsen, Xich Le, Marty LeFave, Michelle Lightfoot, Paul Litwin, Jim Logerfo, Gianna Malo, Jill Marsden, Chuck Maynard, Jim Moore, Ken Moralee, Carl Morgan, Mark Moulton, Jack Murray, Eugene Nagel, Bill Newbold, Graham Nichol, Bud Nicole, Chris

Niels, Bob Niskanen, Jon Nolan, Irit Nuri, Jeanne O'Brien, Steve Olmstead, Michele Ol-sufka, Gil Omenn, Joe Ornato, Hoke Overland, Steve Perry, Randi Phelps, Judy Pierce, Alonzo Plough, Judy Prentice, Ron Quinsey, Sally Ragsdale, Mike Remington, Karen Rodriquez, Jim Russell, Jim Schneider, Dmitry Sharkov, Larry Sherman, Jenny Shin, Floyd Short, Jennifer Silver, Terry Sinclair, Greg Sinibaldi, Tishawna Smith, David Snyder, Debi Solberg, Gary Somers, Jim Stallings, Susan Stern, Jared Strote, Cleo Subi-do, Ben Stubbs, Jesse Tapp, Dorothy Teeter, the late Tom Torrell, Nicole Urban, Terry Valenzuela, Jeremy Ward, Sam Warren, Rebecca Watson (who provided several figures for the book), Roy Waugh, Douglas Weaver, Mary Weirich, Barbara Welles, Lindsay White, Roger White, Adrian Whorton, Mary Won, Lihua Yin, and Jean Yoshihara.

Special acknowledgment goes to a handful of people. First of all, my thanks to Leonard Cobb and Michael Copass; our EMS system and its high standards would not exist without these two remarkable individuals, and I could not wish for better men-tors, teachers, and colleagues. Another special thanks to Tom Hearne, who for three decades supported and nurtured the partnership between University of Washington faculty members and the EMS Division of Public Health—Seattle and King County. After Tom's untimely death in 2010, Michele Plorde stepped in to keep a steady course as interim director. Beginning in 2011, Jim Fogarty's leadership continues the strong bond between the University and the EMS Division. I also owe a huge debt of gratitude to Sheri Rowe, who coordinated our research projects for thirty years, and to Linda Becker, who has managed the cardiac arrest surveillance system for thirty-six years (and who provided the data from King County that are used in the book); we have shared much as we've watched our system evolve from its infancy to its current matu-rity. I am fortunate to work side by side with Mike Helbock, who has transformed EMS education in King County; I admire his skills as a master educator, and I value his ex-perience and wisdom. Hendrika Meischke has taught me the skills of health services research; her social science perspective has added a new dimension to our research, for which I am grateful.

I am lucky to count as the closest of my colleagues Tom Rea and Peter Kudenchuk, two physicians whom I greatly respect; Tom and Peter represent the next generation of researchers, educators, and medical directors who will maintain and even improve the culture of excellence in our system, and I am confident that they will help define the standard of care for resuscitation in the coming decades. A very special thanks to Tore Laerdal, a fellow traveler in the quest to reverse sudden death, for unwavering support and friendship over the past three decades. I greatly admire his recent efforts to reduce infant mortality and perinatal mortality in developing countries.

And last, let me offer heartfelt thanks to the leadership of the Resuscitation Acade-my. In addition to Drs. Copass, Cobb, Rea, and Kudenchuk, Jonathan Larsen and Norm Nedell (captain and senior paramedic, respectively, in the Seattle Fire Department) provide strong leadership in the Academy and help cement the partnership between

Seattle Medic One and the King County EMS Division. Jan Sprake, executive director of the Seattle Medic One Foundation and also faculty for the Academy, provides keys insights in how to fund the extra margin of excellence for any EMS program. Michael Sayre, a recent transplant from Columbus, Ohio, adds new enthusiasm and ideas to the Academy. Ann Doll, who is the executive director of the Resuscitation Academy and also manager of the Medical QI Section in the EMS Division, brings competence and vitality to everything she tackles. She is a joy to work with. It is conceivable we could have an Academy without her leadership but it would be a pale comparison to the one she has helped create.

Our research over the past thirty-six years would not have been possible without generous grant support from the National Heart, Lung, and Blood Institute, the Agency for Healthcare Research and Quality, the Medic One Foundation, the Medtronic Foundation HeartRescue Program, and the State of Washington Life Sciences Development Fund. I am also most appreciative of the Laerdal Foundation for Acute Medicine, Philips Healthcare, and Physio Control for unrestricted grants in support of our research efforts.

Special thanks to the University of Washington Press, especially to Pat Soden, who believed in the value of this project, and to Xavier Callahan, Jacqueline Ettinger, Beth Fuget, Dustin Kilgore, Rachael Levay, Ashley Saleeba, and Marilyn Trueblood who helped turn a sow's ear into (dare I say?) a silk purse.

And last, first, and always, thanks to Jeanne—my partner in this amazing journey called life.

Guide to Terminology

ACS — acute coronary syndrome. An unstable condition ranging from increasing or unstable angina to acute myocardial infarction. ACS usually occurs in individuals with underlying coronary artery disease.

AED — automated external defibrillator. AEDs are used primarily by EMTs and first responders (see below) such as police. They are increasingly being found in public locations such as airports, malls, exercise facilities, etc.

ALS — advanced life support. Refers to the level of care provided by paramedics (see below).

Asystole — without contraction and synonymous with flat line. There is no electrical signal or heart muscle contraction.

BLS — basic life support. Refers to the level of care provided by basic EMTs (see below).

CAD — coronary artery disease. Other terms with the same meaning are atherosclerotic heart disease or ischemic heart disease (which implies that the patient has symptoms of angina).

Dispatchers are specifically designated by their role within a communications center. The call receiver speaks with the person calling 911 and offers telephone CPR instructions. The dispatcher receives the location information from the call receiver and dispatches the proper units. In small centers both roles are wrapped up in one individual. I use the term dispatchers for both roles since this is how the general public thinks of these individuals. The term **telecommunicators** is also used for dispatchers and call receivers. In King County dispatchers receive 40 hours of training, specifically in medical emergencies (this is above the training required for general dispatching) and must complete 8 hours of emergency medical continuing education every year. Many community colleges and private companies offer preparatory training for employment in public safety emergency communications centers. Because of differing computer-aided dispatch systems, most communication centers offer their own extensive in-house training program.

DOA — dead on arrival. EMTs and paramedics (see below) are allowed not to begin resuscitation in patients for whom there is no chance of success. These patients are termed DOA. They are cool to the touch and have pooling of blood in dependent portions of the body. This pooling and discoloration of the skin is termed lividity.

DNR — do not resuscitate. Patients who express end-of-life wishes and choose not to be resuscitated in the event of a cardiac arrest are DNR patients. Whenever possible EMTs and paramedics attempt to determine whether the patient has expressed end-of-life wishes and to respect these desires. See chapter 8 for further discussion of DNR.

EMS — emergency medical service(s). EMS involves the spectrum of community-based emergency services ranging from emergency dispatch centers and prehospital emergency response agencies to emergency departments, as well as to the communication links that bind all these components into a system. Though EMS comprises the totality of care from 911 to hospital emergency department, in common use it refers to the prehospital components of the larger spectrum. This book uses the more common definition for EMS to denote the prehospital component of emergency care.

EMT refers to a basic emergency medical technician, sometimes called **EMT-B**. The training for an EMT-B consists of a 110-hour national curriculum published by the Department of Transportation. EMTs can provide CPR, manage an airway with oral airways and bag valve masks, and defibrillate using automated external defibrillators. There are also intermediate EMTs (EMT-I) who are trained in IV skills, medication administration (such as nitroglycerine), and airway control beyond what basic EMTs can provide. In Seattle and King County, intermediate EMTs are not part of the EMS system.

First responders is an ambiguous term because it can refer to uniformed individuals with a duty to respond to emergencies when they encounter them. Thus, police and security guards are often referred to as first responders, especially when they arrive at the scene prior to EMTs or paramedics. The term also refers to uniformed individuals who have completed a formal 40-hour training program using a curriculum published by DOT. These individuals are certified as First Responders (capital F, capital R). Though police may be called first responders, they usually have not completed the First Responder training or certification.

MI and **AMI** are used interchangeably and denote myocardial infarction and acute myocardial infarction, respectively. Technically, an MI can be old or acute and the context usually clarifies the matter. "He is having an MI" refers to an AMI. "He has a history of an MI" means he has an old MI.

Paramedics are trained to the highest level and can do all that EMTs can do, as well as start IVs (peripheral and central lines), administer medications, intubate, and take 12-lead electrocardiograms. The term **EMT-P** also refers to paramedics. The above categories are not perfectly demarcated and will vary from state to state. For example, some communities authorize basic EMTs to take 12-lead ECGs or perform glucometry (determining blood glucose using a drop of blood and a glucose meter).

PEA — pulseless electrical activity. PEA is one of the three major rhythm disturbances associated with cardiac arrest (the others being VF and asystole). PEA is defined as organized electrical activity as seen on the ECG or cardiac monitor but no pump function. The patient has no pulse or blood pressure and the prognosis is terrible.

PSAP — public safety answering point. This is where your call to 911 goes. There are dfferences between the primary and the secondary PSAP. The primary PSAP answers the 911 call and sometimes may send it to a secondary PSAP for the proper vehicles to be dispatched. For example, in Seattle the primary PSAP answers the 911 call and determines if it is a police, fire, or medical emergency. If it is a fire or medical emergency, the PSAP transfers the call to the secondary PSAP, which is located at a different site. Often the call-receiving function (answering the 911 call and determining the nature of the emergency) and the dispatching function (actually sending the units) are located within a PSAP but handled by two different individuals.

QI — quality improvement. QI is synonymous with quality assurance (QA). The QI process is straightforward—namely, to objectively examine performance and see if improvements are needed. Once the improvements are in place, reexamine the performance to see if things are better. In this regard QI is a continuous process—measure, improve, measure, improve. . . . Medical QI merely means the QI effort is applied to medical matters.

Resuscitation is an attempt to revive a person in cardiac arrest. It is also used to indicate a successful outcome from cardiac arrest. I will try to be clear as to which meaning is being used in the text. For example, "he was resuscitated" is ambiguous unless further clarified. Better to state, "He was successfully resuscitated."

SCA and **SCD** — sudden cardiac arrest and sudden cardiac death. These terms are used interchangeably. Unless otherwise indicated, cardiac arrest also refers to sudden cardiac arrest.

Seattle Medic One is the term for the Seattle paramedic program. The Medic One name has been co-opted by the other paramedic providers in King County. Medic One has become a generic term for paramedic services and is used by other paramedic services throughout the country.

Seattle is the largest city in **King County**, Washington. There are approximately 600,000 people in Seattle and another 1,400,000 in the surrounding suburban and rural areas of King County. Seattle is the industrial and commercial hub for the county, although several suburban cities such as Bellevue, Redmond, and Renton have growing industrial and office complexes. Boeing (technically, Boeing moved its headquarters to Chicago), Microsoft, Amazon, Starbucks, Costco, and the University of Washington all have their homes here. During business hours the population of Seattle swells by approximately 100,000 because of workers traveling downtown and because of students and staff heading to the University of Washington (located in the north part of Seattle) and other colleges in the city.

The Seattle Fire Department administers the Seattle paramedic program. The King County paramedic program is a mixed fire department/health department system. There are four fire department based paramedic agencies, and one health department paramedic agency in the county. The health department helps administer all regional services for the county including the coordination of BLS services with the thirty county fire departments. Though the EMS systems in Seattle and King County are administered differently they are essentially identical. Seattle's program began in 1970 and the King County program was implemented sequentially over six years from 1973–1979. The King County program purposely replicates the Seattle program. The paramedics in the city and county are trained the same, use the same standing orders, have the same continuing education requirements, have similar medical control, and provide the same care. In fact, the survival rate from cardiac arrest is almost identical in the Seattle and King County systems. In this book I use the two systems synonymously since they are for all practical purposes one system.

Success is defined in this book as "discharged alive." Thus "successfully resuscitated" or "a successful resuscitation," as used in this book, means an effort was undertaken to revive the person in cardiac arrest, it led to the person being revived, and the person was discharged from the hospital. Just to be perfectly clear, discharged from hospital is used in the conventional sense to mean discharged alive. I suppose a patient could be discharged to a morgue or funeral home but this is a rather unconventional use of the term.

Survived cardiac arrest or survivor of cardiac arrest means that a person was discharged alive from the hospital. Being successfully resuscitated only to die in the hospital is a pyrrhic victory.

VF — ventricular fibrillation. VF is the most common rhythm associated with cardiac arrest and is also the rhythm with the highest likelihood of successful resuscitation. I will try to make the distinction throughout the text between VF cardiac arrest (also VF sudden cardiac arrest and VF sudden cardiac death) and cardiac arrest in general (which includes all rhythms associated with cardiac arrest, VF, and other rhythms). This is important because the possibility of survival is much greater with VF SCA. Clearly it would be misleading to compare survival rates from VF SCA in one city to SCA survival (from all rhythms) in another, since the denominators would be completely different and have different possibilities of success.

ONE

How We Die Suddenly

CARDIAC ARREST

REDMOND, WASHINGTON

Peter A. had been doing fine, considering. He and his wife, Joanna, had been enjoying his retirement from Boeing, and they found the suburban community of Redmond, Washington—close to Seattle and its urban attractions, but with the advantage of quiet streets and large lots—perfect for them. Their yard was big enough for Joanna to pursue her hobby of butterfly- and bird-attractive gardening.

For Peter, on this afternoon, lifting heavy bags of steer manure for Joanna's garden had directly triggered another episode of the vague, intermittent ache that he had been experiencing in his upper left arm, mostly when he climbed stairs. This episode, though, was more severe than previous ones, and Peter felt somewhat nauseated. He also felt the ache radiating into the left side of his jaw. But it was his overwhelming sense of fatigue that prompted him to go back inside and lie down on the couch in the living room.

One month before, Peter's doctor had told him that his cholesterol had crept up to the "needing treatment" point, and that his blood glucose now placed him in the prediabetic range. But more disturbing had been his doctor's concern that the ache in Peter's left arm might be related to his heart. Peter's cardiogram had been normal, a result in which he had taken some solace, so he had continued to put off the treadmill test recommended by his doctor. He wanted to believe that the statin medication he had started taking to lower his cholesterol must be working—it certainly cost enough! And though he hadn't lost any weight, as his doctor had also recommended, it seemed to him that the ache in his arm had become less frequent.

Joanna, from her vantage in the den, saw Peter enter the house, and she knew from his slow gait and the way he half-collapsed into the couch that something was wrong. She rushed to his side and tried to control her panic as she noted his limp body, the pasty coloring on his face, and the bluish cast of his lips.

"Peter!" she shouted, shaking him by the shoulders.

He didn't respond.

With great presence of mind, Joanna brought the portable phone to Peter's side as she called 911.

"911 operator," came the voice on the other side of the line. "What are you reporting?"

"My husband has collapsed. He's not moving."

The emergency dispatcher quickly asked Joanna where she was calling from. Thanks to his training, he knew right away that he should send a full medic response, which he accomplished by typing the directions to Peter's house into his computer console and pressing several buttons on a "tone out" dispatching machine. As he did all this, the dispatcher continued to ask questions.

"Is he conscious?"

"No," Joanna replied.

"Is he breathing normally?"

Joanna looked at her husband. Peter was taking breaths that were more like slow grunts—definitely not normal. She told the dispatcher what she was seeing and hearing. From Joanna's description, the dispatcher knew that she was reporting agonal respirations—the kind of breathing associated with cardiac arrest, a sign of the brain's last-gasp effort to send breathing signals to the lungs. He also knew that there was little air moving in or out.

"Do you know CPR?" he asked Joanna. "Cardiopulmonary resuscitation?"

Joanna did not.

"OK," the dispatcher said. "I'm going to give you some instructions. First, pull on his feet, and drag him onto the floor. Now lift his chin, so his head tilts back. Pinch his nose shut, seal your lips over his, and blow two deep breaths into his lungs, just like you're blowing up a balloon. Watch his chest rise. Now move your hands to the center of his chest, one hand on top of the other, right between the nipples, and press down firmly, fifteen times. I'll count for you.[1] That's it. Keep doing it, now. Two more breaths."

In the background, over the phone, the dispatcher heard the Redmond Fire Department's sirens, and he told Joanna to open her front door. She did, and she saw the fire department's emergency medical personnel already running up the driveway, carrying heavy suitcases. It had seemed like an eternity to Joanna, but the two emergency medical technicians, or EMTs, had arrived within four minutes of the dispatcher's "tone out." The regional Medic Unit, staffed by paramedics, was also on the way.

It was obvious to the EMTs that Peter was in cardiac arrest—an experienced firefighter in the EMT role doesn't really need to shake the person or even check for a pulse, though protocol does require a pulse check. The EMTs placed their cases next to Peter and knelt down, one on each side of his head. One of the EMTs started CPR. He positioned Peter's head, placed a face mask attached to an air bag over Peter's mouth and nose, compressed the bag to push two deep breaths into Peter's lungs, glancing sideways to make sure his lungs were rising, and then repositioned himself to administer fifteen chest compressions. Meanwhile, the other EMT unzipped a smaller case. Inside was a gray plastic box about the size of a hardcover book—an automated external defibrillator, or AED. He opened the box, which contained two small square pads, and pressed a green button. The button lit up. Joanna was surprised to hear a commanding voice come from inside the box.

Attach the two pads to the chest, the mechanized voice said.

The EMT did as instructed.

Plug in the connector.

The EMT did so.

Assessing rhythm. Do not touch the patient.

Both EMTs moved back. After ten seconds, the voice spoke again. *Shock required. Stand back. Press the flashing orange button.* An orange button, labeled with a bolt of lightning icon, began to flash insistently.

Again the EMT followed the instructions. Joanna was startled to see her husband's chest jump up an inch as electricity flowed from the AED and passed between the two pads.

The EMTs allowed the defibrillator to make another assessment of the heart's rhythm. This time the machine's message was different.

No shock required. Check pulse. Check breathing. If needed, begin CPR.

The EMT who had been doing CPR placed his fingers on Peter's neck. "I've got a pulse," he said to his partner.

Joanna finally allowed herself to take a breath. One minute later, the paramedics arrived, and the EMTs briefed them on what had happened.

NEW YORK CITY

Clarence B. had not been doing well lately. His doctor had been treating him for heart failure due to longstanding coronary artery disease, and Clarence's weekly tray of medications contained a rainbow of pills compartmentalized into six separate "feedings" over the course of each day.

Earlier in the week, Clarence's doctor had e-mailed him about a recent study showing that a patient like Clarence might benefit from an implantable defibrillator. The doctor suggested that Clarence schedule an appointment to talk about it. Clarence had read about these devices in the newspaper, and he knew that they cost a fortune. He wondered how much of the cost would be covered by Medicare. He had asked his doctor about a heart transplant at one point and had not really been surprised to learn that his age disqualified him. He had wondered at the time if the decision was based on chronological or biological age—Clarence looked and felt a decade older than his seventy years.

When Clarence's symptoms began, their onset must have been very gradual—almost imperceptible initially. Perhaps he just had a little more difficulty breathing. At first he may have attributed the trouble to a mild stomach upset. But as it got worse and worse, he would have found himself leaning forward to try to take in more air. Soon beads of perspiration would have been covering his forehead.

However his symptoms began, Clarence managed to ring his neighbor and ask for help. By the time his neighbor got down the corridor to Clarence's apartment, there was no answer, and the neighbor had to run back to his own apartment to get the key Clarence had given him. When he finally entered, Clarence was on the floor. The neighbor dialed 911 and waited fourteen minutes for the paramedics to arrive. When they hooked Clarence up to the defibrillator, Clarence's heart was already flatlining. There was nothing to be done.

PLATTSBURG, MISSOURI

Margaret and Sidney J. were retired from farming, but they still lived on their farm, renting most of the land to other farmers who grew alfalfa and wheat. It was only a ten-minute drive from the farm to Main Street in Plattsburg, a town with a population of 5,000 that lies halfway between Kansas City and St. Joseph.

Plattsburg's fire department was staffed by full-time professionals during the day shift, but the evening and night shifts were staffed by volunteer firefighters and volunteer EMTs. This arrangement was typical of small towns that simply do not have the tax base or volume of calls to support full-time staffing around the clock, seven days a week.

Margaret had just cleaned up after dinner and was settling into the recliner to work on the crossword puzzle in the newspaper. But as she sat down, Sidney, out of the corner of his eye, saw her not so much collapse as do a slow slide into total limpness. Margaret had never had any symptoms. There was no warning at all.

Sidney called his wife's name twice. He went to her and shook her by the shoulder. An overwhelming sense of dread flooded his mind, and for a moment he couldn't think of what to do. Then his mind cleared enough for him to dial 911.

When the dispatcher received Sidney's call, he activated the paging system for the EMT on call that evening. This system gave the volunteer EMT the address of the emergency and the nature of the call. Because the address was not in his immediate vicinity, the volunteer EMT followed protocol by heading to the station and waiting for a second EMT to arrive. It took the first EMT four minutes to reach the station, where he waited three more minutes for his partner to arrive. The two of them then drove the rescue vehicle to Sidney and Margaret's farm, a trip that took eight minutes.

When they arrived, one EMT started CPR while the other attached Margaret to the automated external defibrillator and stood back as it cycled though its analysis: *No shock indicated. Check pulse. Check breathing. If needed, begin CPR.*

After five minutes of CPR at the scene, the EMTs decided to load Margaret into the rescue vehicle and drive the twenty-five minutes to St. Joseph Mercy Hospital. Margaret had no heart activity upon arrival. The emergency department's physician heard the story, saw Margaret's lack of heart rhythm, and told everyone to stop CPR.

MAGNITUDE OF THE PROBLEM

Regrettably, sudden deaths like those of Clarence and Margaret occur hundreds of times a day in the United States. Heart disease—with its most common manifestation, sudden cardiac arrest—is the leading cause of death among adults in Western countries. In the United States, heart disease accounts for 1.2 million deaths per year, twice as many as those attributable to all cancers, and ten times as many as those accounted for by all accidents. Of deaths due to heart disease, approximately half occur outside hospitals, and half of these are sudden and unexpected. Indeed, sudden death due to heart disease strikes 250,000 times a year in the United States.

The emotional cost of sudden death is incalculable. These deaths happen in the community, usually in people's homes, and often with little or no warning. Death comes unexpectedly to mothers and fathers, grandmothers and grandfathers, sisters and brothers, daughters and sons, wage earners and retirees—in short, to ordinary people. The average age for sudden death in men is the mid-sixties, with a six-decade range from age thirty to ninety. Women, by contrast, tend to die suddenly about a decade later than men do. This age difference is due to the fact that heart disease begins about ten years earlier in men than in women.

The economic cost of heart disease is staggering, too—an estimated $156 billion per year. For example, if heart disease were to miraculously disappear, the savings would be triple the money spent annually on education. But this otherwise thoroughly depressing picture contains one good element: between 1950 and 1999, the overall death rate from heart disease decreased by 59 percent, and the number of sudden cardiac deaths fell by 49 percent.[2] No single factor explains why heart disease has fallen so dramatically. Undoubtedly, many factors have contributed. These include improved diet; decreased rates of smoking; better control of blood pressure, cholesterol, and diabetes; better therapy for coronary heart disease, including medications, surgery, angiography, and stents; and improved emergency medical services. But such good news—which is indeed worthy of celebration—cannot erase the cold fact that heart disease is still, far and away, the leading cause of death in the United States.

Are there reasons why Peter lived but Clarence and Margaret did not? Absolutely. That's what this book is all about. In the chapters to come, I pose two simple questions, which I hope to have answered. First, why is it that in some communities there is excellent survival after cardiac arrest, but in others there is not? And, second, what can be done to improve the chances of survival?

CHANCES OF SURVIVAL

It would be nice to think that your chances of surviving cardiac arrest are approximately the same whether you suffer a heart attack in New York, Seattle, Miami, or Detroit. Unfortunately, that is not the case. If you live in certain communities, you are forty-six times more likely to survive a cardiac arrest than if you live in others (see figure 1.1). The term "survive," as used here and throughout this book, pertains to a patient discharged from the hospital after sudden cardiac arrest. In 2003, a series of articles published in *USA Today* surveyed the medical directors of twenty-eight emergency medical services (EMS).[3] The reported survival rates for patients who suffered a witnessed cardiac arrest with ventricular fibrillation ranged from 3 percent, in Omaha, to 45 percent, in Seattle. An additional eighteen communities either didn't know their survival rates or refused to report them. And in 2004, an article published in *Resuscitation*, a leading journal of research on cardiac arrest, found that survival rates in thirty-four communities among patients who suffered ventricular fibrillation ranged from 3.3 percent, in Chicago, to 40.5 percent, in Rochester, Minnesota.[4] Since then, two more studies have defined the high end of the curve: the 2005 report of a thirteen-year study from Rochester, Minnesota, showing a 46 percent rate of survival for patients who had suffered witnessed ventricular fibrillation; and, equally impressive, a 2006 article in *Circulation*, the main scientific journal of the American Heart Association, which likewise reported a survival rate of 46 percent in King County, Washington, the suburban community surrounding Seattle.[5] The low end of the curve was defined by a 2007 study in *Resuscitation* that reported the survival rate for cardiac arrest in Detroit—a nearly hopeless rate of less than 1 percent.[6]

A 2008 study in *JAMA* reported survival from ventricular fibrillation cardiac arrest among six U.S. and three Canadian cities. The range of survival was 8 to 40 percent. This prospective study used common definitions and methodologies among the communities and was part of the Resuscitation Outcomes Consortium.[7] The message of all these studies seems clear. There can be tremendous difference in survival from cardiac arrest. The community you reside in to a very large extent determines whether you will live or die.

Would we accept such differences in the ability of fire departments to put out house fires? in the ability of police departments to solve crimes? in the potency of antibiotics? in how effectively poultry is protected from contamination by salmonella? in the quality of automobiles' air bags? Or consider hospitals' efforts to control hospital-acquired infectious, a reporting requirement of the Joint Commission on Accred-

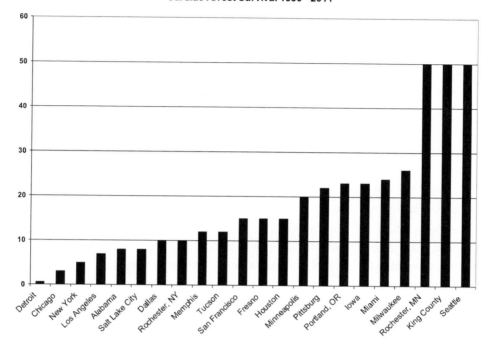

Cardiac Arrest Survival 1990 - 2011

1.1 Comparative survival rates, by percentages, for ventricular fibrillation across communities. Survival is defined as discharge from a hospital. The data are derived from peer-reviewed scientific literature (see Notes 5-19 for Chapter 1). Not all articles distinguish between witnessed and unwitnessed VF. The peer-reviewed literature for Rochester, MN and and King County report rates of 46% (page 6 and Note 5). For these communities, as well as for Seattle, survival rates have been updated with personal communications from Drs. Roger White, Leonard Cobb, and Tom Rea, respectively.

itation of Healthcare Organizations. Inevitably, a certain number of such infections will occur, though monitoring and control procedures can keep the rate extremely low. But what if a hospital doesn't even know its rates of infection? What if a hospital knows that it has a problem but doesn't do anything about it?[8]

Whatever the service or product, we expect a reasonable standard of quality and a reasonable level of consistency from community to community. For some products and services, we actually have national standards and national enforcement. But when it comes to cardiac arrest, we have no such standards, no agency monitoring the quality of service, no political groundswell demanding improvements, and no public outcry for change. The typical community doesn't even know its rate of survival for cardiac arrest. Some communities do know but are doing little to improve their systems. But a few communities are aware of how they perform, and they keep making improvements. So when I advise you to have your heart attack in Seattle or King County or the Minnesota city of Rochester, I'm not just being flippant.

TERMINOLOGY AND THE CONTINUUM OF HEART DISEASE

The term "heart attack," of course, is too imprecise to convey much real meaning. Presumably, a heart attack is something bad (an attack) that happens to the heart. The popular image associated with this term is that of someone, usually a man, clutching his chest and falling over. But this "attack" may take the form of a cardiac arrest, or an acute myocardial infarction, or an episode of angina, or even chest pain not necessarily related to the heart. In short, the term "heart attack," even though I used it earlier, is too general and all-inclusive to be useful in the context of emergency medical services because it can mean anything from death to a twinge of chest pain. The term's imprecision is reinforced in part by people in the media who may not want to learn about the differences among the various kinds of "heart attacks," or who may assume that their audiences simply don't care. Yet important differences do exist. For example, if I read in the newspaper that Senator Jones had a heart attack and was taken to Bethesda Naval Hospital, I want to know if the senator is in a coma after a cardiac arrest or is recovering from a myocardial infarction or was hospitalized as a precaution after a bout of angina. In the first case, he is at death's door. In the two others, he is watching cable TV in his private room.

In other words, heart disease, like most other kinds of disease, exists on a continuum. For heart disease, the continuum runs from total absence of symptoms to sudden death. In the passages that follow, let's start with the mildest form of heart disease and proceed to its most severe manifestation. As you read, bear in mind that the distinctions among terms like "angina," "unstable angina," and "myocardial infarction" are blurred and not always as clearly demarcated in the real world as they are in the examples to come. That's because the pathological process within the coronary artery can be exacerbated and may undergo rapid change. For example, the artery may occlude (be blocked) but then partially reopen, or the blockage may lessen or worsen within a relatively short period. Think of the process as one that is unstable, dynamic rather than fixed (one term that reflects this instability is "acute coronary syndrome," useful in describing the situation of a person whose underlying coronary artery disease, or CAD, is just beginning to produce symptoms). And from now on, let's throw out the term "heart attack."

Heart Disease without Symptoms

The mildest form of heart disease is disease without symptoms. The medical term used to describe disease with no symptoms is "subclinical." In other words, there are no signs or symptoms of the illness.

The most definitive way to determine the presence of heart disease is to look at the heart's arteries, called "coronary arteries." This can be done with a procedure called a "coronary arteriogram" or "arteriography," which is an X-ray study in which dye is injected into the coronary arteries. Newer generations of high-speed computerized tomography (CT) can also help identify disease. In high-speed CT, calcified areas of coronary arteries "light up," and these areas are highly correlated with atherosclerotic deposits. The main advantage of high-speed CT is that the test in noninvasive. The gold standard, however, is still the coronary arteriogram.

There is another way to identify disease before symptoms appear—namely, the treadmill exercise test. This inexpensive test is considered to be a good screening procedure before a coronary arteriogram. The patient walks and runs on a treadmill while hooked up to an electrocardiograph that records the heart's rhythm and traces electrical images (electrocardiograms, or ECGs) of the heart. If certain portions of the heart have a reduced blood supply, the stress of running will show characteristic changes on the ECG. As the treadmill speeds up, however, the patient's only symptom may be tiredness.

Heart disease without symptoms can be present for decades. Unfortunately, in approximately 30 percent of sudden cardiac arrests (the percentages are higher in some studies), cardiac arrest is the first manifestation of heart disease. In other words, the patient was unaware of having coronary artery disease until just before he or she dropped dead (if indeed the patient even learned of it—usually his or her relatives are the ones who discover the underlying disease when the autopsy is performed).

Heart Disease with Symptoms of Angina

I may look at someone and say to myself, "He's a myocardial infarction waiting to happen." The person is overweight, huffing and puffing at the slightest exertion. He smokes, has high blood pressure (hypertension), diabetes, and high cholesterol, and he leads a stressful life. And the clincher—he has chest pain when he climbs a flight of stairs. The term "angina" is derived from the Greek word *anchein*, meaning "to strangle." The word describes the sensation experienced when a portion of the heart does not receive an adequate blood supply. When the heart is at rest, the demands made on it are few, so a partially blocked artery will be symptom-free. With activity or exertion—or a large meal, emotional stress, extreme cold or heat, or smoking—the heart beats faster and requires additional blood. But the partial blockage won't allow additional blood through, so the downstream heart muscle cramps up, just as other muscles do. This cramping is what is called "angina." Angina can take a variety of forms. Typically, it is felt under the sternum (breastbone), in the center of the chest, but sometimes it may be experienced as pain radiating to the left side of the chest, the jaw, the back, or the upper left arm. If the person experiencing angina rests or takes a nitroglycerine tablet, the symptoms usually subside within a few minutes. Bouts of angina do not lead to permanent damage of the heart muscle.

Heart Disease with Imminent Myocardial Infarction

The same person, overweight with symptoms of angina, may note a change in the character of his angina. Now the angina seems to be present when he is just walking, and even sometimes when he is at rest. Climbing stairs is an ordeal, and he has to stop for a while between steps. If you could look into this person's coronary arteries, you would see a partial blockage that is expanding in size but hasn't yet closed the coronary artery completely off. This condition has a variety of names, including "pre-infarction angina," "crescendo angina," and "unstable angina." These terms describe an unsteady state—namely, a worsening that may soon lead to an infarction. Typically, the patient with this condition will have a coronary angiogram to identify the location and extent of the blockage. Then, depending on the location of the partial blockage, surgery or an angioplasty procedure will be performed.

Heart Disease with Acute Myocardial Infarction

Middle-aged men sometimes joke about having "the big one," meaning a myocardial infarction. But it is no joking matter. I have never seen anyone who was experiencing an acute myocardial infarction and also wanted to banter. There is usually crushing pain in the center of the chest, with pain radiating down the left arm. The person is pale, nauseated, and profusely sweating and often has a dreadful sensation of impending doom. Maybe jokes about "the big one" are a defense against such a catastrophe.

In an acute myocardial infarction, one of the coronary arteries has become completely blocked. The patient's symptoms result when heart-muscle fibers downstream from the blockage start to die. But there is hope. Clot-dissolving drugs can eliminate or reduce the damage if taken in a timely manner, as can emergency procedures like coronary angioplasty, stenting, laserectomy, and immediate bypass surgery if they are performed in time. If the blocked artery can be reopened within sixty minutes of an acute myocardial infarction, the damage will be minimal. The damage will also be less if the artery can be reopened between one and six hours from the time of the infarction. After six hours, the damage is largely irreversible.

Heart Disease with Cardiac Arrest

This is the worst-case scenario. The most dramatic form of sudden death, and its most common cause, occurs when the heart goes into the fatal rhythm of ventricular fibrillation (VF). This happens literally in an instant. The heart is beating normally, and then—*wham!* All hell breaks loose as the heart's electrical signaling system goes berserk. It is as if a harmoniously performing orchestra were to suddenly revolt against the steady rhythm of the conductor's baton. Instantly, all the musicians begin to play random and cacophonous notes. The beautiful melody ceases at once.

If you could look at a heart at the moment of fibrillation, it would appear to wiggle chaotically. A heart in ventricular fibrillation has been described as a sack of undulating worms. The moment fibrillation begins, the pulse is lost, and the blood pressure falls to zero. The goal of a defibrillatory shock is to jolt all the muscle fibers into contraction. This jolt is followed by a momentary standstill and, if the shock is successful, a return of the heart's normal rhythmic contractions. Picture again the cacophonous orchestra, and imagine that the conductor can jolt every musician's seat with an electric shock and cause all the performers to stop for a second. Now the conductor has a chance to get back in charge.

DEFINING SUDDEN CARDIAC ARREST

The term "sudden cardiac arrest" is fairly descriptive. The event appears to happen all at once. It is caused by heart (cardiac) disease. Its manifestation is an arrest (the heart ceases pumping blood). Unless the ventricular fibrillation can be reversed and a normal blood pressure be restored, the event is always fatal. But more qualifications are needed. Let's consider each of the three words in the term "sudden cardiac arrest."

What is meant by "sudden"? Does the word refer to an event that is instantaneous, or to one that occurs over a period of less than twenty-four hours? Most researchers define "sudden" as referring to events taking place within a range of time that is anywhere between an instant and less than one hour. The cardiac arrests that befell Peter, Clarence, and Margaret, the people we met earlier in this chapter, all fit this definition of "sudden": these people either had no warning symptoms at all (Margaret) or experienced symptoms of cardiac arrest that arose and dramatically worsened or accelerated within just a few minutes (Peter and Clarence). To take another example, someone can be having mild to moderate symptoms of acute myocardial infarction for several hours, but then her symptoms can suddenly grow worse, causing her blood pressure to fall and leading her to collapse over the course of only twenty minutes. This sort of event is very different from a situation in which someone is on a slow downhill course toward death. For example, someone dying of emphysema may experience an increase in symptoms over a period of days, with a gradual onset of coma. Death from cancer is often a slow slide into coma, and death from sepsis or pneumonia occurs slowly over a period of days. In fact, most deaths happen over hours or days. That's why the death scenes in Hollywood films are so unrealistic—a realistic movie, if it contained a death scene, would go on for hours. Likewise, people admitted to the hospital for symptoms of heart disease do not tend to die there of sudden cardiac arrest. It's possible, of course, to die suddenly and unexpectedly of cardiac arrest in the hospital, but the term "sudden cardiac arrest" is generally reserved for community settings outside the hospital. A heart patient already admitted to a hospital is there for evaluation of his symptoms, for cardiac therapy, or for a procedure like open-heart surgery. But usually someone who is experiencing the sudden onset of cardiac symptoms, particularly when those symptoms herald ventricular fibrillation, cannot get to the emergency room in time to be treated and admitted.

As for the term "cardiac," it refers to the cause of death. In sudden cardiac arrest, the heart most commonly shows underlying coronary artery disease. By contrast, it is possible to die suddenly from noncardiac causes. For example, a person with a ruptured aortic aneurysm—an abnormally widened aorta whose bursting can lead to a massive internal hemorrhage—may die within minutes, but the cause is not the heart. And, of course, traumatic deaths can be extremely sudden.

The word "arrest" simply points to the absence of pulse or blood pressure. The heart has arrested—in a word, it has stopped. There are three primary heart rhythms that can cause the heart's pumping function to stop: ventricular fibrillation, pulseless electrical activity (PEA), and asystole (flatlining).[9] In ventricular fibrillation, the most common rhythm associated with cardiac arrest, the heart instantaneously goes from a normal rhythm to this fatal one. It is difficult to know what percentage of sudden cardiac arrests may be associated with ventricular fibrillation, but estimates are 75 percent or higher. The precise number is unknown mostly because of the delay between a person's collapse and the time when EMTs or paramedics arrive to assess his or her heart rhythm. VF, if untreated, deteriorates to asystole within approximately twenty minutes. Therefore, if the patient's heart rhythm is determined after this twenty-minute period has elapsed, it will appear that the patient flatlined (that is, that his or her heart rhythm went to asystole), even though the rhythm actually associated with the arrest was VF. A few studies have reported on sudden out-of-hospital deaths in patients who were being monitored at the time of arrest (they were wearing a device called a Holter monitor, which continuously records the heart's rhythm). Virtually all of these patients suffered VF-associated arrest, typically with a very brief bout of ventricular tachycardia that preceded the VF.[10]

Though VF is the most common cause of sudden cardiac arrest, other frequently encountered fatal rhythms are asystole, described earlier, and pulseless electrical activity, defined as an organized rhythm seen on an electrocardiogram but with no pumping activity—the heart muscle is so terminal that it has lost its ability to contract. It is possible in some instances for a heart to go in a matter of minutes (sometimes even seconds) from a normal-appearing rhythm directly to asystole or PEA. This usually occurs in the context of a massive myocardial infarction or severe heart failure. Both asystole and pulseless electrical activity are almost impossible to treat successfully, since there is so much underlying structural damage to the heart. If the rhythm of VF is like that of a complex machine seizing up because of a tiny malfunction in a fuse, the rhythms of asystole and pulseless electrical activity are like that of a machine that stops because its motor has burnt out. Occasionally, however, paramedics encounter correctable causes of PEA, and they are taught to always search for such causes before terminating a resuscitation.[11]

Another key feature defining sudden cardiac arrest is that the heart was not expected to stop. At the final moment of every death, of course, the heart stops, but in sudden cardiac arrest, it stops unexpectedly. People who are gravely ill with various diseases cannot be said to die of sudden cardiac arrest even when their hearts suddenly stop beating, since the gravity of their illnesses makes death likely and therefore expected. Likewise, someone whose vital signs (such as blood pressure) have fallen gradually and terminally cannot be considered to have died unexpectedly. Thus, to define the term "sudden cardiac arrest" more precisely, we should say that it is a rapid, fatal (unless the normal rhythm can be quickly restored), unexpected cessation of heart contraction caused by underlying heart disease. The key point is that the event must be both sudden and unexpected. When the heart stops beating in patients who have most other diseases, death is gradual or expected or both.

So let's reduce the preceding paragraphs to a one-sentence definition: *Sudden cardiac arrest leads to the rapid and unexpected death, in an out-of-hospital community setting, of someone who had underlying heart disease but either had no symptoms at all or had symptoms for less than one hour.* There are many qualifiers in this definition, I know, but its essence can be summarized in five key terms: *rapid, unexpected, death, community*, and *underlying heart disease.*

Though sudden cardiac arrest may be associated with VF, asystole, or PEA, this book focuses on VF. As already mentioned, asystole and pulseless electrical activity have almost no chance of reversal. Each is also less likely to be of sudden onset and is often the terminal event of a more chronic condition. VF, by contrast, meets the very definition of "sudden," since it manifests almost instantly. I emphasize VF throughout this book because the management of asystole and PEA, which both have such poor survival rates, sheds little light on the quality of an EMS system, whereas ventricular fibrillation and its therapy allow me to focus incisively on what is right and what is wrong with EMS programs. Furthermore, international consensus recommends that survival rates for cardiac arrest in communities be reported on the basis of cases of ventricular fibrillation. Throughout the book, I use the terms "sudden cardiac death" and "sudden cardiac arrest" synonymously. When I report community survival rates for sudden cardiac arrest, I make clear whether those rates pertain to all cardiac rhythms or only to ventricular fibrillation.

THE MOMENT OF SUDDEN DEATH

Is it a tautology to state that sudden death is fatal? Not entirely. Sudden death can be reversed—*if* a defibrillatory shock reaches the victim in time.

When the heart fibrillates, events happen fast, and death's stopwatch begins its countdown. With the onset of ventricular fibrillation, the body is clinically dead. A person becomes totally unresponsive, and there are no vital signs—no pulse, no blood pressure, no breathing. The body becomes a mass of dying cells.

The ideal resuscitation restarts the heart before any permanent organ damage occurs. But the window of opportunity is very narrow indeed. With every passing minute, the likelihood of resuscitation diminishes. If nothing is done for four to five minutes, the condition of clinical death will begin to turn to biological death. And after ten to fifteen minutes, biological death will be complete. The person will be *dead* dead, and the return to a living state is impossible.

With ventricular fibrillation, the heart's blood-pumping activity ceases. There is no forward flow of blood though the lungs and therefore no opportunity for oxygen to be delivered to the organs and cells. There is also no delivery of nutrients, such as sugar (glucose) and electrolytes, nor is there any means to carry off the products of cell metabolism, such as acids and carbon dioxide. Imagine a conveyor belt in a factory. If it stops because of a power outage, every station along the production line backs up, and the whole factory comes to a stop.

Certain organs of the body are more sensitive than others to lack of oxygen. The brain is by far the most sensitive. If the brain is deprived of oxygen, consciousness is lost almost right away—all the oxygen stores in the brain are used up in ten seconds. Normally, atoms of sodium, potassium, and calcium travel back and forth across the cell membranes, maintaining the proper chemical balance between the inside and the outside of each cell. But when oxygen is lacking, the circulation of these atoms ceases, and calcium begins to accumulate within the cells. Chemical chain reactions begin. They break down the DNA within each cell's nucleus, a process that leads to irreparable damage. A by-product of this damage is the production within the cells of acid that enters the bloodstream. Normally, blood contains the proper balance of acids and bases within a narrow range. Too much acid or too much base is fatal. With cardiac arrest, the acid reaches a fatal level within ten to fifteen minutes. Glucose is almost as crucial as oxygen and is needed to fuel all the chemical reactions within the cells, but the glucose in the brain cells is depleted within five minutes. And once their glucose is depleted, the destruction of the brain cells accelerates. The brain is such a fragile structure—millions of years of evolution have created its glorious complexity, but a few brief minutes without oxygen can utterly destroy it.

With cardiac arrest, the heart also dies, but at a slower rate than the brain. Initially, the fibrillatory waves are very coarse. This is because the heart's muscle fibers, at the moment of VF, still have energy and a full load of oxygen. The heart, like all other muscles, requires a fresh supply of oxygen, glucose, and nutrients. With VF, however, the coronary arteries at the base of the aorta receive no forward flow of blood, and so these vital supplies are rapidly depleted. The strength of each muscle fiber's contraction weakens, and the contractions disappear completely within approximately twenty minutes. If you could look at an electrocardiogram during this process, you would see that the fibrillatory waves at first appear chaotic and tall (these are the coarse waves, about half an inch high), but they gradually lessen in amplitude (after ten minutes, they become fine waves, about one-sixteenth of an inch high), and after twenty minutes the ECG shows flatlining.[12] A Swedish study has estimated that fine VF may last even beyond twenty minutes, though there have been virtually no survivors of long-duration VF.[13] The potential of the heart to convert from fibrillation to a normal rhythm is directly related to the duration of fibrillation. The coarser the waves, the more easily an electric shock can convert the rhythm to normal. It is estimated that for every minute of delay in defibrillation, the odds of survival fall by approximately 10 percent.[14]

THE VITAL ROLE OF CPR

Consider two scenarios. In the first, a patient collapses in VF at work and receives CPR from his office colleagues. Paramedics arrive ten minutes after the patient's collapse and shock his heart into a normal rhythm. The patient leaves the hospital seven days later, neurologically intact. In the second scenario, a patient collapses at work and receives no CPR. The paramedics arrive in the same amount of time, and after four shocks and a difficult resuscitation effort, they bring the patient's heart back to a normal rhythm. Three weeks later, the patient is discharged from the hospital to a nursing home. He has significant neurological impairment and is unable to feed himself or speak coherently. The difference in outcome between these two scenarios is due primarily to the rapid initiation of CPR in the first one.

CPR slows the dying process, buying time for the defibrillator to arrive and shock the heart into a normal rhythm. CPR delays the onset of irreversible damage to the brain and the heart by keeping a flow of oxygenated blood circulating to the vital organs. Even with the help of CPR, however, the flow of blood is far from normal and probably achieves only 10 to 30 percent of normal cardiac output. But this trickle of oxygenated blood is enough to delay the death of cells, especially the sensitive cells of the brain.[15] CPR by itself cannot restart a heart—for that, an electric shock is needed —but it can buy as much as four to eight minutes, time enough for the defibrillator to arrive. Shocking a fibrillating heart four minutes after the patient's collapse, with no preceding CPR, would be roughly equivalent to shocking the heart eight to twelve minutes after the patient's collapse, with proper CPR performed before the arrival of the defibrillator.

CPR and defibrillation work in tandem. Imagine yourself in a boat rapidly sinking, tossing you into in the ocean—fortunately you are wearing a flotation device and another boat comes along for the rescue. CPR is like that flotation device, and the defibrillator is like the boat. If the boat comes right away, you don't really need the flotation device. In the same way, CPR isn't needed if a defibrillator is instantly available. But let's be realistic. Defibrillators, though relatively common, are not yet as ubiquitous as cell phones, personal digital assistants, or iPods.

THE ROLE OF DEFIBRILLATION

If CPR slows the dying process, defibrillation stops it. By delivering an electric current across the heart, the defibrillator stops the heart from fibrillating so that, one hopes, a normal heart rhythm can resume. Defibrillation is somewhat like rebooting a computer that has gone haywire—by turning it off and then on again, you hope to disrupt the bad signals being relayed within the device and make it work properly again. Similarly, by using a blast of electricity to "turn off" the fibrillation signal in the heart, you hope to reset the heart's internal workings to their proper level of functioning.

But defibrillatory shocks do not always work. The most important determinants of success are how much time has elapsed between the patient's collapse and delivery of the shock, whether CPR has been performed, and the underlying condition of the heart. Clearly, the more quickly the shock can be delivered after fibrillation begins, the greater the likelihood of success. And if the heart's underlying condition is reasonably good, then the shock will have an excellent chance of "rebooting" the heart. If the heart has been severely weakened, however—say, by multiple myocardial infarcts or long-standing hypertension or chronic heart failure—then defibrillation will be less likely to succeed. Defibrillation can get an old car running again, but it can't turn a Honda Civic into a Lexus.

DID CAVEMEN AND CAVEWOMEN DIE OF SUDDEN CARDIAC ARREST?

Yes—when saber-toothed tigers chewed them in half. Ancient men and women died suddenly from all kinds of trauma, including accidents, drowning, and battle injuries in addition to animal attacks. But it is very unlikely that they died of sudden cardiac arrest related to coronary artery disease. We cannot know this with absolute certainty, of course, since autopsies have been done for only the last few hundred years, but it seems likely that CAD is a disease of modern Western civilization. The syndrome of coronary artery disease was first described a mere century ago, and the cause of acute myocardial infarction—blockage of a coronary artery—was identified only in 1980. It is possible that our extended life expectancy has allowed the epidemic of CAD to emerge. Several hundred years ago, when the average life expectancy was fifty years, coronary artery disease may not have been very apparent. And yet, even though our comparative longevity offers what may be a partial explanation, I think that lifestyle changes account for the bulk of the epidemic. These changes include three very obvious ones in the typical American style of life over the past century—increased smoking, reduced physical activity, and a diet rich in saturated fats.

THE HOLLYWOOD HEART ATTACK

In the 2001 movie *The Deep End*, one of the leading characters has a sudden cardiac arrest. With no prior symptoms, he collapses on the kitchen floor. His daughter begins CPR—not very effectively—but soon gets help from a trained bystander. He takes over the chest compressions and orders her to give mouth-to-mouth ventilations. Meanwhile, he orders another person to call 911.

Watching this movie, I expected to see paramedics rush in and defibrillate the patient. But, much to my surprise, the patient began to regain consciousness after two minutes of CPR. He looked great on his way to the hospital. I cringed while I watched this scene—another botched Hollywood portrayal of a cardiac arrest. For such a key dramatic scene, you'd think that the movie's two codirectors, between them, could have found a way to pay for a medical consultant.

As you can tell, I have a beef with Hollywood, and it's at several levels. First, movie and television scriptwriters create unrealistic images of how successful resuscitation efforts actually are. According to a study published in the *New England Journal of Medicine*, 68 percent of the cardiac arrests portrayed in the entertainment media have successful outcomes.[16] The reality, however, is closer to 8 percent.[17]

Second, films and TV shows rarely if ever explain the relationship of CPR to defibrillation. The fact is that CPR alone cannot definitively treat cardiac arrest. A defibrillator is needed. Every time a movie or TV show portrays CPR saving a life, an opportunity is missed to educate the audience about defibrillation.[18] I realize that Hollywood executives view their mission to be entertainment, not education, but I don't buy that excuse. Depictions of defibrillation can be just as dramatic as depictions of CPR, and little extra effort is needed to write an accurate script.

Third, I'm frustrated by how Hollywood productions always show the victim of cardiac arrest collapsing with few if any premonitory symptoms. He clutches his chest, grimaces, and then succumbs. Cardiac arrest certainly can happen this way, but one can easily get the impression that this is the only way for someone to die suddenly, whereas warning indicators, such as chest pain, actually precede collapse most of the time. People should realize that chest pain calls for action.

And, fourth, only men are portrayed as suffering cardiac arrest. You could be excused for concluding that women never suffer cardiac arrest. No wonder the public is confused!

THE BIG PICTURE

Cardiac arrest represents about 1 percent of the EMS calls in any given community, but the management of this 1 percent encapsulates everything good and bad about a community's EMS system. In this regard, cardiac arrest is a surrogate for the entire system. A community that can successfully respond to and manage this emergency is likely to perform well on the other 99 percent of emergencies. Every step, large or small, to improve therapy for cardiac arrest—faster response times, better training and continuing education, tighter medical control, better data management, higher expectations, and a host of other factors—will raise the entire system to a higher level. If you improve resuscitation, you improve the care for every patient needing emergency medical care. And that's likely to be any one of us at some point in our lives.

TWO

A History of Resuscitation

ANCIENT RESUSCITATION

50 BCE, SEA OF GALILEE

Jacob ben C. hauled the small fishing boat onto the shore. The catch was good. As Jacob mentally estimated the weight and calculated the extra shekels he'd have for Sarah's pendant, the headache struck like a hammer blow—a blast of searing white light, knife blades down the neck and into the back, and a tidal wave of nausea. Jacob had but a moment to reflect how different this was from the minor aches he had been feeling deep behind the eyes over the previous two days.

His fellow fishermen saw his collapse play out in slow motion—first Jacob fell to his knees, and then he fell over backwards. Three of them rushed to help him, but Jacob did not respond to their shouts or vigorous shakes. When they looked into his face, they were surprised to see that one of his eyes was widely dilated. One of the fishermen ran to get Sarah. When she arrived, twenty minutes later, all she could do was hold Jacob and cry over and over, "God, God, why did you do this? Give him back! Give him back!"

Death is invariably wrenching. But although death with an antecedent illness can seem inevitable, almost acceptable, sudden death—the transition from life to death in an instant—assaults our sense of the universe. Sudden death has always seemed incomprehensible.

In biblical times, sudden death was not caused by heart disease—lifestyle factors and a short life expectancy made this a rare phenomenon. Instead, sudden death came

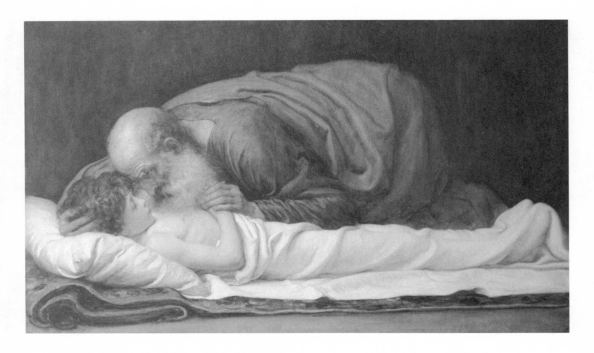

2.1 *Elisha Raising the Son of the Shunamite*, by Lord Frederick Leighton (1830–1896). Oil on canvas, 1881. Courtesy Leighton House Museum, The Royal Borough of Kensington and Chelsea, London/The Bridgeman Art Library.

through accidents and catastrophic illnesses, such as the cerebral aneurysm suffered by Jacob in this fictional case history. But even though heart disease is of relatively recent origin, the desire to resuscitate is as old as recorded history itself.

In biblical times, it was believed that only God or God's agents could reverse death. That is why Sarah, Jacob's wife, implores God to return her husband—only God and his agents were believed to have that power, as has been well described in the Bible. Even to attempt resuscitation without being an agent of God was to blaspheme God.

In the first of the Hebrew Bible's resuscitations, the prophet Elijah plays the leading role. A grief-stricken mother has brought her lifeless child to him ("And the son of the woman became ill; and his illness was so severe that there was no breath left in him"). The woman begs Elijah for help. Elijah carries her son to his own bed and prays to the Lord. Then he stretches himself over the child three times: "And the Lord harkened to the voice of Elijah, and the soul of the child came into him again, and he revived." Elijah, with the assistance of God, brings the child back to life.

The Bible gives an even more detailed account of another resuscitation, this one performed by the prophet Elisha, a disciple of Elijah. Elisha has befriended a Shunamite couple, and one day the couple's child is found to be suffering from a severe headache. The boy cries out, and then he collapses. Is this heatstroke? Is it an aneurysm, like the fictional Jacob's? The Bible gives no further clues.

The boy is carried to his mother, and he dies several hours later. The frantic mother then quickly rides to a neighboring village, where she finds Elisha, and together they return to the boy. Elisha enters the house and sees the boy laid out on his bed (figure 2.1). First he prays to the Lord. The Bible tells the rest of the story:

> [Elisha] placed himself over the child. He put his mouth on his mouth, his eyes on his eyes, and his hands on his hands, as he bent over him. And the body of the child became warm. He stepped down, walked once up and down the room, then mounted and bent over him. Thereupon, the boy sneezed seven times, and the boy opened his eyes.

Some authorities speculate that Elisha's weight must have compressed the child's chest, and that the prophet's beard tickled the child's nose and caused the sneezing. (Perhaps this is the origin of the custom of saying "God bless you" after someone sneezes.[1]) The resuscitations performed by Elijah and Elisha are physiologically unsound, but the point of these biblical stories was not to teach proper mouth-to-mouth technique. It was to show the power of God or his agents to reverse sudden death.

RESUSCITATION IN THE EIGHTEENTH CENTURY

JULY 25, 1771, AMSTERDAM

Maarten M. was ecstatic. Annika had said yes to his proposal of marriage, and she had shyly kissed his lips. Maarten was so overjoyed. He climbed onto the railing of the canal bridge and attempted a silly celebratory jig. His fall into the canal was almost inevitable.

Maarten knew how to swim, but as he fell he struck his head on the edge of the roadway. Annika stared, horrified, at his still body, floating face down.

One of the bystanders on the bridge was a member of Amsterdam's Society for Recovery of Drowned Persons. Since he was well dressed and spoke with authority, the other bystanders listened to him as he directed the rescue effort. A few of them pulled Maarten from the canal and positioned him face down. They lifted his legs repeatedly. Someone ran to a nearby house to get a fireside bellows, which someone then placed in Maarten's mouth, pressing its sides together as though trying to ignite a fading spark of life. After several minutes, there was a cough and a spurt of water, and Maarten reentered the land of the living.

The Enlightenment, which began around 1750, was a remarkable time in human history—a time of scientific discovery, political democracy, and a growing consciousness

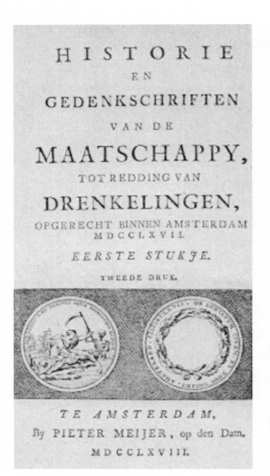

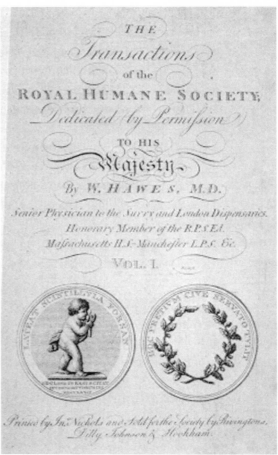

2.2 (*left*) Front cover of the Amsterdam rescue society's first annual report, published in 1768, the year after the society was founded; note the figure of the rescuer poised over a drowning victim while pushing back the Grim Reaper. (*right*) Dedication page of *Transactions of the Royal Humane Society*, vol. 1. (1794), illustrating both sides of the lifesaving medal awarded by the society. Courtesy Royal Humane Society, London.

that humans could unravel the mysteries of the universe. The nascent belief in the power of science challenged death itself. Could death be reversed? Could the secrets of life be discovered? In this climate of scientific ferment, it was inevitable that people would conceive of resuscitation as a human endeavor rather than as the strict province of divine intervention.

The first city to teach and promote resuscitation was Amsterdam, in the heart of the European Enlightenment. Known as the Venice of the North, Amsterdam paid dearly for its many canals with up to 400 drownings every year. Death from cardiac disease was still not prevalent, and most other sudden deaths resulted from accidents.

In August 1767, a few wealthy and benevolent gentlemen in Amsterdam gathered to form the Society for Recovery of Drowned Persons (fig. 2.2). This endeavor marked the first organized effort to respond to sudden death.

Rescue societies soon sprang up in most European capitals, and all these societies were established with the goal of finding a way to successful resuscitation. In 1769, one German city, Hamburg, even passed an ordinance that effectively mandated training of the general population in resuscitation techniques. The ordinance called for notices to be read in churches, describing the types of assistance possible for people who had been drowned, strangled, and frozen or overcome by noxious gases. A few years later, in 1774, the Royal Humane Society was founded in London.[2] It served as the model for similar societies in New York, Philadelphia, and Boston.

Within four years of its founding, Amsterdam's Society for Recovery of Drowned Persons was claiming that 150 people had been saved by its recommendations.[3] The society's resuscitation techniques consisted mostly of common sense coupled with a

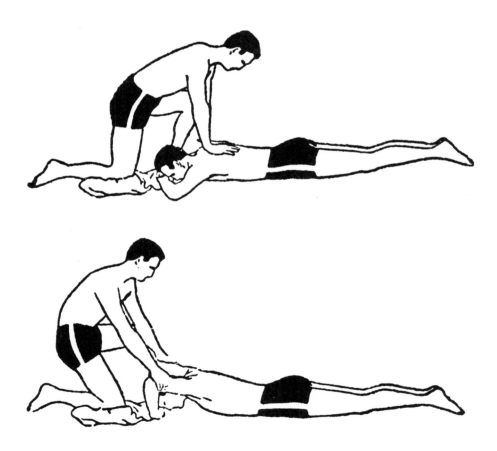

2.3 Back-pressure/arm-lift method of artificial respiration, showing technique for expiration (*top*) and for inspiration (*bottom*).

few methods for stimulating the body. The recommended measures were warming of the victim; positioning of the victim's head lower than his feet, application of manual pressure to his abdomen, and tickling of the victim's throat to promote removal of swallowed or aspirated water; stimulation of the victim by such means as rectal and oral fumigation with tobacco smoke; using a bellows to blow air down the throat; and bloodletting.[4] Although the practice of blowing smoke into the rectum seems bizarre today, it is possible that the nicotine was enough of a stimulant to engender a response in someone who was nearly dead.

These early techniques of resuscitation seem almost quaint today, and somewhat pathetic by our standards. What is important for us to note here, however, is not the scientific merit of these techniques but rather the collective belief that resuscitation was possible—that the suddenly dead could be revived. The rescue societies of the eighteenth century were the precursors of today's emergency medical services.

For the next century and a half, scientists—not to mention quite a few quacks—advocated literally hundreds of resuscitation techniques.[5] Some of these were even partly effective in respiratory emergencies. For example, the back-pressure/arm-lift method ("out goes the bad air, in goes the good air"), taught to countless thousands of Boy Scouts until the late 1950s, could occasionally save a drowning victim (fig. 2.3). But the technique was of no benefit in the case of cardiac arrest, since it resulted in a suboptimal amount of air exchange and did nothing for circulation.[6]

MODERN RESUSCITATION

AUGUST 15, 1955, TACOMA, WASHINGTON

Jack C. was a heart attack waiting to happen. He was overweight. Having put on an extra pound or two every year since his high school graduation, in 1920, he now tipped the scales at 213. He rarely exercised—demonstrating vacuum cleaners at Sears hardly burned off the calories. And he loved his meat and potatoes, preferably slathered in butter or gravy. Bacon and eggs were daily fare, too. Jack also smoked—unfiltered Luckies.

Jack's first hint that something might be wrong came while he was at work. He had been feeling a nagging ache located on the inside of his left arm. Now he climbed a flight of stairs, and it got worse.

Suddenly Jack felt a crushing pain in his chest. He was nauseated and sweating profusely. All these things happened at once, and before Jack could even stub his cigarette out, he collapsed, almost hitting his head on the latest Eureka model.

Jack's co-workers saw him go down. One of them scrambled to find the seven-digit number for the Tacoma Fire Department. Another asked if anyone knew how to do the back-pressure/arm-lift lifesaving maneuver, but no one did.

It took about eight minutes for the fire department to arrive. The firefighters carried in heavy breathing apparatus and large oxygen cylinders, which they assembled and strapped to Jack's face. One performed the back-pressure/arm-lift maneuver. Then they loaded Jack onto their gurney and proceeded to Tacoma General Hospital.

The emergency room—literally just a room—was adjacent to the admitting office. A doctor was paged, and when he got there he took one look at Jack and pronounced him dead.

Jack, sadly, was stricken a few years too early. He never really had a chance—in 1955, CPR hadn't even been discovered. Defibrillation wasn't yet practical, and prehospital emergency care was mostly a load-and-go operation. More often than not, once the patient reached the hospital, the doctor took one look and declared the victim dead.

Jack died at the peak of the epidemic of heart disease, but if his collapse had occurred fifteen years later, the outcome might have been different. In the 1950s and 1960s, though, Americans chained-smoked, ate diets high in saturated fats, and didn't exercise much. Cholesterol levels were sky high, and high blood pressure was rampant. Sudden cardiac arrest was the single most prevalent cause of death, and no one could do anything but tally the rising statistics.

The management of cardiac arrest defied simple solutions; there was no quick fix in sight. How could the problem be attacked? It would require an across-the-board strategy of developing new medications, devising new surgeries and techniques, identifying risk factors, educating the population about preventive measures, and discovering ways to treat cardiac arrest. Key discoveries had to be made, and crucial therapies had to be developed. All of this would take decades. And once therapies had been developed, there would have to be a means of delivering them quickly enough for them to work.

Doctors speak about the "natural history" of a disease—that is, the time that elapses between a patient's acquiring a disease and his or her death from that disease.[7] This characterization promotes an understanding of how therapy can alter the disease's usual progression. For example, the natural history of untreated breast cancer can be measured in months, but when the disease is treated with surgery or chemotherapy, its natural history can be measured in years, or the disease may even be cured. Sudden cardiac arrest, viewed as a disease, is one with an extremely brief natural history, one measured in minutes, and with an inevitable outcome. But when sudden cardiac arrest is treated with CPR, the course of death can be extended, since CPR delays the dying process, and if the arrest is treated in time with defibrillation, the dying process can be aborted.

For sudden cardiac arrest, the elements of resuscitation became cardiopulmonary resuscitation (CPR, comprising mouth-to-mouth ventilation and chest compression); defibrillation; and mobile intensive care, or emergency medical services (the means of quickly bringing these interventions to the patient). Each of these elements has its own history.

Cardiopulmonary Resuscitation

The Breath of Life: Mouth-to-Mouth Ventilation

MAY 17, 1958, CHICAGO

The two firefighters had just carried the victim out of her apartment building. She was not breathing. As soon as they had placed her in the ambulance, face down on the gurney, one of them began to perform the back-pressure/arm-lift method of artificial ventilation. The woman's face was purple, and it was obvious after four minutes that there was no improvement.

Another firefighter arrived and offered to help, saying that he wanted to try something new. He turned the woman onto her back and began to deliver mouth-to-mouth ventilations. His partners stood slack-jawed, wondering what their colleague was up to. And then, three minutes later, to the amazement of the first two firefighters, the woman began breathing on her own.

Where had this firefighter learned to do this? It turned out that his wife was a proofreader for the *Journal of the American Medical Association* and had brought some work home with her. In the latest issue of the journal was a description of this new technique for rescuing victims of drowning and smoke inhalation.

James Elam, an anesthesiologist, deserves honor for rediscovering mouth-to-mouth ventilation. I say "rediscovered" because it had been known for many centuries that this technique could be useful in resuscitating newborns. Elam's (re)discovery occurred in Minneapolis in 1946, in the middle of a polio outbreak. Here is how Elam describes what happened:

> I was browsing around to get acquainted with the [hospital] ward when along the corridor came a gurney racing—a nurse pulling it and two orderlies pushing it, and the kid on it was blue. I went into total reflex behavior. I stepped out in the middle of the corridor, stopped the gurney, grabbed the sheet, wiped the copious mucus off his mouth and face . . . sealed my lips around his nose and inflated his lungs. In four breaths he was pink.[8]

The evening before, Elam had been reading a book that contained a chapter on the history of resuscitation. In that chapter the technique of covering the baby's nose and mouth with the rescuer's mouth and exhaling into the baby's lungs had been described. Elam credits the chapter for his "reflex behavior." Elam originally recommended mouth-to-nose ventilation for adults but soon advocated the mouth-to-mouth technique as being equally effective and easier to perform. He set out to prove that exhaled air was adequate to oxygenate people who were not breathing. To accomplish this goal, he obtained permission from his chief of surgery to do studies on postoperative patients before their ether anesthesia wore off. He demonstrated that normal oxygen saturation could be maintained if air was blown into the patient's endotracheal tube (that is, the plastic tube placed in the patient's throat and inserted into the trachea during surgery to keep the patient ventilated).

Several years later, Elam met Peter Safar, also an anesthesiologist, and Safar joined Elam's effort to convince the world that mouth-to-mouth ventilation was effective. Safar set out on a series of experiments using paralyzed individuals to show that the mouth-to-mouth technique could maintain adequate oxygenation. Safar recounts the experiments as follows:

> Thirty-one physicians and medical students and one nurse volunteered. . . . Consent was very informed. All volunteers had to observe me ventilate anesthetized and curarized patients without a tracheal tube. I sedated the volunteers and paralyzed them for several hours each. Blood O_2 and CO_2 were analyzed. I demonstrated the method to over 100 lay persons who were then asked to perform the method on the curarized volunteers.[9]

These experiments provided compelling data in support of abandoning the back-pressure/arm-lift method of resuscitation in favor of mouth-to-mouth ventilation. The United States military accepted and endorsed the mouth-to-mouth method in 1957, and the American Medical Association followed suit in 1958. The May 17, 1958, issue of the *Journal of the American Medical Association* contains the following endorsement:

> Skillful performance of expired air breathing is an easily learned, lifesaving procedure. It has revived many victims unresponsive to other methods and has been proved in real emergencies under field conditions. Information about expired air breathing should be disseminated as widely as possible.[10]

The Pulse of Life: Chest Compression

OCTOBER 15, 1960, BELLEVUE HOSPITAL, NEW YORK CITY

The ambulance driver brought the cyanotic patient through the double doors of the emergency room.

"Looks like a heart attack," he said.

The intern on duty managed to place a breathing tube into the patient's trachea. The senior resident arrived and began chest compression.

No one on the scene had ever seen chest compression before. Everyone stopped momentarily and stared. Now the resident showed the intern how to position his hands and press on the patient's chest. The intern counted and grunted with each chest compression. The resident, meanwhile, was amazed to feel a strong femoral pulse on each of the intern's downstrokes. But the electrocardiograph attached to the patient showed that the patient had flatlined. The resident ordered the resuscitation to stop, and at 4:52 P.M. he declared the patient officially dead. According to the ambulance driver, the patient had collapsed at about 4:15 P.M. The senior resident wondered privately what the outcome would have been if CPR had been started sooner.

Unlike cessation of respiration, which is an obvious sign of sudden death, the stoppage of circulation, and particularly the rhythm of the heart, are invisible to an observer. Perhaps as a result, the development of artificial circulation lagged considerably behind the obvious need for artificial respirations. Moreover, even if scientists in the post-Enlightenment period did appreciate the need to circulate blood, there was simply no effective means of doing so. Closed-chest massage was described in 1904, but its benefits were not appreciated, and anecdotal case reports did little to promote them. Instead, the prevailing belief was that physicians were powerless to reverse a patient's stopped circulation.

It would be nice to believe that all scientific discoveries result from the painstaking accumulation of small facts whose accretion leads to a grand synthesis. The truth, however, is that the role of accident cannot be discounted. Chest compression was actually a serendipitous discovery made by William Kouwenhoven, G. Guy Knickerbocker, and James R. Jude at Johns Hopkins University in 1958 (figure 2.4). They had been inducing ventricular fibrillation in dogs when they noticed that they could achieve a pulse in a dog's femoral artery by forcefully applying the paddles to its chest. In other words, they discovered that rhythmic pressure on the chest led to the forward flow of blood. Further meticulous experimentation involving dogs answered such basic questions as where the compressions should be applied as well as how fast and how deep they should be. When the technique had been refined, it was ready for use on humans. Jude recalls the first person to be saved with this technique, "rather an obese female who . . . went into cardiac arrest as a result of flurothane anesthetic. . . . This woman had no blood pressure, no pulse, and ordinarily we would have opened up her chest. . . . Instead, since we weren't in the operating room, we applied external cardiac massage. . . . Her blood pressure and pulse came back at once. We didn't have to open her chest. They went ahead and did the operation on her, and she recovered completely."[11]

In 1960, in the *Journal of the American Medical Association*, the three investigators

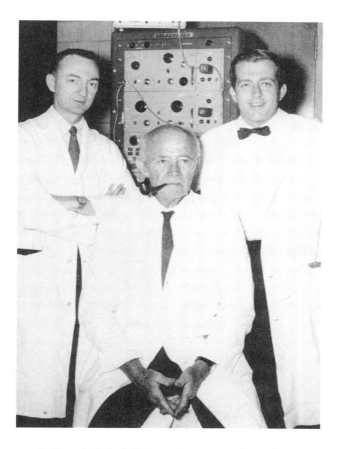

2.4 Dr. James R. Jude (*left*), Dr. William Kouwenhoven (*center*), and Dr. G. Guy Knickerbocker (*right*) in Dr. Kouwenhoven's laboratory at Johns Hopkins Hospital, 1961. From P. Safar, ed., *Advances in Cardiopulmonary Resuscitation* (New York: Springer-Verlag, 1977), 291. Used with permission of Springer Science and Business Media.

reported their findings on twenty cases of in-hospital cardiac arrest. Fourteen of the twenty patients (70 percent) survived and were discharged from the hospital. Many of these patients had been in cardiac arrest as a result of anesthesia. Three had been documented as being in ventricular fibrillation. The duration of chest compression varied, from less than one minute to sixty-five minutes. The message of these investigators' findings was very straightforward concerning patients in VF: chest compression buys time for an external defibrillator to arrive on the scene. As the authors wrote, "Anyone, anywhere, can now initiate cardiac resuscitative procedures. All that is needed is two hands."[12] But their published research gave relatively little attention to respiration—many of the twenty patients had been intubated, so there had been no need for mouth-to-mouth ventilation. Soon, however, chest compression was formally "married" to mouth-to-mouth ventilation, and the couple's new name was CPR.

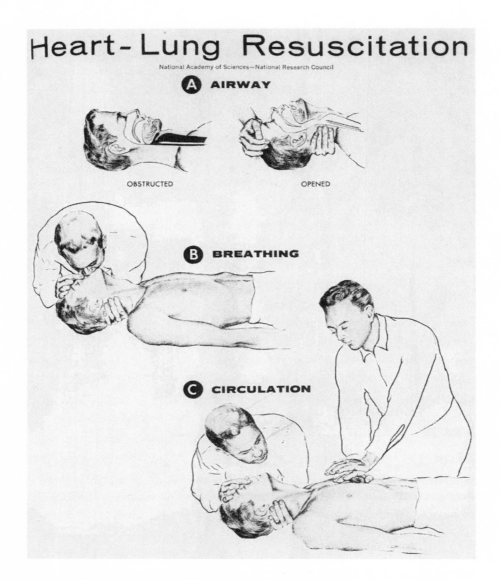

2.5 The ABCs of CPR. Reproduced from Committee on CPR of the Division of Medical Sciences, National Academy of Science–National Research Council, "Cardiopulmonary Resuscitation," *Journal of the American Medical Association* 198 (1966), 372–79. Copyright 1966, American Medical Association. Used with permission.

Mouth-to-Mouth Ventilation Plus Chest Compression Equals CPR

NOVEMBER 30, 1960, CARDIOLOGY CLINIC, BALTIMORE CITY HOSPITAL

Brian N. had almost made it to the clinic's waiting room when he collapsed. Someone inside alerted the receptionist, who called out for help as she dialed the hospital operator and asked for a "Doctor Blue" page to the clinic.

The clinic doctors placed Brian on his back, and the code team arrived shortly thereafter. One member of the team placed himself at Brian's head and bent over to provide mouth-to-mouth ventilation. Another knelt by Brian's chest and began chest compression. Brian was then placed on a gurney and quickly rolled into the hospital's emergency room. There a large and ungainly defibrillator was used to defibrillate Brian's heart.

Brian, discharged to his home two weeks later, was the first out-of-hospital survivor of sudden cardiac arrest—technically, he had collapsed outside the clinic's doors.

The formal connection of chest compression with mouth-to-mouth ventilation, to create CPR as it is practiced today, occurred when Safar, Jude, and Kouwenhoven presented their findings on September 16, 1960, in a panel at the annual meeting of the Maryland Medical Society. In his opening remarks, the moderator said, "Our purpose today is to bring to you . . . this new idea." It was so new, in fact, that it was still without a name. The moderator stated that the two techniques could not "be considered any longer as separate units, but as parts of a whole and complete approach to resuscitation."[13] Safar, in his own remarks, stressed the importance of combining ventilation and circulation. He presented convincing data that chest compression alone did not provide effective ventilation—mouth-to-mouth respiration had to be part of the equation.[14]

To promote CPR, Jude, Knickerbocker, and Safar began a worldwide speaking tour. In 1962, Archer Gordon, along with David Adams, produced a twenty-seven-minute training film, *The Pulse of Life*, which was used in CPR classes and viewed by millions of students. For their film, Gordon and Adams devised the easy-to-remember mnemonic "A, B, and C," which represented the sequence of steps in CPR—airway, breathing, and circulation (fig. 2.5). In 1963, the American Heart Association formally endorsed CPR, and in 1966 the National Research Council of the National Academy of Sciences convened an ad hoc conference to establish standardized training and performance standards for CPR. In the same year, recommendations from this conference were reported in the *Journal of the American Medical Association*.[15]

The Spark of Life: Defibrillation

JULY 7, 1964, EMERGENCY ROOM, CHARITY HOSPITAL, NEW ORLEANS

It was the intern's first night on duty. She had been briefed on the equipment and on how to order X-rays and blood work, request charts, and complete patient records.

Her hopes for a quiet night were shattered when an ambulance crew rolled in with a patient in cardiac arrest. One nurse and an aide started CPR while another nurse attached ECG leads to the patient's chest.

The rhythm strip showed a chaotic line, and the intern hesitated. Was this VF? (She had read about VF but never seen it in an actual patient.) Could it be artifact? Perhaps it was 60-cycle electrical interference? She'd never live it down if she shocked artifact.

With considerably less than 100 percent confidence, she grabbed the defibrillator paddles, placed them on the patient's chest in what she hoped was the right position, and shocked him. Amazing! In twenty seconds there was an organized rhythm, and in sixty seconds she perceived a faint pulse. But she was embarrassed to see the large red circular burn marks where the paddles had been applied.

"Damn," she said to herself, "guess I forgot the conducting gel."

Still, this wasn't bad for her first night.

Claude Beck, professor of surgery at Western Reserve University[16] in Cleveland, worked for years on a technique for defibrillation of the human heart. By the 1930s, it was known that electric shocks, even small ones, could induce ventricular fibrillation in a dog's heart, and that more powerful shocks could erase the fibrillation.[17] Beck believed that electricity could be of equal benefit to surgical patients whose hearts fibrillated during surgery or induction of anesthesia.

It was probably in 1922 that Beck witnessed his first cardiac arrest, while he was an intern on the surgery service at Johns Hopkins Hospital in Baltimore. During a urological operation, the anesthetist announced that the patient's heart had stopped. To Beck's amazement, the surgical resident removed his gloves, went to a telephone in a corner of the operating room, and called the fire department. Beck remained in total bewilderment as, fifteen minutes later, the fire department's rescue squad rushed into the operating room and applied oxygen-powered respirators to the patient's face. The patient died, but the episode left an indelible impression on Beck. He went on to develop techniques for taking the management of cardiac arrest away from fire departments and placing it back into the hands of surgeons.[18]

Beck realized that ventricular fibrillation often occurred in hearts that were basically sound, and he coined the phrase "hearts too good to die." In 1947, using open-chest massage and internal defibrillation with alternating current, he had accomplished his first successful resuscitation on a fourteen-year-old boy (fig. 2.6) The boy was being operated on for a severe congenital malformation of the chest, but in all other respects he was normal. During closure of the large incision in his chest, the boy's pulse suddenly stopped, and his blood pressure fell to zero. He was in cardiac arrest. Beck immediately reopened the boy's chest and began manual heart massage. As he looked at and felt the heart, he realized that ventricular fibrillation was present. Massage was continued for thirty-five minutes, and then an electrocardiogram was taken. It confirmed the presence of ventricular fibrillation. Another ten minutes passed before a defibrillator was brought to the operating room. The first shock, using electrode paddles placed directly onto the sides of the heart, was unsuccessful. Beck then adminis-

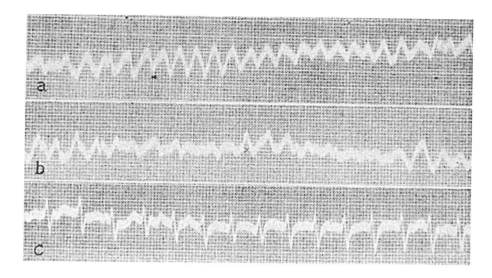

2.6 Actual electrocardiograms for a fourteen-year-old boy, the first human being ever to have been successfully defibrillated. The top two panels show the boy's heart in ventricular fibrillation before the lifesaving electric shock delivered by Dr. Claude Beck. The bottom panel shows a life-sustaining supraventricular tachycardia after the shock. Reproduced from C. S. Beck et al., "Ventricular Fibrillation of Long Duration Abolished by Electric Shock," *Journal of the American Medical Association* 135 (1947), 985. Copyright 1947, American Medical Association. Used with permission.

tered procainamide, a medicine used to stabilize the heart's rhythm, and gave the boy's heart a second shock, which wiped out the fibrillation. Within seconds a feeble, regular, fast contraction of the heart was occurring. The blood pressure rose from 0 to 50 millimeters of mercury. Beck noted that the heartbeat remained regular, and he watched the boy's blood pressure slowly begin to rise. Twenty minutes after the successful defibrillation, he closed the chest wound for the second time. After three hours, the boy's blood pressure had risen to a normal level, and he awoke and was able to answer questions. The boy made a full recovery, with no neurological damage.[19]

Thus Claude Beck pioneered internal defibrillation of the heart. In other words, during this procedure the chest was open, and the defibrillator paddles were placed directly onto the heart. It was groundbreaking work, but it was soon to be eclipsed by devices that could defibrillate the heart externally, through the closed chest.

For Paul Zoll, well aware of Beck's accomplishment, the development of an external defibrillator had been a natural extension of his earlier work with an external cardiac pacemaker. In 1955, a sixty-seven-year-old man had survived several episodes of ventricular fibrillation, thanks to Zoll's external defibrillator, and had gone home from the hospital a month later. Over a period of four months, using external defibrillation and shocks ranging from 240 to 720 volts, Zoll successfully stopped ventricular fibrillation eleven times in four more hospitalized patients. The following year, Zoll published his landmark findings.[20]

Zoll's defibrillator, like earlier versions invented by Kouwenhoven and Beck, utilized alternating current (AC) and was run off line current (the electricity from any wall socket). The decision to use alternating rather than direct current had been a practical one—in the 1950s, capacitor technology, driven by direct current, powerful enough to do the job and portable enough for practical use, did not exist. An AC defibrillator was very large and heavy, primarily because it contained a transformer to step up the line current from 110 volts to 500 or 1,000 volts. Although a defibrillator like this was far too massive to carry, it could be mounted on wheels and pushed down a corridor from one part of the hospital to another. Still, unless the problem of the AC defibrillator's inherent nonportability could be solved, not many lives would be saved.

The portability problem was solved by Bernard Lown, who devised a defibrillator that utilized direct current (DC) instead of alternating current. A series of experiments on dogs in 1960 and 1961, along with clinical use with patients in the early 1960s, established that DC shocks were extremely effective in defibrillating the heart.[21] What's more, it was clear that DC was actually safer than AC when a shock was delivered through the chest wall. With direct current, it was possible to use power supplied by a battery to charge a capacitor in just a few seconds. The capacitor stored the energy until it was released in one massive jolt to the chest wall. The availability of new, smaller capacitors considerably reduced the size and weight of the device. No longer would defibrillators require bulky transformers, and no longer would they be tied to line current. The cord was cut—the defibrillator could travel to the patient.

Mobile Intensive Care

MAY 3, 1966, ROYAL VICTORIA HOSPITAL

The call that came in to the nursing station on the cardiology ward was from a general practitioner. He reported that one of his patients had phoned him, complaining of chest pain, and was too weak to make it in to the hospital on his own. The patient needed an ambulance, and he needed it now.

The ward nurse took down the patient's address and rang the ambulance bay. Then she gathered up the other team members, who were scattered throughout the ward. The team—a doctor, a medical student, and an ECG technician in addition to the nurse— hurried to the hospital's front entrance, where an ambulance was waiting.

It took the team members fourteen minutes to reach the patient's home. They lugged a medicine box, a small oxygen tank, and a twenty-pound electrocardiograph machine up two flights of stairs and found the patient on his bed, sweating profusely.

The bulky, 12-lead electrocardiograph confirmed what the team already suspected—

a large myocardial infarction. The ambulance driver ran to retrieve the defibrillator, just in case. As the team helped the patient off his bed and onto a transport chair, he went limp. The ambulance driver quickly reappeared, huffing and puffing from his quick trip up the stairs, and set the defibrillator down.

Now the doctor reattached the ECG leads to the patient's chest, and a squiggly chaotic line coursed across the paper—the unmistakable sign of ventricular fibrillation. The ambulance driver, reaching to plug the defibrillator in, groaned as he saw that its adaptor would not fit into the socket on the patient's bedroom wall. He ran back down to the ambulance and back upstairs again, this time carrying two 12-volt car batteries.

Meanwhile, the team had started CPR. As soon as the ambulance driver produced the batteries, the team members wired them to the defibrillator. Then, holding their breath, they delivered the shock, and the patient's upper body twitched in response. The ECG showed twenty seconds of flatlining, then a contraction, and then another. Soon the ECG showed real improvement, and the patient started to moan. Everyone knew that the worst was over.

For many years, all that a civilian ambulance service could do was to take a patient to the hospital. The driver may have had a little first aid training; for all practical purposes, though, all he could offer was lie-down taxi service. It is true that in a few cities interns rode in ambulances as part of their training, but they provided little medical care at the scene.

During the 1930s and 1940s, municipal fire departments in some cities, including Los Angeles, Columbus, Baltimore, and Seattle, began to provide rescue, first aid, and resuscitation care. In 1966, the United States National Academy of Sciences and the President's Commission on Highway Safety issued reports decrying the unevenness in ambulance personnel's competence and the lack of standard procedures. The commission, for its part, described the carnage resulting from traffic accidents as a neglected disease of society. The subsequent National Highway Safety and Traffic Act of 1966 authorized the Department of Transportation to establish a national curriculum for prehospital personnel, and this act in turn led to the training and certification of a newly created group of medical professionals—emergency medical technicians.

EMTs did much to upgrade the general performance of ambulance services throughout the United States. The eighty-hour course and certification, which included training in CPR, ensured that victims of motor vehicle accidents and other emergencies would at least have access to proper care. For example, EMTs could provide artificial ventilation and closed-chest massage at the scene of an accident and en route to the hospital. Nevertheless, EMTs were neither trained nor authorized to provide definitive care for cardiac arrest. They could not provide defibrillation, intravenous medications, or advanced airway control, such as endotracheal intubation. The sad reality was that EMTs saved few if any victims of sudden cardiac arrest. The time required for EMTs to be dispatched, arrive at the scene, load the patient into the ambulance, and transport the patient to the closest emergency room was too long for resuscitation efforts to be successful. Not even letter-perfect CPR can save a life if it takes too long to begin defibrillation and other advanced procedures.

In the mid-1960s, hospitals began to open coronary care units (CCUs) in response to data showing that more patients in those units survived cardiac arrest than did patients in regular wards. The causes were attributed to many factors, but an obvious one was rapid treatment with a defibrillator when the heart went into VF. I suppose that such early successes may have led a few cardiologists to dream of moving CCUs into the community. That dream became reality in Belfast, Northern Ireland.

In 1965, Frank Pantridge, a cardiologist at the Royal Victoria Hospital, turned his attention to the vexing problem of heart attacks and sudden cardiac death. His sensitivity to the problem had two sources. First, he had heard frequent comments from personnel in the hospital's emergency department about the number of patients who were coming in dead on arrival. Second, Pantridge had recently read a telling study in a medical journal, which indicated that among middle-aged or younger men with acute MI, more than 60 percent died within one hour of the onset of symptoms. Pantridge realized that the problem of death from acute MI had to be solved outside the hospital, not in the emergency room or the coronary care unit. As he later wrote, "The majority of deaths from coronary attacks were occurring outside the hospital, and nothing whatever was being done about them. It became very clear to me that a coronary care unit confined to the hospital would have a minimal impact on mortality." Pantridge wanted his coronary care unit in the community—or as he put it, "We must go out and get these people."[22]

Pantridge's solution was to develop the world's first mobile coronary care unit, or MCCU. He staffed it with an ambulance driver, a physician, and a nurse. Sometimes a medical student and an ECG technician rode along, too. Pantridge encountered numerous obstacles to the creation of the MCCU. He dealt with them in his typical fashion—head-on, with bulldog determination to succeed, and with transparent contempt for politicians and authority figures who opposed him. Even his cardiology colleagues were skeptical. "My noncardiological medical colleagues in the hospital were totally unconvinced and totally uncooperative," Pantridge said. "It was considered unorthodox, if not illegal, to send hospital personnel including doctors and nurses outside the hospital."[23] Pantridge's new program began service on January 1, 1966.

John Geddes, a resident in cardiology at the Royal Victoria Hospital, also worked on Pantridge's service. As a junior member of the team, he was responsible, along with four other residents, for riding along in the ambulance when it was called into action. Why had this breakthrough in cardiac care occurred in Belfast, of all places? Geddes thought he knew the answer. As he said in 1990, there were "two reasons":

One was Pantridge himself. He is a remarkable personality who is very persuasive. He can persuade people to do things, and . . . actually make them enjoy doing things that he has made them do because they are successful. So there was his tremendous enthusiasm behind the system. Then there was the fact that the layout of the [Royal Victoria] hospital was flat and it was quick and easy to get to people and resuscitate them. I didn't realize this at the time, but I subsequently visited hospitals in various parts of England. They had slow elevators and so on, and you could never move around the hospital quickly with any kind of emergency apparatus.[24]

Their success in the hospital wards led Pantridge and Geddes to believe that success in the community was also a possibility. As Geddes observed, the leap from the hospital to the community owed its inception to a hospital's architectural layout combined with a physician's driving and persuasive personality. But one cannot discount the resuscitation infrastructure already in place: mouth-to-mouth ventilation, chest compression, and portable defibrillation. Without each of these three elements, the Belfast program would have been a waste of time and effort.

In August 1967, Pantridge and Geddes published the initial results of their program in *The Lancet*, reporting their findings on 312 patients seen over a fifteen-month period. Half the patients had experienced MI, and there were no deaths during transport to the hospital. Of groundbreaking importance was the information on ten patients who had experienced cardiac arrest. All of these patients had ventricular fibrillation; six of the arrests occurred after the arrival of the MCCU, and four occurred shortly before its arrival. All ten patients were resuscitated and admitted to the hospital. Five were subsequently discharged alive.[25]

The Belfast system was established to reach patients who had suffered acute myocardial infarction. The patients who were resuscitated were those whose hearts had fibrillated either after the ambulance arrived or while it was on the way. But the system was too slow to resuscitate people whose hearts fibrillated before the ambulance was called. In 1966, it was still assumed that most cardiac deaths in out-of-hospital community settings resulted from acute myocardial infarction. It was not yet appreciated that ventricular fibrillation can occur without myocardial infarction, and that it can take place with only seconds of warning—or with no warning at all. To tackle sudden death due to VF, a new model of care was needed. And one was developed in the United States.

PARAMEDICS TAKE TO THE STREETS

MAY 30, 1971, SEATTLE

Greg S. was a graduate of the first class of paramedics to be trained in the Seattle area, and he loved his new job. He and his colleagues were actually bringing in live patients!

The patients had been defibrillated in the field, with their IVs started and their trachea tubes in place. Their meds had already been administered, and they were coming in with a bounding pulse and blood pressure. These outcomes were very different from what Greg had known when he was a firefighter. In those days, he could never get a pulse, and dragging the patient to the emergency room had been an exercise in futility. In fact, the only advantage of transporting the patient had been that the hospital would declare him dead, so Greg wouldn't have to wait in the patient's room until the mortuary van arrived to pick up the body. That had been the worst part of the job.

The extensive international readership of *The Lancet* helps to explain why Pantridge's idea spread so rapidly to other countries. Within two years, similar physician-staffed MCCU programs had begun in Australia and Europe. The first such program in the United States was begun in 1968 by William Grace of St. Vincent's Hospital, in the Greenwich Village neighborhood of New York City. The program was a clone of the Belfast program and utilized specially equipped ambulances with physicians on board to provide advanced resuscitation care directly at the scene of cardiac emergencies. Medical emergency calls in which chest pain was a complaint were passed on from the police operator to the hospital. From the hospital, an ambulance would fight New York traffic to arrive at the scene. Grace has described the rather full ambulance and how the team was assembled and dispatched:

> The personnel includes an attending physician, resident physician, emergency room nurse, ECG technician, as well as a student nurse observer, in addition to the driver and his assistant. This team is summoned from various points in the hospital to the emergency room by a personal paging system which each member of the team carries. This team has four and one half minutes to get to the emergency room, obtain their equipment and board the ambulance. Anyone who is not there within this time is left behind.[26]

In a scientific report on the program at St. Vincent's, Grace described the program's experience with its first 161 patients. In only two instances had the physician failed to reach the emergency room in time to board the ambulance, which usually reached the patient within fourteen minutes of leaving the hospital, for a total of eighteen and a half minutes from the time the call came in to the time the MCCU arrived at the scene (one call had taken twenty-five minutes because of heavy traffic). Among the first group of patients seen by the MCCU were three who had been treated for ventricular fibrillation. One of the three survived.[27]

Grace had taken an innovative concept imported from overseas and made it work in his own community. By the standards of 1968, it was quite unusual to have physicians with defibrillators rushing through the city to reach nonbreathing, unconscious people whose hearts had stopped. But the program was limited in its vision, and although it was feasible in some urban communities that had large teaching hospitals, it was not a program that could be applied at the national level.

Pantridge, Geddes, and Grace had broken through the conceptual block that had confined resuscitation to hospitals. Now someone had to break through the conceptual block that was still keeping resuscitation in the hands of physicians. The next stage would call for a major change in the personnel who were allowed to perform resuscitation. An evolution in prehospital emergency care was needed.

The new model would require a specially trained individual, a "physician extender"—someone who was not a physician but could perform some of the physician's resuscitation procedures. In the United States, the evolution from physician-staffed mobile intensive care units to paramedic-staffed units occurred independently and almost simultaneously in several communities. Two communities that led the way were Miami and Seattle, but others included Portland, Oregon, Los Angeles, and Columbus, Ohio. Not only were paramedics used instead of physicians, but these programs, from their inception, had also been established to deal with the problem of sudden cardiac arrest. By contrast, Pantridge's program had been established primarily to reach MI victims quickly and thereby prevent death during the early, vulnerable stage of an MI; as a result, cardiac arrest could be treated successfully only if it occurred as a complication of MI and only if the ambulance was either already at the scene or on the way. But the new paramedic-staffed programs in American cities were far more nimble than the earlier physician-staffed programs, and they were specifically designed not only to treat the early stages of MI but also to attempt resuscitation for sudden cardiac arrest wherever and whenever it occurred. Indeed, reversal of death itself would be a major purpose and goal of the new paramedic programs. Beck's vision of treating "hearts too good to die" was becoming a reality.

Eugene Nagel, an anesthesiologist at the University of Miami, had become aware of Pantridge's work in 1967. He believed that the physician-staffed model of prehospital care was not going to work for the United States in general, or for Miami in particular. For one thing, it cost too much to hire physicians to sit around in fire stations waiting around the clock for calls. For another, if physicians had to be picked up at hospitals, it would take too long for them to arrive at the scene. When Nagel or his colleague James Hirschman rode along in the ambulances, they could defibrillate and provide medications, of course, but they could hardly be present for all shifts. And, much as they liked riding with the firefighters, they did, after all, have regular jobs at the hospital. Nagel became convinced that it was time to move away from programs using physicians and to adopt programs staffed by firefighter paramedics. He considered firefighters to be perfect candidates for the job of paramedic. Firefighters had a long tradition of first aid and rescue, and fire stations were strategically located throughout the city.

Nagel moved incrementally. He did not think that it would be possible initially to sell the idea of paramedics working alone, even if they had the training to perform medical procedures that had been authorized in writing by physicians. Therefore, his first step was to establish a radio link and telemetry (that is, electronic transmission of a patient's ECG signal to a receiving monitor) between paramedic firefighters and hospitals.[28] Nagel had a hidden agenda in promoting telemetry—for him, it was the Trojan horse that would allow him to step around the legal impediments to firefighters' ability to defibrillate patients and administer medications. Nagel reasoned that if the fire department could send an ECG signal to a hospital via telemetry, then the firefighters, with special training, could be authorized by the physician in charge to administer the needed drugs and perform the necessary procedures before arriving at the emergency room. He believed that a paramedic at the scene should be considered a legal extension of a physician. As he recalled later, "We saw telemetry as the key to extending our treatment to outside the hospital, where hitherto trying to legislate it was the dark side of the moon in those days. The telemetry looked like it might be the 'open sesame' to doing some treatment prehospital."[29]

Nagel had hoped to find support for his position from the medical community; instead, he encountered only discouragement. (Opposition to innovation seems to have been a recurring theme.) As Nagel recalled, "It was a rare doctor that favored us doing any of this stuff—very rare. We had incidents in the street when we were just sending an ECG, where doctors on the scene would tell the paramedics to quit fooling around and haul the victim in."[30]

It should not be surprising, then, that the medical directors of the various paramedic programs remember the first resuscitation in their city. Nagel himself vividly recalled the first save of the Miami paramedic program. The collapse had occurred near Station 1, on the fringe of downtown Miami, where, as Nagel puts it, "the good part meets the bad part":

> There was a guy named Dan Jones who was then about 60 years old, who was a wino who lived in a fleabag [hotel] in the bad part of town. Jones was well known to rescue. In June of '69 they got a call—man down—it was Jones. They put the paddles on him, he was in VF, started CPR, zapped him, he came back to sinus rhythm, brought him in to ER and three days later he was out and walking around. In gratitude, about a week later, he came down to Station 1, which he had never done before, and he said he would like to talk to the men who saved his life. They told me they had never seen Dan Jones in a clean shirt and sober, both of which he was that day. He would periodically come to the firehouse and just say hello and he seemed to be sober. In my talks in those days I said this was the new cure for alcoholism. That was our first true save.[31]

Pantridge's work had also energized Leonard Cobb, a cardiologist at the University of Washington, who was working at Harborview Hospital in Seattle. Cobb knew that the Seattle Fire Department was already involved in first aid, so he approached the fire chief, Gordon Vickery, and proposed a new training program to treat cardiac arrest. Seattle's fire department had already become one of the first in the United States to use a computerized system for documenting first aid runs. Cobb realized that this system could provide scientific documentation for the efficacy (or lack thereof) of Pantridge's ideas, and he suggested to Vickery that they pool their knowledge and resources. Cobb and his colleagues then provided instruction and training to firefighters in cardiac emergencies, including cardiac arrest. The firefighters all freely volunteered to become trained as paramedics.

The Seattle program, known as Medic One, became operational in March 1970, nine months after Nagel's first save in Miami. The mobile unit—and there was only one at first—was stationed outside Harborview's emergency department. As Cobb himself has pointed out, the mobile unit staffed with firefighter paramedics was not the real innovation; rather, it was the program's concept of a tiered response to medical emergencies, using the fire department's existing aid units, which were quickly followed by a secondary response from the mobile intensive coronary care unit. The beauty of the tiered-response system was its efficient use of the fire department's personnel—and, as in Miami, the strategic locations of the fire stations made this rapid response possible. Firefighter EMTs staffing the aid unit reached the scene quickly— on an average of three or four minutes—to start CPR. Then a few minutes later the paramedics arrived to provide more definitive care such as defibrillation. (For the first twelve years of the program only paramedics were authorized to use defibrillators, but in the early 1980s EMTs were also trained to defibrillate patients.) Under this tiered-response system, the patient's brain could be oxygenated and kept alive until an electric shock converted the heart to a normal rhythm. After the patient was stabilized, the paramedics transported him or her to the hospital.[32]

Seattle's program made pioneering use of paramedics, and it promoted the use of a tiered-response system. But it did more than that—it was the first program in the world to make citizens an element of emergency response. Cobb was familiar with the data that the program had collected, and he knew that the sooner CPR was started, the better the chances of the patient's survival. He reasoned that the best way to ensure early initiation of CPR was to train anyone who might one day become a bystander. And so Cobb, with the support of Vickery, began a program in 1972 called Medic Two. Its goal was to train more than 100,000 people in Seattle in how to do CPR. Cobb recalled how this idea had first been proposed:

> One day [Vickery] said, "Look, if it's so important to get CPR started quickly and if firemen come around to do it, it can't be that complicated that other

folks couldn't also learn—firemen are not created by God to do CPR. You could train the public." I said, "That sounds like a very good idea." Shortly afterwards things started.[33]

Cobb decided to use an abbreviated course of training:

> We weren't going to do it by traditional ways where they had to come for 20 hours [of training]. So they had to do it at one sitting—how long will people participate?—well, maybe three hours and that's pretty much the way it was.[34]

Cautiously, Cobb did not say how long it would take to train 100,000 people. He had no idea. In fact, however, it took only a few years, and by the twentieth anniversary of the establishment of the citizen training program, more than 500,000 people in Seattle and the surrounding suburbs had received training in CPR.

Some people were skeptical about mass citizen training in CPR; indeed, many felt that the potential for harm was too great to put such a procedure in the hands of laypersons. The skeptics also had the support of national medical organizations. But the alarmist voices were stilled by some fortunate saves. Cobb recalled one resuscitation that had been carried out soon after the citizen training program began. "In March 1973 there were these kids playing golf at Jackson Park. They came across a victim a quarter of a mile from the clubhouse." The man was unconscious and not breathing; later it was confirmed that he was in ventricular fibrillation. "But these kids had taken the [CPR] course over at the local high school. Two or three of them started doing CPR and the other kid ran off and phoned the fire department. Shortly they came with the aid car and Medic One screaming over the fairways." Cobb concluded, "They got him started up again. He survived; he's alive today [1989]. That was a very convincing story. I didn't mind it being written up in the *Reader's Digest*."[35]

The development of CPR had begun in the 1960s. By the end of that decade, paramedic programs were operating in Miami, Seattle, Portland, Columbus, and Los Angeles. The common denominator in all these cities was a physician who had seen the problem of out-of-hospital cardiac deaths, decided not to accept the irreversibility of death, and championed doing something about it. Just as important was the willingness, shared by all these innovating physicians, to buck the system and challenge the idea that only physicians are entitled to perform certain medical procedures. They questioned the conventional wisdom, and they moved the practice of medicine out of the hospitals and into the streets, people's homes, and the community. By the early 1970s, as a result of these groundbreaking efforts, all these cities had programs in place to provide CPR, defibrillation, and rapid prehospital care. The structure for resuscitating the victims of sudden death had been built, and the programs were proving successful. Paramedic services began to spread across the nation.

The story of resuscitation does not end with the early 1970s. In 1980, the first program to train EMTs to perform defibrillation began in King County, Washington, and this kind of training was then taken up by other communities. It required ten hours, and in the first demonstration project, the survival rate for ventricular fibrillation increased from 7 percent to 26 percent.[36]

Also in King County, the first program to train firefighter EMTs in the use of automated external defibrillators began in 1984. The use of AEDs simplified the training of EMTs and thus allowed the procedure to spread more rapidly throughout the United States. It requires considerably less time to train someone to use an automated external defibrillator than to use a manual defibrillator, since the EMT using an AED does not have to interpret the cardiac rhythm.[37] Training in the use of automated external defibrillators is now part of the national EMT curriculum.[38]

In 1983, a program to provide telephone instructions in CPR began in King County.[39] This program trained emergency dispatchers to tell callers how to perform CPR while the fire department's EMT personnel were on the way. The demonstration project increased the rate of bystander-provided CPR by 50 percent, and it improved the survival rate for out-of-hospital cardiac arrest.[40] Dispatcher-assisted telephone CPR is strongly endorsed by the American Heart Association and is now standard in dispatcher centers throughout the United States and in other countries, such as Israel, Great Britain, Sweden, and Norway.

The American Heart Association uses the metaphor of a four-link chain to name the elements of successful resuscitation. These links are *early access* (recognizing that a cardiac arrest has occurred, and calling 911), *early CPR*, *early defibrillation*, and *early advanced care* (such as medications and endotracheal intubation). The first paramedic programs were all designed to provide CPR, defibrillation, and advanced care quickly enough to resuscitate patients in cardiac arrest, but innovations over the past several decades have allowed advanced care to be delivered even more quickly.

Thus our ancient quest for resuscitation, which began with the biblical prophets, reaches fulfillment—at least some of the time—in our own day.

THREE

Causes of Sudden Cardiac Death

This chapter describes in greater detail the common and uncommon heart-related causes of sudden death as well as the non-heart-related causes.[1] In King County, Washington, 72 percent of people who experience cardiac arrest and who receive care from emergency medical services have underlying heart disease as the cause of cardiac arrest. The remaining 28 percent suffer from a variety of causative conditions. Among them are respiratory disease (7 percent); stroke and aneurysm (3 percent); cancer (4 percent); drug overdose and alcohol intoxication (3 percent); sudden infant death syndrome (2 percent); renal disease (1 percent); drowning (1 percent); other conditions, including anaphylaxis (6 percent); and unknown causes (1 percent; see figure 3.1).

HEART DISEASE AS THE CAUSE OF CARDIAC ARREST

As figure 3.1 illustrates, underlying heart disease is by far the leading cause of cardiac arrest.[2] The term "underlying heart disease" refers in general to problems of the heart. The specific causes of heart disease that may lead to cardiac arrest are listed in table 3.1. Myocardial ischemia and myocardial infarction are responsible for 70 to 75 percent of all cardiac arrests connected with underlying heart disease. The remaining 25 to 30 percent of such cardiac arrests are caused by a variety of other heart conditions, including congestive heart failure, dilated and hypertrophic cardiomyopathy, primary electrical diseases (long Q-T syndrome, Brugada syndrome, and Wolff-Parkinson-White syndrome), valvular heart disease, and commotio cordis, all of which are described in this chapter.

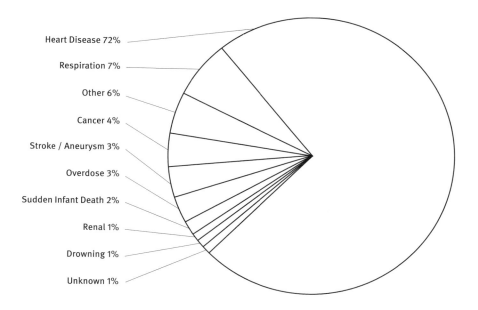

Heart Disease 72%
Respiration 7%
Other 6%
Cancer 4%
Stroke / Aneurysm 3%
Overdose 3%
Sudden Infant Death 2%
Renal 1%
Drowning 1%
Unknown 1%

3.1 Causes of cardiac arrest, by percentage in King County, Washington, 1980-2010, for cases in which EMS personnel attempted resuscitation.

CORONARY ARTERY DISEASE AND ISCHEMIA

At first William A., a retired pharmacist, thought it was his typical angina—a squeezing sensation under his breastbone, radiating into his upper left arm. The pain tended to be triggered by eating a large meal or making a strenuous effort, such as climbing stairs too fast or mowing the lawn on a hot day. William's doctor had told him about some angina-prevention medications he could take before such activities, but William hadn't yet filled the prescription. (Ironically, this former pharmacist didn't like taking medications.)

William's angina usually let up if he rested and took a nitroglycerin tablet or two. But this time the pain was still there after three tablets. William wondered if he should take a fourth, or call 911 as his doctor had told him to do if his symptoms persisted after three tablets. He decided to do neither. Instead, he would just wait and see if the pain subsided. The last thing he wanted was an ambulance racing up to his house with lights flashing and sirens blaring.

Over the next fifteen minutes, the pain and pressure in his chest did seem to lessen somewhat, and it occurred to William that it might be a good idea for him to start taking the medications his doctor had mentioned. And that was his last thought. As his heart fibrillated, he instantly lost his pulse and blood pressure.

That evening William's daughter, after phoning him repeatedly, found him slumped on one side of his favorite chair. He looked peaceful, she said later.

Table 3.1. Causes of heart disease that may lead to cardiac arrest

Cause	Estimated Frequency
Coronary artery disease and ischemia	40–50%
Acute myocardial infarction	10–20%
Primary ventricular fibrillation	10–20%
Congestive heart failure	10–20%
Dilated cardiomyopathy	< 10%
Hypertrophic cardiomyopathy	< 5%
Primary electrical diseases	< 2%
Valvular heart disease	< 5%
Commotio cordis	< 1%

William's death from sudden cardiac arrest was due to underlying coronary artery disease (also known as "atherosclerotic heart disease" or "ischemic heart disease"). The actual trigger of ventricular fibrillation was the ischemia in his heart muscle. The term "ischemia" means a condition in which insufficient blood and oxygen are reaching the heart muscle. It leads to the symptom of angina, which is like a muscle cramp.[3] Ischemia is the most common cause of sudden cardiac death, probably accounting for 40 to 50 percent of all sudden deaths due to underlying heart disease. The symptoms of angina typically occur before the heart fibrillates. They may be brief, perhaps lasting only seconds or minutes, or they may go on for hours. Clearly, the fact that an area of the heart is receiving insufficient blood and oxygen is the trigger for the VF episode. What is not so clear is why a particular episode of angina has triggered VF, especially when the victim may have had dozens and dozens of anginal episodes without any long-term harm. What separates the fatal bout of ischemia from the routine one? The answer is not known.

ACUTE MYOCARDIAL INFARCTION

Harold R.'s wife had called an ambulance, and Harold was actually relieved to hear the sirens—anything to stop the pain, the sweating, the nausea, the feeling of utter exhaustion. He could barely lift his left arm, and the vise-like pain in his chest was the worst he had ever experienced. This was no bout of angina! And yet, as terrible as the pain was, he could almost stand it, because there was something even worse—a feeling deep inside, an awful sense of doom. He was going to die!

Harold's wife let the two paramedics in and described her husband's symptoms as she led the way to the couple's bedroom. When they entered, they found Harold unconscious, with no pulse or blood pressure. The paramedics pulled him to the floor, and while one started CPR, the other attached the leads from their defibrillator/monitor. Harold's heart rhythm was slow, and it appeared to be organized, but the paramedics still couldn't get a pulse.

They knew this rhythm well—pulseless electrical activity, often seen in massive myocardial infarctions. They knew that Harold's prognosis was grim, but they put in thirty-five minutes of effort—continuous CPR, endotracheal intubation, and intravenous medications, including four doses of epinephrine. In the end, though, their efforts were fruitless; they had to stop. And Mrs. R had watched it all, inconsolable.

What Harold experienced was an acute myocardial infarction. Myocardial infarction (MI) is the underlying cause of sudden death in approximately 15 to 20 percent of cases of sudden and fatal cardiac arrest. One can think of an MI as the most severe form of angina.

Angina is due to reduced blood flow to a coronary artery; MI is due to the artery's complete or near complete blockage. Think of the heart as a large twelve-ounce muscle. If small portions of the muscle are damaged, there is still enough power to pump blood. But if 40 percent or more of the muscle is damaged, the heart cannot pump sufficient blood to maintain adequate circulation, and everything downstream of the blockage will die unless the artery is rapidly reopened. In the case of MI, sudden death is due either to massive pump failure or to VF.

This is the situation in which we see the condition known as a massive MI, like the one that killed Harold. If you had been able to see inside Harold's chest, you would have seen a complete blockage of his left coronary artery, the one that supplied his heart's large left ventricle. Only if it had been possible to reopen the artery in a matter of minutes could Harold's death have been prevented. An MI can also be small, as when a minor branch of one of the main coronary arteries is blocked. In that case, the downstream damage may be to only 2 or 3 percent of the heart muscle—not enough to cause death through pump failure. But there is still a risk of ventricular fibrillation, since even a small MI can irritate the muscle within the affected zone. In that case, the irritated area can trigger VF.

MIs do not always lead to sudden death. In fact, most MIs do not. Typically, the patient is admitted to the hospital and may or may not undergo certain procedures, such as coronary angioplasty (wherein a catheter with a balloon is placed in the blocked coronary artery and used to open it) or stent placement (a stent is a small tube that is placed over the balloon used in coronary angioplasty, and left in place to keep the artery open after the balloon has been removed). A patient who has suffered an MI will be discharged 90 percent of the time. But in some instances (approximately 10 percent of admissions for MIs), the patient does not recover and dies in the hospital. Often the patient's death is due to ongoing pump failure, which occurs over hours or days rather than as a sudden, unexpected event. A person who has suffered an MI, reaches the hospital, and dies after admission still dies in the hospital. His or her death does not fit this book's definition of sudden cardiac death occurring in an out-of-hospital, community setting.

PRIMARY VENTRICULAR FIBRILLATION

Lihua B., a trim sixty-nine-year-old, was jogging slowly (mostly walking, actually) around Green Lake on a beautiful Seattle day made to order for exercise enthusiasts. The path around the lake, nearly three miles, was a great place for people watching, and Lihua usually managed to complete the circuit in fifty minutes. Today as she made her way along the path, she saw the usual runners, bikers, walkers, and rollerbladers along with lots of dogs on leashes, two ferrets, and even a parrot.

Near the parking lot, she stumbled a few steps forward and then fell face first onto the asphalt. Quite a few people had seen her stumble and fall. One of them was a retired fire-fighter on a walk with his granddaughter. He rushed over to Lihua, shook her, and then turned to a bystander.

"Call 911," he directed. "Tell them it's a cardiac arrest."

He took a clean handkerchief out of his pocket and wiped the blood off Lihua's mouth. Then he gave her mouth-to-mouth respirations, followed by chest compressions.

There was a fire department only a few blocks away, and its aid vehicle was there in three minutes. The EMTs attached Lihua to an automated external defibrillator, and her heart, after only one shock, returned to a normal rhythm.

Lihua woke up in the hospital shortly after being admitted, with no memory of any of the day's events. Five days later, she left the hospital with an implantable defibrillator in place.

Primary ventricular fibrillation is the most mysterious cause of sudden heart-related death, and it was Lihua's good fortune that she survived. With primary VF, there is absolutely no warning or premonition. In what is literally an instant, the heart goes into arrest. Primary VF gets its name from the fact that it is not secondary to another clear cause, such as ischemia or acute myocardial infarction. It accounts for approximately 10 to 20 percent of all sudden cardiac arrests. Even without a precipitating event like ischemia or acute MI, silent coronary artery disease is often present in up to half of those with primary VF. The rest of these victims appear to have perfectly normal hearts and coronary vessels.

CONGESTIVE HEART FAILURE

When Mary H., seventy-six, failed to appear for her volunteer job at the hospital gift shop, a concerned friend called Mary's number several times throughout the day but got no response. Finally Mary's friend called the police, who went to Mary's apartment building and had the manager open the door to Mary's apartment. Mary, lying in her bed, was clearly dead, but she looked very peaceful.

The medical examiner's office called Mary's doctor and asked if he would be willing to sign the death certificate. He agreed. Mary, whom he had been treating for stable congestive heart failure, had been his patient for fifteen years. The cause of death, as listed on the certificate, was cardiac arrest due to long-standing congestive heart failure.

Congestive heart failure (CHF), sometimes simply called "heart failure," is a definite risk factor for sudden cardiac arrest. In congestive heart failure, the ventricles of the heart are weakened and unable to pump blood adequately. As a result, blood backs up in the lungs. This backup leads to congestion in the lungs as well as to swollen feet and legs.[4]

There are two main types of heart failure: systolic and diastolic. In systolic heart failure, the heart's ability to contract is diminished. In diastolic heart failure, the heart muscle is abnormally stiff, cannot relax adequately between contractions, and the amount of blood pumped with each contraction is decreased. Both types of heart failure can cause fluid to back up in the lungs and/or in the feet and ankles. There is often considerable overlap between systolic and diastolic heart failure.

Heart failure affects 5,000,000 Americans, and 400,000 new cases are diagnosed every year.[5] The condition is twice as common among African Americans as among whites. CHF directly accounts for 39,000 deaths a year and is a contributing factor to an additional 225,000 deaths. Just in the period between 1970 and 1990, the death rate increased 64 percent. The condition now affects 1 percent of people over the age of fifty and about 5 percent of people over the age of seventy-five. This reported increase in deaths from heart failure probably explains the fall in the proportion of sudden cardiac deaths with associated VF that occur in community settings. Often in deaths from heart failure, there is asystole or pulseless electrical activity, whereas there is more VF in sudden cardiac deaths associated with ischemia or acute myocardial infarction.

The person with CHF experiences limitations on usual kinds of activity, such as walking, and more readily feels shortness of breath and fatigue. The most common cause of CHF is coronary artery disease. Even so, there may be few or no symptoms of angina, and there may be no history of myocardial infarction.

CARDIOMYOPATHY

The term "cardiomyopathy" is defined as disease of the heart muscle itself. In cardiomyopathy, the heart loses its ability to pump blood adequately, as discussed earlier in connection with congestive heart failure. Cardiomyopathies are classified according to the appearance or physical characteristics of the heart. The heart may be enlarged (a dilated cardiomyopathy), abnormally thickened (hypertrophic cardiomyopathy), or abnormally stiff (restrictive cardiomyopathy).

If known, cardiomyopathies (whether dilated, hypertropic, or restrictive) can also be classified according to their specific cause. For example, an ischemic cardiomyopathy, as already discussed, is caused by underlying coronary artery disease. To qualify as an ischemic cardiomyopathy, heart function must be impaired. That is, in ischemic heart disease the muscle may be episodically affected by ischemia but otherwise has normal or near normal function. An ischemic cardiomyopathy develops when the heart muscle has been damaged by ischemia or infarction to the degree that its pumping function is weakened. Typically, this results in heart enlargement, or what is called an ischemic dilated cardiomyopathy. Nonischemic cardiomyopathy is also fairly common and is said to affect 50,000 Americans. Any type of cardiomyopathy places a person at increased risk for sudden cardiac arrest.

Dilated Cardiomyopathy

Linda S. did not drink or smoke. She was something of a hypochondriac, but her doctor had little doubt about Linda's diagnosis of dilated cardiomyopathy. It was moderately severe, and it was likely to progress.

Linda was already on maximal medications. The best explanation for her condition was that it had been caused by a viral illness, perhaps one she had contracted as a child. Other than the usual colds and bouts of flu, however, Linda could not remember having had any serious viral infections.

Linda's doctor knew that cardiomyopathy placed Linda at high risk for sudden death, but he had never spoken to her about that possibility. What good, he reasoned, would it do?

Dilated cardiomyopathy (from either ischemic or nonischemic causes) is the most common form of cardiomyopathy and the leading reason for heart transplants. In dilated cardiomyopathy from whatever cause, the heart expands (enlarges) as a result of diseased muscle fibers and fluid accumulation in the body. A vicious cycle ensues, which in turn eventually leads to the development of symptoms and signs of heart failure, such as shortness of breath and edema. By the time heart failure is diagnosed, the disease has reached an advanced stage. Once failure occurs, the five-year survival rate is only 50 percent.

More than half of persons with dilated cardiomyopathy have no identifiable explanation for it, and are said to have an idiopathic dilated cardiomyopathy (this is a fancy medical way of saying that the cause is unknown). But some factors—such as alcoholism, or a viral illness leading to a heart inflammation—have been linked to the disease (alcohol has a direct suppressant effect on the heart). The condition can occur in pregnancy as well, although that is rare. Among the other less common causes are the medications used to treat some cancers and toxins. Hereditary causes of dilated cardiomyopathy—such as right ventricular cardiomyopathy, in which the muscle in the right ventricle is replaced with fibrous and fatty tissue—have also been identified, but they too are rare.

Hypertrophic Cardiomyopathy

Jared R. played basketball with a passion that had made him the star center on his high school team. Tall and agile, he was a natural athlete, and smart enough to know that basketball was his ticket to a college scholarship.

With four minutes left, Jared's team was up by fifteen. The coach, deciding to pull Jared for the final minutes of the game, rose from the bench to signal him. But, with bizarre symmetry, just as the coach stood up, Jared collapsed—three wavering steps, then a hard fall. Everyone in the stands heard Jared's head hit the court.

CPR was started almost immediately, and eleven minutes later the paramedics arrived. They worked on him for thirty minutes before rushing him to the hospital, continuing CPR all the way. But to no avail. The autopsy revealed hypertrophic cardiomyopathy.

Sudden cardiac arrest in a young person, especially an athlete, is often due to hypertrophic cardiomyopathy. The term refers to abnormally thickened diseased heart muscle.

Hypertrophic cardiomyopathy is a common form of nonischemic cardiomyopathy, and the most common cause of cardiac arrest in young athletes. This is an inherited condition and affects about 1 in 500 persons (0.2 percent of the population). In this condition, the heart muscle is abnormally thickened. In addition, the outflow tract of the heart may be abnormally narrowed because of an overgrowth of muscle, and thus the heart's ability to pump blood is diminished. With extreme exertion, the heart can fibrillate because the coronary arteries are not receiving enough blood, or because of abnormalities in the hypertrophied (abnormally thickened) muscle itself. Typically, there are no symptoms, or only mild ones. Sudden collapse is frequently the first indication of the problem—and, sadly, also often the last.

Restrictive cardiomyopathies results from abnormal stiffness in the heart muscle. It it caused by a variety of conditions such as amyloidosis, sarcoidosis, post-radiation therapy, and other relatively uncommon causes. Patients with restrictive cardiomyopathy are candidates for heart transplantation.

PRIMARY ELECTRICAL DISEASES

Even when there is no evidence of disease in the heart muscle, the coronary arteries, or the heart valves, some people may be at risk for life-threatening problems with heart rhythm. Many of these conditions are hereditary, caused by genetic abnormalities that affect the flow of electrical currents in the heart muscle.[6] Examples of such abnormalities include long Q-T syndrome and Brugada syndrome. In other cases, a person may be born with an extra electrical connection in some region of the heart. This extra connection, when activated by a precisely timed heartbeat, may cause a disturbance in heart rhythm. An example of this type of problem is Wolff-Parkinson-White syndrome.

Long Q-T Syndrome

At first there didn't seem to be any reason why Melissa T. kept fainting. Her mother thought it was just nerves, so she tried not to overreact, not wanting to make her nine-year-old daughter even more anxious. But after the third episode—Melissa had fainted during soccer practice—Mrs. T. took her daughter to the family's pediatrician.

As part of the workup, Melissa's doctor ordered an electrocardiogram, and the diagnosis of long (or prolonged) Q-T syndrome was made. Melissa's grandfather had died at an early age, and the cause of his death had never been determined. Maybe he, too, had suffered from this disorder.

The pediatrician discussed the treatment options with Melissa's family. Melissa was too young for an implantable defibrillator, so the doctor prescribed an automated external defibrillator instead and arranged for all of Melissa's family members to be trained in its use. The AED had to accompany Melissa to school as well. Her teachers and classmates were very supportive, and school staff were taught how to use it. Melissa's doctor also placed her on beta-blockers, to lower the likelihood of her experiencing ventricular fibrillation.

In prolonged Q-T syndrome, the ability of the heart's electrical system to recover (or reset itself) after each heart beat is abnormally slowed. As a result the heart becomes more likely to suddenly fibrillate. The most common initial manifestation is syncope (fainting), for which an ECG is part of a medical workup. In young people, however, sometimes the first manifestation is sudden collapse in cardiac arrest. Among young athletes, for example, prolonged Q-T syndrome is the second most common cause of sudden death after hypertrophic cardiomyopathy.

The therapy for long Q-T syndrome depends on the severity of the symptoms. Many patients with this condition are placed on beta-blockers. For high-risk patients—those with cardiac arrest or frequent fainting episodes—an implantable defibrillator is recommended.

Brugada Syndrome

Brugada syndrome, less common than long Q-T syndrome, is an inherited disease in which the heart's conduction system goes haywire, with little warning. This is a newly characterized condition, and it may be responsible for some primary VF events in young men (the average age of onset is thirty-eight). Brugada syndrome may be preceded by fainting spells. Abnormalities on a routine ECG may suggest the disease. An individual with this condition should receive an implanted defibrillator.

Wolff-Parkinson-White Syndrome

A person with Wolff-Parkinson-White syndrome (WPW) has a conduction abnormality in the pathways between the atria and the ventricles. It can lead to a very fast heart rate, which in turn can sometimes trigger VF. The underlying cause of this condition —an extra electrical circuit, called an "accessory pathway"—can be eliminated through a procedure known as "catheter ablation," in which a catheter is placed into the heart and the location of the accessory pathway is identified and then electrically zapped.

VALVULAR HEART DISEASE

Maria B.'s doctor used ultrasound to diagnose a prolapse of her mitral valve. The doctor had heard the heart murmur during a routine physical and wanted to be certain that it wasn't due to a more serious cause. Once the cause was known, the doctor reassured Maria that the murmur was benign. The only thing the doctor recommended was for Maria to take antibiotics during dental procedures to prevent valvular infection.

Although it is very treatable, valvular heart disease can lead to sudden death. Aortic stenosis, in which the aortic valve's failure to open completely is the cause of decreased cardiac output, is the valve problem most likely to be associated with sudden death. Mitral valve prolapse, in which the mitral valve balloons out when it shuts, is a common condition affecting over 1 percent of the population. Most authorities consider the condition to be benign, but some investigators have noted an association between mitral valve prolapse and sudden death. If there is such an association, it is probably very small.

COMMOTIO CORDIS

Jimmy L., a twelve-year-old Little Leaguer, had been playing first base all season, so the play that brought him down, a simple grounder fielded by the second baseman, shouldn't have been complicated. But the runner was barreling toward first inside the baseline, and Jimmy, momentarily distracted, missed the ball fired at him by the second baseman. It struck him full in the chest, and he collapsed.

By the time the paramedics arrived, their defibrillator/monitor showed fine ventricular fibrillation. They were unable to resuscitate Jimmy, probably because it had taken them thirteen minutes to reach the scene.

Commotio cordis (the term means "commotion in the heart") is a rare but well-described cause of cardiac arrest, usually in children, when a direct blow to the chest triggers ventricular fibrillation. There is no underlying heart disease.

The average age of death from commotio cordis is thirteen. Such items as baseballs and hockey pucks are the most common culprits, but direct bodily contact can also cause the cardiac arrest.

To trigger VF, the blow must strike the chest at the precise moment of vulnerability in the heart's cycle. This period of vulnerability, which lasts a few milliseconds, occurs immediately after the heart contracts. Because children's chests are probably more compliant than those of adults, the force of the blow is also more likely to be transmitted directly to the heart.

NON-HEART-RELATED CAUSES OF SUDDEN AND UNEXPECTED DEATH

Just over a quarter of all sudden out-of-hospital cardiac arrests are caused by conditions other than heart disease. At the top of the list of non-heart-related causes of sudden death are respiratory diseases, but other causes include brain aneurysms, strokes, cancer, drug reactions, kidney failure, sudden infant death syndrome, and anaphylaxis.

Respiratory Diseases

Just as there are multiple heart-related causes of sudden death, so are there many respiratory causes of sudden death. Probably the most common ones are emphysema and chronic obstructive pulmonary disease (also called chronic bronchitis). Others are asthma, pulmonary hypertension, and restrictive lung disease. Less common respiratory causes are occupational lung disease and conditions that lead to lung impairment, such as drug toxicity, infectious diseases, and cystic fibrosis.

When sudden and unexpected death is caused by a respiratory condition, the lung fails before the heart does. In the terminal stages, the lung cannot oxygenate the body, and this failure ultimately leads to respiratory arrest, which in turn, after a period of several minutes, leads to cardiac arrest. Typically, the rhythms associated with primary respiratory arrest are asystole or pulseless electrical activity rather than VF.

Aneurysms

A brain aneurysm is another non-heart-related cause of sudden death. Indeed, about the only ways in which true sudden death can happen are for the heart to stop pumping blood, as it does in ventricular fibrillation, or for a vessel in the brain to burst. The latter phenomenon is caused by an aneurysm—a small outpouching in an artery.

A burst aneurysm in the brain can be catastrophic. If only a small amount of blood leaks out, the victim may survive. But if the rent in the vessel is large enough, and if the bleeding is fast enough, death will be almost instantaneous. Sometimes the event is heralded by one or more intense headaches.

But an aneurysm can occur in any artery. If it occurs in a major artery, such as the aorta, death can be fairly sudden, though not as rapid as with a brain aneurysm. The victim hemorrhages internally, and if the tear in the vessel is large enough, death can come in just a few short minutes. Aortic aneurysms—especially where the aorta leaves the heart, as well as in the abdominal portion of the aorta—are not uncommon, particularly in the elderly.

A variation on brain aneurysm is an arterial-venous malformation (also called "A-V malformation"). This developmental abnormality results when a small artery connects directly to a vein without the usual capillary interface. In such a case, the high-pressure artery eventually causes the vein to weaken, and eventually the vein may rupture. The signs and symptoms of an A-V malformation are very similar to those of a brain aneurysm.

Strokes and Clots

A stroke is another way to die suddenly. A stroke is caused by blockage of an artery so that insufficient blood reaches a portion of the brain. If the stroke is large enough, or if a vital part of the brain is affected, death can come rapidly.

Related to strokes is a condition known as "pulmonary embolus." In this condition, a large blood clot develops in the veins of the pelvis or upper leg. If the clot is dislodged, it may travel through the right side of the heart and then lodge in the pulmonary artery. Such a clot, if large enough, can be fatal. The reasons for the clot's formation are abnormally high coagulability of the blood (underlying cancer and other conditions can lead to this condition, as can certain medications, such as birth control pills) and inactivity (causing stasis of the blood in the veins and making coagulation more likely). Pulmonary embolus is a known risk of long flights or automobile trips. Some airlines now urge their passengers to reduce the likelihood of clot formation by getting up occasionally and walking up and down the aisle of the plane.

Cancer

Cancer deaths typically are not unexpected. They are usually associated with asystole or pulseless electrical activity, and the likelihood of successful resuscitation is exceedingly low. Nevertheless, not all cancer patients are in the terminal stages of their disease, and so it may be very appropriate to attempt to resuscitate these individuals. At some point, however, the cancer does progress to its final stage, when death, even if it comes suddenly, is expected.

Drug Reactions

Many drugs—including some very common ones, such as certain antibiotics, antihistamines, antidepressants, antipsychotics, antifungal medications, and antihypertensive medications—have been associated with cardiac arrest. Fortunately, however, the "side effect" of sudden death is very rare in people taking these medications. Among recreational drugs, cocaine has been the one most implicated in sudden death. Its harm comes from its excitatory effects on the heart muscle. Other recreational drugs, such as heroin, can lead to death, but the cause is typically respiratory depression leading to cessation of breathing.

Kidney Failure

Kidney failure is another condition that can lead to sudden death. Patients with kidney failure are unable to produce sufficient urine (in fact, usually no urine is produced) to excrete and filter the body's waste products, and therefore a dialysis machine (or kidney transplantation) must do the job. There are now 275,000 Americans on chronic dialysis. The causes of kidney failure are multiple and include diabetes, autoimmune diseases (such as lupus and rheumatoid arthritis), and infections as well as causes that are idiopathic. Dialysis can keep people alive for many years, but dialysis is not without risk. The process of dialysis causes large shifts in fluids as the dialysis machine filters out urea, potassium, and other electrolytes. Rarely, ventricular fibrillation may occur.

Sudden Infant Death Syndrome

Nothing is more tragic than the death of a child or infant. Sudden infant death syndrome (SIDS) occurs in infants up to one year old, and a specific cause has yet to be determined. Fortunately, the incidence of SIDS has been falling for almost two decades, and it is now a very uncommon cause of sudden death. In King County during the 1980s, there were approximately twenty attempted resuscitations in SIDS cases per year. In the last few years, the annual average has fallen to six.

Anaphylaxis

Anaphylaxis—a severe allergic reaction—is yet another way to die suddenly. Certain foods (such as peanuts and shellfish) and medications, as well as bee venom, can trigger fatal anaphylaxis. Severe allergic reactions to peanuts, for example, have become so common that manufacturers of commercially prepared foods are now required to provide packaging that lists the presence of peanuts and other nuts.

In anaphylaxis, the allergen stimulates a massive release of histamine, which in turn can lead to upper-airway swelling, to dilation of vessels, and to shock, skin hives, and severe gastroenteritis. Death can occur in a matter of minutes as the swollen throat and soft palate block the airway. Typically, people subject to anaphylaxis know of their allergic conditions and may even have been prescribed epinephrine in the form of a vial from which they can inject themselves in the event of encountering an allergen.

If this chapter has led you think that the heart can stop beating at any second, be reassured—it is actually rather difficult for a healthy person to die suddenly. You can't will yourself to die. You can't hold your breath as a means to die. If you try, you may black out, but breathing will resume. This is because the body's autonomic nervous system, which operates in the deep background without conscious control, is what causes the heart to beat and the lungs to inhale. Millions of years of evolution have fine-tuned this system to make the basics of life—blood circulation, breathing, digestion, and sentience—durable and reliable.

In summary, the causes of cardiac arrest are many. Three-quarters of cardiac arrests are due to underlying heart disease (comprising, for the most part, coronary artery disease and ischemia, acute myocardial infarction, and cardiomyopathy), and one-quarter of cardiac arrests are due to a variety of other causes. Whatever the cause, once the heart goes into arrest, treatment is fairly straightforward. The priority is to regain a normal cardiac rhythm, with a pulse and blood pressure. Then attention can be directed toward the cause of the arrest. This is a simplification, of course, since some causes may require unique therapy (for example, dialysis patients in cardiac arrest may require specific therapy to lower potassium in the blood). But for the most part, the task of EMTs and paramedics is to deal with the immediate situation—namely, a heart that has stopped beating. And if they can reach the patient quickly enough, there is a decent chance of snatching life from the jaws of death.

FOUR

A Profile of Sudden Cardiac Arrest

Paul M., a firefighter, is grumbling to his lieutenant about all the extra work involved in a cardiac arrest, for himself and everyone else. But Paul and his lieutenant both know that his complaints are for show. Despite the detailed reporting requirements, these calls give him the most satisfaction.

After every such event, Paul completes his single-page incident report, and then he returns to the station to complete the online report. The report for a cardiac arrest requires far more detailed information than a routine call does, with extra questions about the circumstances of the patient's collapse, about any bystanders who performed CPR, and about the patient's heart rhythm and response to defibrillatory shocks.

One good thing, as far as Paul is concerned, is that the online report form automatically downloads the scene information—the address, the time of the call, the time of the dispatcher's response, and the time of the EMTs' arrival. Paul must also download the digitized AED record containing all the patient's rhythms as well as voice recordings of everyone who spoke during the resuscitation. The AED record also reports when CPR occurred, the rate and depth of compression, and when ventilations were given. Paul then sends this digital tape file via a secure Web site to the cardiac arrest registry maintained by the King County EMS office, where all the information about a patient's cardiac arrest flows. In addition, after every cardiac arrest, Paul has to call an 800 number to give information to a research nurse who records it for two ongoing studies of cardiac arrest.

But this is only the beginning. In addition to the firefighter's online report and the digital recording from the AED, the King County EMS office receives an online report of the care provided by paramedics. Since paramedics are able to provide more advanced care than EMTs, their reports contain a detailed flowchart of all clinical interventions—including medications, additional defibrillations, airway interventions, and the response of the patient—in an almost minute-by-minute account. The King County EMS office also requests a digital recording of the call from the dispatch center. If the patient has been admitted and discharged from the hospital, the patient's hospital record is requested. And if the patient has died, a copy of the death certificate is obtained from the health department's office of vital statistics.

The totality of information from all these sources comprises hundreds of variables and data points—all this for one cardiac arrest.

THE KING COUNTY REGISTRY: THREE DECADES OF CARDIAC ARREST SURVEILLANCE

Seattle and King County have the longest continuing cardiac arrest surveillance programs and registries of cardiac arrest in the world. Both registries were established when the paramedic programs began—1970 in Seattle, and 1975 in the county.[1]

The registries have become a font of scientific information about cardiac arrest and its circumstances. What is more important, the registries provide a baseline for measuring the effects of new and pilot interventions for treating cardiac arrest. The information contained in the registries has provided material for more than 250 published scientific articles. When special studies are under way (and they always are), additional information is requested from firefighters and/or paramedics, and interviews are often requested with surviving patients or family members. Also in connection with the surveillance programs and registries, there have been more than a dozen clinical trials to study new medications, new methods of defibrillation, and new resuscitation techniques.[2] Several innovative programs that began in Seattle and King County have been endorsed nationally and serve to define current standards of care; for example, as mentioned in the previous chapter, Seattle initiated widespread training of citizens in CPR, and dispatcher-assisted telephone CPR and defibrillation by EMTs were first studied in King County. Now these programs have been instituted in every American city and in many other places around the world.[3]

The previous chapter explained the causes of sudden cardiac arrest—the "what." This chapter takes a different approach, describing the "who," the "when," and the "where"—the characteristics of the victim, and the circumstances of the collapse. It describes several key factors associated with either survival or death. These are the presence or absence of witnesses to the victim's collapse; the presence of absence of particular heart rhythms, especially ventricular fibrillation; the presence or absence of bystanders who can perform CPR; the time and place of the victim's collapse, as well as the activities in which the victim is engaged when it occurs; and the time it takes for EMS personnel to respond to the emergency.

Most of the data reported in this book are derived from the King County registry of cardiac arrests for 1977 through 2011. Unless otherwise indicated, information is presented for all thirty-one years. Some of the variables included in the registry have been fairly constant, whereas others have changed over the years.

Most of the cases of cardiac arrest discussed in this chapter and throughout the book involved adults over the age of eighteen whose arrest was due to underlying heart disease rather than to noncardiac causes (see chapter 3); the exclusion of noncardiac causes allows the facts about the bulk of cardiac arrests to emerge more clearly. Moreover, in the cases discussed in this and other chapters, a firefighter EMT or a paramedic initiated or continued CPR; cases of cardiac arrest in which the victim was judged to be dead on arrival, or in which a bystander initiated CPR but an EMT subsequently judged the victim to be dead on arrival, are not discussed. In other words, here and elsewhere, the only cases discussed are those in which a professionally trained EMT or paramedic determined that there was some possibility of successful resuscitation.[4]

CHARACTERISTICS OF PEOPLE WHO SUFFER SUDDEN CARDIAC ARREST

Mildred P. lived alone at Campus Place, an assisted living facility for retired schoolteachers. Her heart failure confined her mostly to her one-bedroom apartment. The facility provided dinner and also arranged for deliveries of food. She had family members living nearby and, despite her eighty-nine years, cooked a meal for her granddaughter almost every Sunday.

Recently Mildred had been experiencing troublesome palpitations, and she had just seen her doctor about them. The doctor found signs of increasing failure—Mildred's lower legs were more swollen, her neck veins were up, and her chest congestion was worse than it had been the last time he'd seen her. He had increased the dosage of the diuretic she was taking, and he'd adjusted two of her other medications. But Mildred herself had not been very optimistic that these medication changes would help.

The Campus Place manager, in his office, phoned Mildred the second he heard her MedicAlert go off. When she didn't pick up her phone, he immediately dialed 911. Eight minutes later the paramedics arrived and found Mildred in cardiac arrest, with a heart rhythm showing pulseless electrical activity. The manager informed the paramedics that Mildred was a full code—she wanted everything to be done in the event of a cardiac arrest. They worked for thirty minutes trying to get a pulse, but to no avail.

The paramedic wondered why the woman's heart had stopped. Her husband had told him that she was only fifty-eight. Anne wasn't a smoker, he said, and she didn't have high blood pressure or diabetes. But as the paramedic continued asking about her history, he learned that when she was thirty-one she'd had a hysterectomy, with both ovaries removed.

The King County registry since 1977 contains information on more than 26,0000 cases of cardiac arrest in which care was provided by EMTs and paramedics. The average number of attempted resuscitations per year is 700. King County's population increased during that period, and when that figure is adjusted for the increase in population, the incidence of heart-related cardiac arrest is seen to be falling—a decrease consistent with national figures on cardiac mortality.

The male-to-female ratio for cardiac arrest is 2 to 1; 69 percent of cardiac arrests occur in men. Furthermore, men experience cardiac arrest at a younger age than women do: the average age for men is sixty-six; for women, it is seventy-two. This six-year difference reflects the comparatively delayed onset of coronary artery disease in women. Estrogen appears to be cardioprotective in premenopausal women, though the mechanism is not entirely clear (for example, if you give estrogen to a man, you will not protect him from heart disease, but you will cause breast enlargement).

CIRCUMSTANCES OF CARDIAC ARREST

Witnesses

Charles R., the head of new product development for a medical biotech company in Seattle, was listening to a panel of experts at the American Heart Association's annual conference on new developments in cardiac resuscitation. He tried to pay attention but found his thoughts drifting.

There must be a way, he mused. If only an alarm could be devised to go off when the heart stopped beating! Then almost every cardiac arrest could be witnessed. The spouse downstairs, the caregiver doing laundry, the manager at the adult care home—any one of them could hear the alarm and, within just a few seconds, check on the victim and call 911. Charles knew that about 50 percent of all cardiac arrests are witnessed. But if this gizmo could be produced, the rate of witnessed collapse would climb to almost 100 percent, maybe doubling the survival rate.

How should the device work? Should it measure impedance changes via two electrodes? Monitor the flow in the carotid artery? Use sound to detect the heart's contractions? Detect cellular function subcutaneously?

The panelists' voices droned on, and Charles continued to ponder his revolutionary alarm. What a technological breakthrough it would be!

A witnessed cardiac arrest is defined as one in which a bystander sees or hears the victim collapse. According to thirty-one years of data in King County's cardiac arrest registry, cardiac arrests are witnessed, on average, 55 percent of the time. In the first few years when data were recorded, the figure was about 60 percent, but it has fallen to 50 percent over the past decade. This decrease is probably due to an increase in the number of elderly people living alone.

Most of the time when a cardiac arrest is unwitnessed, the victim cannot be resuscitated—it takes too long for therapy to begin, and there is simply too much cellular death in the brain and the heart. An individual who has been in cardiac arrest for six minutes and has not had CPR has virtually no chance of survival (even if a resuscitation attempt is successful, there is likely to be severe neurological damage). Unwitnessed cardiac arrests in which resuscitation efforts have been successful constitute a tiny minority of all cases. These are probably situations in which the victim collapsed only minutes before being discovered.

Newspapers had been piling up outside Mabel F.'s door. Finally her neighbor called 911.

When the fire department's EMTs arrived, they had to break the lock on Mabel's door. They found Mabel in bed, cold and still. There were purplish splotches on the sides of her thighs, caused by pooled blood, and rigor mortis was present.

The EMTs called the duty officer in the medical examiner's office, who in turn contacted Mabel's doctor. Since her doctor had agreed to sign Mabel's death certificate, there was no need to involve the medical examiner. The EMTs stayed with Mabel's body until the private mortuary's van arrived.

When a cardiac arrest has been unwitnessed, the decision about whether to attempt resuscitation is based on the presence or absence of signs of irreversible death. These signs include a cold body, lividity (pooling of blood), and rigor mortis. If there is any uncertainty about these signs, EMTs and paramedics are trained to begin a resuscitation attempt: "When in doubt, resuscitate."

In an unwitnessed arrest, the situation is especially challenging for the dispatcher, who must figure out whether to offer the caller CPR instructions over the phone. The dispatcher has to interview the caller and try to determine when the victim was last seen alive. In some instances, the dispatcher even has to ask the caller to touch the victim's body and report whether or not it is cool. In this situation, the emergency dispatcher's job is tougher than the EMT's or the paramedic's—at least they can see and touch the victim.[5]

Heart Rhythms

In the early days of the paramedic program in Seattle and King County, there was a patient who had ten episodes of ventricular fibrillation over a three-year period. Fortunately, he lived only a block from the fire department. Every time he collapsed, he was found to be in VF, and every time the firefighters responded, they used their new defibrillator to shock him.

The firefighters came to know this patient well, and they nicknamed him Resusci-Jimmy. They knew that Jimmy was being considered for an experimental therapy at Johns Hopkins Hospital—a defibrillator that would be implanted directly in his chest. Regrettably, though, Jimmy died before the new technology could help him.

Most victims of cardiac arrest are found to be in ventricular fibrillation (fig. 4.1). But this is good news, since VF is the rhythm disturbance most likely to be associated with a chance of successful resuscitation. The bad news, however, is that the incidence of VF is falling. In King County, for example, over the twenty-two years shown in figure 4.1, 43 percent of patients, on average, were found to be in VF, but in the late 1970s the VF rate was 60 percent, whereas it fell to 33 percent in the years from 2001-2011. This recent decline in VF has also been reported by other investigators.[6] The reasons for the decline are not clear, though there are some likely explanations. One is the changing spectrum of heart disease. There are proportionately more patients with heart failure as the cause of cardiac arrest, and this condition is more likely to be associated with pulseless electrical activity (see chapter 3), whereas death due to ischemic heart disease is more likely to be associated with VF. Another possible reason for the lower rates of VF is the effectiveness of therapy for heart disease—the number of patients who have had bypass surgery, have coronary artery stents, and are taking cardiac medications is far greater today than thirty years ago. Moreover, high blood pressure and diabetes, two of the biggest contributors to heart disease, are certainly better controlled today than they were three decades ago. Other possibilities are decreased rates of smoking, better control of cholesterol and blood pressure (beta-blockers are commonly used for high blood pressure and may also lead to a lower incidence of VF), and better diet (ingestion of fish oils is associated with a lower incidence of sudden

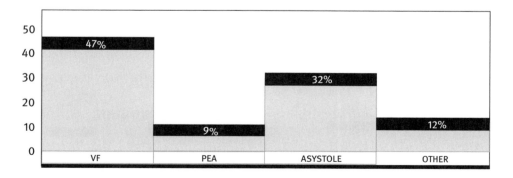

4.1 Rhythms, by percentage, associated with cardiac arrest due to underlying heart disease, King County, 1990-2011.

cardiac death). Today it is unusual for a patient to have repeated episodes of ventricular fibrillation, since the patient who survives such an episode usually receives an implantable defibrillator.

Asystole (see chapter 1) is associated with 33 percent of all cardiac arrests, and pulseless electrical activity (see chapter 1) is seen in 12 percent of arrests. Other rhythms are associated with 12 percent of cardiac arrests.

Asystole and, to a lesser extent, PEA are terminal rhythms. There is virtually no chance of reviving a patient in asystole, and there is only a very small chance of reviving someone who has PEA. In other words, they represent the very end stage of cardiac arrest. VF eventually degrades to asystole, usually within twenty minutes. PEA usually represents a severely dysfunctional heart, with death the usual outcome. There are a few instances, however, in which PEA is associated with a correctable cause. Therefore, paramedics are taught not to abandon a resuscitation attempt for a patient in PEA without checking for such treatable conditions as pneumothorax (a collapsed lung), low blood volume, cardiac tamponade (blood in the sac surrounding the heart), low body temperature, drug overdose (for example, from beta-blockers, calcium-channel blockers, or digitalis), high potassium, and severe acidosis. Other causes of PEA, such as massive myocardial infarction and massive pulmonary embolus, clearly cannot be treated in the field.

There is a very strong relationship between, on the one hand, the heart rhythm of someone who has suffered cardiac arrest and, on the other, the presence or absence of witnesses to the victim's collapse (see fig. 4.2). When there are witnesses, VF is present 61 percent of the time. When there are no witnesses, VF is present only 27 percent of the time. By contrast, most patients who are found to be in asystole have collapsed without witnesses. Asystole is found in only 11 percent of cases in which the victim's

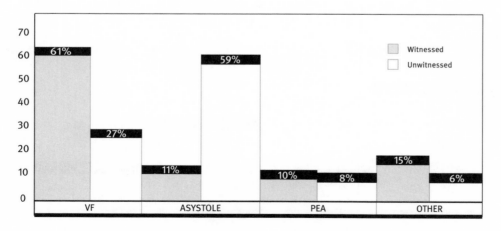

4.2 Rhythms, by percentage, that caused collapse in witnessed and unwitnessed cardiac arrest due to underlying heart disease, King County, Washington, 1990-2011.

collapse is witnessed, but it is found in 59 percent of cases in which no one has witnessed the collapse. Most of the time, then, when there are no witnesses, VF degrades to asystole. Because of the strong relationship between VF and the presence of witnesses, most programs report survival information on the basis of cases in which the victim collapsed in the presence of witnesses, and they report VF as the first heart rhythm obtained.

CPR-Trained Bystanders

The medical director of the Emerald City paramedic program was leading a panel discussion on how to improve the rates of CPR performed by bystanders. Another member of the panel suggested that citizens who had the courage to undertake this good deed should be rewarded, and she supported her suggestion with a piece of historical trivia. In eighteenth-century London, she said, the rescue society gave a medal to anyone who had attempted to resuscitate a victim of drowning. The medal was embossed with the rescue society's seal—the figure of a cherub blowing on an ember, with a Latin phrase etched on the periphery (its translation was "Perhaps a little spark may yet lie hid").

The medical director thought this was a great idea, but when he presented it to the program's administrative director, she squelched it. The idea was too costly, she said, and finding the name and address of everyone who might deserve such a medal would be a logistical nightmare.

For all rhythms, CPR performed by bystanders doubles the probability of surviving a cardiac arrest. King County is fortunate to have one of the highest rates of bystander CPR in the world. Seattle's Medic Two program (see chapter 2) pioneered CPR training for citizens in 1972, long before national organizations had endorsed that concept. Financial donations to the program are accepted, but the citizen CPR program offers free on-site and in-home training. The program is coordinated by the Seattle Fire Department, and classes are conducted by firefighters who teach on their own time and are compensated out of a donated budget. Every year, the program trains between 12,000 and 13,000 Seattle and King County residents, and it is estimated that almost 800,000 citizens have been trained since 1972. Thus, with more than 50 percent of the population trained in CPR, Seattle and King County have the world's highest proportion of CPR-trained citizens.[7] In addition to massive citizen CPR training, this community began, in 1983, the first program in dispatcher-assisted telephone CPR. The high training rate and the active telephone CPR program are the main reasons for the high rates of bystander CPR. Before the telephone CPR program, bystander CPR was a factor in approximately 30 percent of cardiac arrests in King County. From 1983 through 2006, the proportion of cardiac arrests involving bystander CPR increased to an average of 55 percent.[8] In 2006 alone, that figure was 60 percent.

Seattleites like to joke that a tourist in their city should take care not to trip and fall down on a public sidewalk, since some bystander will be sure to pounce and begin CPR. This has never happened, of course, but the jokesters are half serious. The rate of bystander CPR is far higher in public locations (66 percent) than in private homes (49 percent). Furthermore, bystander CPR is much more likely with a witnessed collapse than one that occurs without being witnessed. For witnessed cardiac arrests occurring in a public place bystander CPR is provided 71 percent of the time compared to 54 percent for unwitnessed cardiac arrests; for arrests in private homes, a witnessed collapse receives bystander CPR 55 percent of the time compared to 44 percent for unwitnessed events.

Timing, Location, and Associated Activities

Timing

Reporter doing a story on the twenty-fifth anniversary of the King County Medic One program: What's it like to come out of a sound sleep and race to the scene of a cardiac arrest? *Paramedic:* It's awful. Fortunately, my adrenaline kicks in just as we pull up to the address.

There are more cardiac arrests in the morning hours than during any other time of day. In King County, the peak hours are between eight in the morning and noon (see fig. 4.3). A similar finding has been reported in Sweden.[9] It is not clear whether this phe-

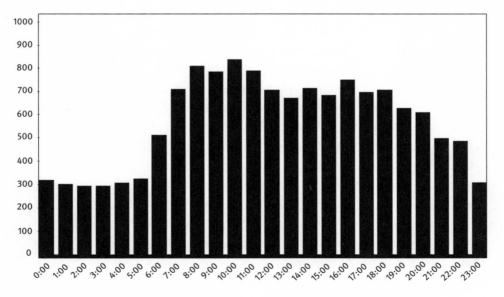

4.3 Cardiac arrests due to underlying heart disease by hour of the day, King County, Washington, 1977–2007.

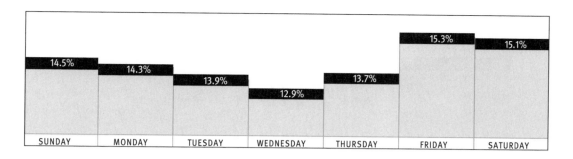

4.4 Percentages, by day of the week, of cardiac arrests due to underlying heart disease, King County, Washington, 1977–2007.

nomenon exists because more cardiac arrests are recognized as family members wake up together or because there may be an early-morning physiological risk. For example, there are known diurnal variations in bodily functions, such as in the amount of cortisol released by the adrenal gland, and this surge in steroids may make the heart more vulnerable to arrest. Other explanations for greater early-morning risk may be increased blood pressure upon awakening, increased activity in the morning, other possible triggers (such as the first cigarette in the morning), and perhaps even stress associated with thinking about the coming day's events.[10] It is more than likely that what seems to be a lower incidence of cardiac arrest during the night is actually an indication that more cardiac arrests go unwitnessed during this period. It is also possible that sleep is cardioprotective.

Moreover, in King County there are approximately 8 percent more cardiac arrests per month during December and January than in the other ten months. The same winter increase has been reported in Sweden.[11] Other authors also report an increase in cardiovascular deaths in cold weather.[12] Is this cold-related stress—temperature-induced changes in platelet function? It is possible, no doubt, to engage in endless speculation. The research from Sweden also reports a slight increase in cardiac arrest on Mondays as compared to other days of the week.[13] Like the research that reports more cardiac arrests in the morning, this finding may reflect not so much a special characteristic of Mondays as a surge in discovery of cardiac arrests when people don't show up for work or fail to arrive at senior centers or are found at home by health care attendants. In King County, we have found that most cardiac arrests occur on Friday and Saturday (see fig. 4.4)—perhaps too much partying?

Location

Reporter: Where was your most unusual resuscitation?

Paramedic: Boy, that's a tough one. I guess it was on a dock. The patient was wedged halfway between the dock and the ramp. Talk about cramped working space! One false

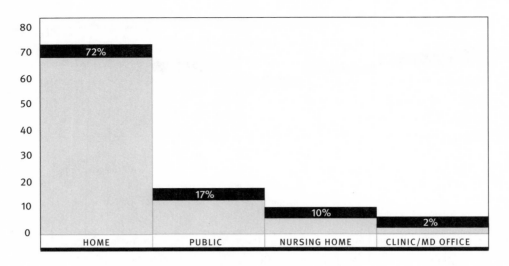

4.5 Percentages, by location of collapse, of cardiac arrests due to underlying heart disease, King County, Washington, 1977–2007.

move, and you'd be in the water. Plus, the thing was bouncing up and down. I'd bend down to shock him, and he'd be four inches below the paddles. We had a doctor with us that day, doing student evaluations. I remember him asking me, "Do you do that often?" "All the time," I said.

The vast majority of sudden cardiac arrests happen in people's homes.[14] This is not surprising, since people, especially retired and elderly people, spend most of their time at home. In King County, 72 percent of cardiac arrests happen in people's homes or in other residences, and similar findings are reported in other cities—10 percent of cardiac arrests happen in nursing homes and extended care facilities, 1 percent occur in doctors' offices,[15] and 17 percent occur in such public places as business offices, outdoor locations like streets and parks, and indoor locations like shopping centers, restaurants, airports, and exercise facilities (see fig. 4.5)

A detailed study in King County reported the incidence of cardiac arrest in various public locations.[16] The sites with the highest incidence included SeaTac Airport, the county jail, sports stadiums, large shopping malls, large industrial sites, golf courses, homeless shelters, ferries,[17] health clubs, and senior centers. For example, there were seven cardiac arrests per year at the airport. There was one per year in the county jail, and there was one every ten years at each of the area's golf courses, on each of the ferries, and at every health club. In other words, an AED at a golf course, on a ferry, or at a health club would probably sit idle for ten years before being used. Other public sites had much lower rates of cardiac arrest. Sites with very low incidence included hotels and motels, government offices, places of entertainment (such as movie theaters), schools, churches, construction sites, and restaurants (the incidence per restaurant was .002 per year).[18] An informed decision would be to place AEDs at the locations where cardiac arrests are most likely to occur. Accordingly, the American Heart Association recommends AEDs for any public site where there is a likelihood of one cardiac arrest every five years.

Associated Activities

Fred L. liked to boast that he was in pretty good shape for his eighty-four years—his prostate was enlarged, and his feet ached all the time, but as far as he knew his ticker was just fine. So he didn't hesitate to grab the snow shovel and start clearing off the driveway.

Thirty minutes later, Fred's wife looked out the kitchen window and saw him lying in the driveway, just outside the garage door.

The paramedics worked on Fred for forty minutes, and though they got a heart rhythm for a few minutes, there never was a pulse. They called their medical control doctor for permission to cease their efforts.

It is widely assumed that physical activity in general triggers cardiac arrest, and many people think that sexual activity in particular is associated with the event. Both assumptions are false. The most definitive study to examine the risk of sudden death in connection with vigorous exertion was published in *The New England Journal Medicine* in 2000.[19] This twelve-year study prospectively followed more than 21,000 physicians who provided information on their own physical activities. The study determined that there was increased risk of sudden death during vigorous exercise, and for up to thirty minutes afterward, but that the overall risk was exceeding small—one sudden death per 1.51 million episodes of exertion. A key finding was that habitual exercise attenuated the risk of sudden death during exertion. In other words, frequent exercise was much safer than the weekend warrior's huffing and puffing. The authors concluded that the benefits of a physically active lifestyle far outweigh the tiny risk of an exercise-associated event. Similarly, a 2006 study reported that exercise-related sudden death in women was extremely rare.[20] The consensus is that exercise is overall a very positive activity, with one qualifier—people who exercise infrequently should use moderation, since the exact mechanism for exertion-related sudden death is not clear.

Sexual activity and physical exertion are often—shall we say usually?—synonymous, but there are no good data on sudden death during sex. In the King County registry, for example, recorded instances of sudden death associated with sexual activity are exceedingly rare. An occasional high-profile event is reported in the media, confirming the stereotype about the risks of sex. It is probably impossible to obtain an accurate account of whether a victim of cardiac arrest was having sex when the collapse occurred, since spouses and lovers are probably unwilling to go on the record.

Perhaps there is an element of embarrassment for the victim's partner, and sex workers fear legal entanglement, although sometimes a 911 call is placed by a sex worker who leaves the scene before the arrival of emergency medical services. The association between sudden cardiac death and sexual activity is a murky one to tease out, whatever the reasons.

Response Time

EMT arriving at the victim's home: Can you tell me what happened?
Victim's wife: I was just talking to him, and then I thought I heard a moan from the kitchen. I couldn't wake him up. I tried reaching his doctor, but the nurse told me to call 911.

It is a real challenge to get accurate measurements of the time intervals involved in a cardiac arrest. Some intervals can be measured precisely, but others are more problematic. Ideally, one would like to know the time of collapse and the timing of key interventions, such as CPR and defibrillation.

The collapse of the patient in cardiac arrest is the anchor time that starts the therapeutic clock. Of course, when the collapse is unwitnessed, it is impossible to determine key time intervals; for this reason, many communities do not attempt to measure

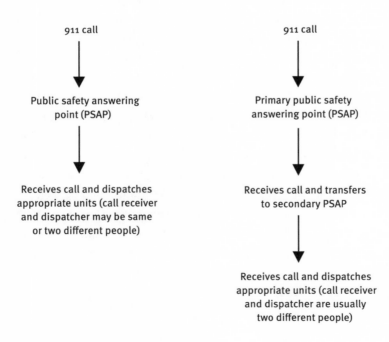

4.6 Types of dispatch systems.

time intervals for an unwitnessed cardiac arrest. But even when there are witnesses to the collapse, it is not possible to know the exact moment it occurred. In King County, we arbitrarily assume that one minute has elapsed between the victim's collapse and the call to 911, unless the caller gives a concrete reason for additional delay (for example, running next door to find a neighbor, or calling a doctor, or being unable to locate a telephone).

Most EMS systems document the time of the call to 911. Nevertheless, this practice may be less straightforward than it seems. For one thing, the dispatch center registers only the time when the 911 operator picked up the phone, but it may have rung repeatedly. For another, many communities route 911 calls to a primary public safety answering point, or PSAP, which then routes the call to a secondary PSAP—the fire department or EMS dispatch center (see fig. 4.6). It is almost impossible to link the call times at both centers, and so the routing time from the primary to the secondary PSAP is usually lost in any time analysis. But let's assume, for our purposes here, that this routing time is thirty seconds or less.

Next is the response time. Again, what should be straightforward is filled with complexity. The response time, ideally, should be equal to the interval between the dispatch center's alerting of the EMTs and paramedics and the latter's arrival at the victim's side. Most communities, however, report the response time as the interval between the EMS personnel's receipt of the alert and their arrival at, or even near, the victim's address. A response time constructed in this way doesn't account for the time needed to assemble the EMS team, or for the time needed for EMS personnel to gather their equipment and carry it to the victim's side after they have reached his or her address.

Next we have the problem of determining when CPR began. When a bystander initiates CPR, it is impossible to anchor this time. Sometimes dispatcher-assisted telephone CPR can define a start time, but few if any centers routinely record this time. Even when EMTs are the ones who start CPR, the precise time is not recorded.

Finally, there is the exact moment when defibrillation occurs. All current defibrillators and AEDs use a time stamp to mark the instant when a defibrillatory shock is provided, so it should be easy as pie to compare this time with the time of the call to 911, and thus accurately calculate the interval between the moment the 911 operator picked up the phone and the moment defibrillation occurs—right? Well, no. Few EMS programs synchronize their AEDs or defibrillators with the times recorded by 911 operators and PSAPs.[21]

Many researchers in EMS make no attempt to determine the down time (that is, the time between the victim's collapse and the call to 911). Instead, they start the clock at the time when emergency medical services were dispatched. There are valid reasons for this practice, not the least of which is the fact that the moment of collapse can only be estimated—better to start with a concrete time than an estimated one. Moreover, the early portions of the 911 call cannot usually be linked or are difficult to obtain, especially if two

PSAPs are involved. But this is regrettable, since exclusion of the down time gives an inaccurate portrayal of the event. Most systems, by making a concerted effort, can at least define the time at which the primary (and, in some cases, secondary) PSAP picked up the call for help (there is usually a time stamp for this event at the alarm center). The pickup time recorded at the primary PSAP defines the front-end anchor of all the other recorded, objective times. For systems without the resources to estimate down time, I think it is reasonable to start the clock at the PSAP pickup time. One has to assume that the down time, on average, was approximately one minute.

When EMTs are known to have initiated CPR, it usually is considered to have begun sixty seconds after they reached the victim's side; that's the fixed interval assigned to the time it is assumed to have taken them to set up their equipment and position the victim. When a bystander initiated CPR, however, estimating that time becomes more problematic for EMS researchers. Since it is impossible to know precisely when the bystander began CPR, an estimate is made that uses half the interval between the time when the 911 call was picked up and the time when EMTs reached the victim. An estimate, of course, is a compromise, but the alternative would be to throw the data out entirely.[22]

Regrettably, most programs continue to report their systems' performance on the basis of simple response times. In many programs, the response time is considered to be the time between the "wheels rolling" point and the EMTs' arrival at the address for which the alarm was phoned in. But this policy completely underestimates the true time intervals between the victim's collapse (or the PSAP pickup time or times) and the key interventions. Building an EMS program that is systematically unable to provide precise measurement of its critical time intervals is comparable to trying to build a 747 aircraft while measuring its parts with a ruler that is accurate to the inch instead of the micron—the plane would fall apart as soon as it began to taxi down the runway. One simply cannot begin to assess the quality of an EMS program without detailed and accurate knowledge of these critical time intervals.

But there are promising developments in the dispatching world. A national effort —championed by the U.S. Department of Transportation, and called "NG911" ("NG" stands for "next generation")—will bring dispatching into the twenty-first century and solve many of the problems inherent in tracking calls between primary and secondary PSAPs.[23] The 911 system of the 1970s, created for voice media only, cannot easily accommodate the new wireless and multimedia technologies. The NG911 network will be able to take voice, text, photographic, and videographic emergency calls from any communications device via Internet-like networks. The enhanced capacity of NG911 will also have the potential to accommodate incident reports (including ECG, physiological, and therapeutic information) and hospital-based clinical information for a particular resuscitation and integrate it into the dispatch database, thus creating a unified and detailed resuscitation report. At present, however, the timetable and funding for this promising technology are still to be determined.

Table 4.1. Times and intervals associated with cardiac arrest

Time	Definition
1. Collapse time	Precise moment of the patient's collapse
2. Down time (access time)	Interval between the patient's collapse and the call to 911
3. Ring time	Interval between when 911 phone rings until it is answered
4. PSAP[a] pickup time	Precise moment when 911 operator answers the phone
5. PSAP process time	Interval between 911 call pickup and transfer of call to secondary PSAP
6. Secondary PSAP ring time	Interval between when secondary PSAP phone rings until it is answered
7. Secondary PSAP pickup time	Precise moment when secondary PSAP dispatcher answers the phone
8. Secondary PSAP process time	Interval needed for dispatcher to decide which EMS personnel to send
9. Dispatch time	Precise moment when EMS personnel receive dispatch order
10. Muster time (also called roll-out time)	Interval needed for EMS team to assemble and for the vehicle to start to move
11. Roll time	Precise moment when EMS vehicle starts to move
12. Response time	Interval between time 3, 4, 7, 9, or 11 and arrival of EMS personnel at address where the patient collapsed
13. Arrival time	Precise moment when EMS personnel reach the address
14. At-patient time (scene time)	Precise moment when EMS personnel reach patient's side
15. Time to CPR	Ideally, interval between time 1 or 3 and start of CPR
16. Time to defibrillation	Ideally, interval between time 1 or 3 and first shock

[a] Public safety answering point

Table 4.1 lists and defines the times and intervals that are frequently associated with cardiac arrest. I have tried to use common terminology, but different terms may be used by various EMS agencies. Figure 4.7 uses a similar set of terms to illustrate the same concepts. There is no universal agreement about precisely how long these intervals are; the intervals shown in the figure are offered only as examples.

DATA FROM KING COUNTY

Response Times

When the heart goes into ventricular fibrillation, bad things happen in a matter of seconds. The pulse instantly disappears, and the blood pressure falls to zero. Con-

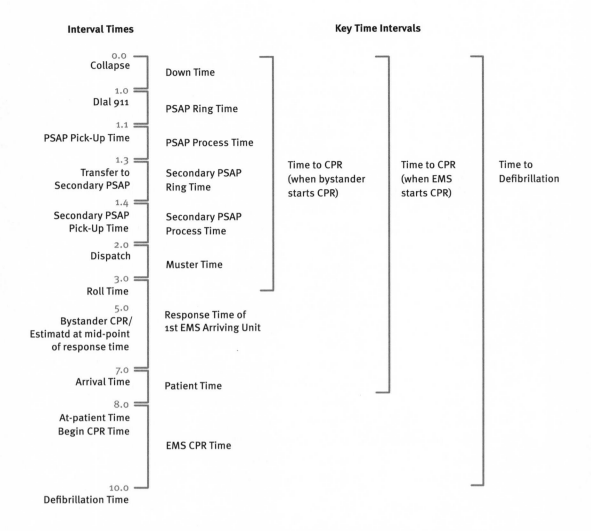

4.7 Key time intervals associated with cardiac arrest. For bystander CPR, the time may be estimated as two minutes after the PSAP pick-up time. For bystander CPR with telephone CPR, the time may be obtained from the recording or estimated as half of the interval from PSAP pick-up to arrival time. For EMS CPR, the time may be approximated as congruent with at patient time.

sciousness is lost in five to ten seconds. Thus a bystander, if one is present, will see the patient slump over or fall down.

Recognition of the event will take a few seconds, with the bystander calling out, "What's wrong? Are you okay?" A few more seconds will be needed to run to the patient and shake him or her. There may or may not be another delay of a few seconds to check for a pulse (pulse checks are no longer taught as part of CPR because of the inability of laypersons to accurately determine the presence of a pulse). Perhaps thirty seconds have now elapsed.

If the bystander is at the victim's home and is not holding a cell phone, he or she will search for a phone (and we all know how a cordless phone has a way of never being in its cradle). The bystander will call 911, expecting the call to be answered on the first ring. But often it will take many rings, each ring taking another few seconds of precious time. Finally, after what seems like an eternity, the 911 operator comes on the line.

When all goes well, the interval between the victim's collapse and the bystander's getting through to the 911 operator takes roughly sixty seconds (this is admittedly an estimate, but it is reasonably accurate). Of course, things can take longer than sixty seconds. The bystander may first call a relative or neighbor or may try to reach the victim's doctor. Or the victim may be in the backyard, and the bystander may need more time to locate a phone. Once the 911 operator picks up, it becomes possible to measure phone time more accurately.

How do we measure time intervals in King County? Ideally, the cardiac arrest clock should start ticking with the exact moment of the patient's collapse, but since it's unlikely there is a stopwatch at the scene, this time must be estimated. For many years our cardiac arrest registry added a minute to response times to take into account this "down time." Though I think a minute is a reasonable approximation of the time interval from a witnessed collapse to dialing 911, one should probably avoid any estimate and stick with exact times. The most accurate time anchor at the front-end of a cardiac arrest is the ring time in the 911 dispatch center (PSAP ring time in fig. 4.7). This starts the cardiac arrest clock. The key time intervals are the time from 911 to start of CPR and the time from 911 to defibrillation. The start of CPR should be further defined as the start of bystander CPR, bystander with telephone CPR, and EMS CPR.

Knowing the exact time of CPR is a challenge—for bystander CPR (without telephone CPR), it must be an estimate. It seems reasonable to code this time at two minutes following the call to 911. (Any good cardiac arrest registry should be able to designate times as accurate or estimated. There is nothing wrong with using estimated times as long as they are defined as estimates.) For bystander with telephone CPR, it is usually possible to accurately define this time by listening to the dispatch recording. We define the start of CPR as the first chest compression. When a tape is not available, define the time as half the interval from the 911 call to "at patient side" (or arrival time if at patient side is not available). When EMS begins CPR, the time may be obtained from the run report or one could use the "at patient side" as a surrogate for this time. Admittedly, EMS crews do not begin CPR instantly upon their arrival at the patient's side, but the time interval is on the order of 30 seconds or so.

Defining the exact moment of a defibrillatory shock is relatively easy assuming the recording is automatically downloaded after the event to the agency office or medical director's office and assuming that the device can auto-synchronize itself. Some AEDs and manual defibrillators are automatically synchronized when the defibrillation download occurs. Thus the exact moment of the shock is known. However, not all defibrilla-tors have this feature, and in this case, the time must be taken from the run report.

Typical Survivors

A single individual in cardiac arrest either survives or dies—his probability of survival is either 100 percent or 0 percent. It is only when you study many events that proba-bility statements make any sense.

There is, of course, no such thing as the typical victim of cardiac arrest, since each such event happens to a unique individual. Nevertheless, given so many events over thirty-one years, we can paint a picture of the average event and the average survivor.

The typical cardiac arrest in King County happens to a man who is sixty-six years old. He has underlying coronary artery disease and high cholesterol. He takes five medications.

The event occurs at home, and most likely his spouse or another relative sees him collapse. He is probably in ventricular fibrillation, and there is a very good chance that the spouse will perform CPR, perhaps with assistance over the phone from the dis-patcher. The victim will be successfully resuscitated with one shock by EMTs using an automated external defibrillator. The paramedics will intubate him, start an IV, and administer cardiac medications. He will be transported to a community hospital's emergency department, where hypothermia therapy will be started.

After twenty-four hours of coma, he will awaken, and on day four he will be trans-ferred from the ICU to a regular bed. Before he is discharged, on day eight, he will receive an implantable defibrillator.

He has some mild memory deficits, but his memory improves considerably over the next several months. By the third month following the cardiac arrest, he has returned to his usual activities, with two exceptions—he has finally given up smok-ing, and he uses an elliptical trainer five times a week. He vows that he will never regain the twenty pounds he has lost.

FIVE

Who Will Live and Who Will Die?

Tom M. and his wife, Janet, walked into the gallery housing Grant Wood's famous painting *American Gothic* at the Art Institute of Chicago. The gallery was crowded, as usual.
Tom and Janet had to work their way over to the painting, and they were gazing at it with
admiration when a wave of nausea broke over Tom. Sweating profusely, he looked for a
place to sit down, but the few seats in the gallery were already taken. He turned to Janet
and motioned toward the gallery's exit.

Janet felt a surge of panic—she had never seen her husband so pale, not to mention
dripping in perspiration this way. They walked together toward the door at the other side
of the room, but even before they reached the next gallery, Tom slumped onto her shoulder. She could feel that he was still partially supporting his own weight, but a few seconds
later that was no longer true. He went completely limp, and before she could call out to
the guard at the door, Tom crumpled slowly to the floor as Janet tried to control his fall.

The guard saw what was happening, but he didn't know exactly what he was dealing
with. Was this a simple faint? No—the man on the floor was lying too still. Could this be
a cardiac arrest, then? No, the guard decided—it must be a seizure. Well, he told himself, at least I won't have to do CPR. That was a relief, since there was blood on the man's
face—probably from hitting the floor a little too hard. All these thoughts passed rapidly
through the guard's mind as he relayed what he had seen over his radio, first asking for
911 to be called, then saying it wasn't necessary, then reversing himself and asking again
for EMS personnel.

While Tom was still lying on the floor, the guard's request for EMS was being routed from the museum's switchboard to the police department's alarm center to the fire department's alarm center and then to the fire station. And while Janet and the guard were waiting for the firefighter EMTs to arrive, Tom received no CPR. The time between his collapse and the EMTs' arrival and application of the automated external defibrillator was fourteen minutes. It took another six minutes for the fire department's paramedics to arrive and take over the resuscitation. (Even though twenty minutes had now gone by, the actual response time of the fire department was listed on the run report as only six minutes.)

Tom received one shock from the AED, but subsequent analyses indicated that no further shocks were necessary. After a total of fifteen minutes at the scene, Tom was lifted onto a stretcher and rushed to Northwestern Memorial Hospital. Physicians in the emergency room determined that Tom was in asystole, and they declared him dead without continuing the resuscitation.

SAN DIEGO

Usually Lorraine J. loved shopping at Macy's. She especially liked the bonus Tuesdays, when she could use her Macy's credit card and receive a 10 percent discount on top of the Macy's Days 20 percent discount. And there was the 5 percent senior discount, too, not to mention the automatic discount on all the clothing hanging on the clearance rack. It was almost like they were giving stuff away, she liked to say.

But on this Tuesday Lorraine was not feeling well, nor had she felt like herself for the past few days. She had noticed increasing fatigue and shortness of breath even when she walked only a short distance. Not being an alarmist, and especially because her doctor had made no adjustments to her medications, Lorraine concluded that what she was feeling must be early symptoms of the flu. Now, already at Macy's, Lorraine regretted her decision to go shopping.

But she wasn't yet ready to contemplate taking the bus back to her apartment at University House, so she asked the sales clerk if there was a seat nearby—her fatigue was overwhelming. Lorraine sat down on an upholstered chair, sighed deeply, and stopped breathing. The clerk didn't hear a thud. It was more of a faint whisper as Lorraine slid off the silk upholstery and onto the carpeting.

Two security personnel arrived within three minutes of Lorraine's collapse. One was carrying an automated external defibrillator. One of the AED's pads was applied to Lorraine's upper right chest, and the other was pressed onto the left side of her chest, below her armpit. By now a small crowd had gathered, and everyone was somewhat surprised to hear the device speak in a firm, commanding voice: *Stand back. Do not touch patient. Shock indicated. Press flashing red button.*

Lorraine's body twitched visibly with the shock. By the time the paramedics arrived, five minutes after the security personnel, Lorraine had a pulse and blood pressure. She was admitted to a hospital and discharged six days later. Her doctors discussed the possibility of an implantable defibrillator, but they told her that since her cardiac arrest had been the result of a myocardial infarction, the risk was low that she would have another cardiac arrest. And Lorraine would not have accepted an implantable defibrillator even if it had been recommended. She was eighty-two, and she had long ago decided that when her time came, she would be ready to go.

These two cardiac arrests, one in Chicago and the other in San Diego, were reasonably similar. Each collapse was witnessed directly, both patients were found to be in ventricular fibrillation, and in both instances a shock was delivered by an automated external defibrillator. But here the similarities end. Tom was in cardiac arrest for fourteen minutes before his heart was defibrillated. Loraine was in ventricular fibrillation for only three minutes before she received a shock. The time between the collapse and the first shock made all the difference in these two cases.

But the story is far more complex; there are actually many factors that determine why some people die and why others live after suffering cardiac arrest. This chapter looks at all the factors associated with surviving cardiac arrest—those that are known, and those that are speculative. Altogether there are fifty such factors. Obviously, if certain factors have been identified as being strongly associated with survival, then it makes strategic sense to focus on them in the attempt to increase survival rates in a community.

WHERE IS UTSTEIN, AND WHAT DOES IT HAVE TO DO WITH CARDIAC ARREST?

We've had prehospital emergency medical services for some forty years, so you'd think we would have lots of data on the survival experience of hundreds and hundreds of communities. But we don't. According to a 2004 review of the scientific literature (already cited in chapter 1), only thirty-five U.S. communities, representing 9 percent of the U.S. population, were reporting their experiences with cardiac arrest when that review was published. Overall, the survival rate for all treated cardiac arrests was 8 percent, and for patients with ventricular fibrillation the rate was 18 percent. That study—using these figures, and extrapolating from them to the entire U.S. population—estimated that approximately 13,000 Americans are discharged from hospitals every year after suffering cardiac arrest.[1]

There are complex reasons why so few communities report their survival rates. Perhaps the biggest one is simply lack of resources. Many small communities can barely pay EMS staff, let alone devote time and resources to gathering information on surviving cardiac arrest. The problem is compounded by hospitals that, invoking privacy laws, refuse to provide discharge information to outside agencies.[2] Furthermore, there are no state or national laws requiring communities to report their experiences with cardiac arrest. Many communities do report figures, but these are often estimates and do not reflect rigorous measurement. For its reported figures to be valid, a community must collect information in a specific fashion and must agree to common definitions. Finally, there is the "shame factor"—a community realizes how few patients it saves and is simply embarrassed to broadcast this information to the world.[3]

Different definitions also have different effects on reported survival rates, as is readily apparent from a 1991 King County study.[4] That study reported rates of survival ranging from 16 percent to 49 percent. The difference was accounted for by how the patients comprising the denominator were defined. For example, when all cardiac arrests from all causes were included, the survival rate (that is, the proportion of patients discharged from a hospital) was 16 percent; but when the only patients included were those who had underlying heart disease, had collapsed in the presence of a witness, and had received CPR within four minutes and definitive care within eight minutes, the survival rate jumped to 49 percent. Same community, different survival rates—magic! Just change your definitions, and you triple your survival rate. Trying to draw cross-community comparisons when all the parties are not using the same definitions is like attempting to organize a tournament in which each team plays by its own rules. A given community, determined to be number one in its rate of survival for cardiac arrest, could simply define its cases as including only those patients who collapsed in front of a witness, had ventricular fibrillation, received bystander CPR, responded to a single shock with a perfusing rhythm (that is, good blood pressure and pulse), and then wondered what was for dinner when they arrived at the coronary care unit. Such a denominator might yield a survival rate close to 100 percent, but that figure would be absurd.

This chaos surrounding definitions was already widely recognized when it led to a major international meeting that was held in the Utstein Abbey just outside Stavanger, Norway, in 1991. The criteria that came out of that meeting are known as the Utstein Criteria. They established a set of common definitions, and they spelled out exactly how data on cardiac arrest should be reported. It was hoped that these criteria would serve as a tool to help EMS leaders and researchers as they sought to understand the reasons for the different survival rates among various communities.[5] In 2004 the criteria were revised, with further clarification of the definitions and the required data elements.[6] Despite this effort to create a consistent case definition (for example, "witnessed cardiac arrest due to presumed underlying heart disease, with the initial rhythm of ventricular fibrillation"), few communities have been able (or willing) to put these criteria to use in publishing accurate survival figures.

WHY DO SOME SURVIVE WHILE OTHERS DIE?

As described in chapter 1, U.S. cities' reported rates of survival for ventricular fibrillation range from less than 1 percent (in Detroit) to 45 percent (in Seattle) and 46 percent (in King County and Rochester). What explains this tremendous range? The remainder of this chapter discusses all the known and speculative factors associated with successful resuscitation and begins to tease out why some communities do well and others do not. If we knew all the factors associated with survival, it would be an easy matter to measure them and begin to understand why some communities succeed and others fail. If only it were that simple!

Hundreds of scientific articles and research studies over the past forty years have shed light on the factors associated with survival after cardiac arrest.[7] Some factors are fairly obvious, such as the time between the victim's collapse and the delivery of critical therapies, but others may not be readily apparent. Some may even come as a surprise. What does socioeconomic status have to do with cardiac arrest? Did the weather influence a cardiac arrest? Did that cheeseburger really cause the heart to stop? Many of the known and speculative factors are beyond the individual's control. A person's age or sex cannot be changed to improve his or her likelihood of being resuscitated. Some factors may result from pure chance. For example, was anyone present to witness the victim's collapse? But many are directly determined by personal and community decisions.

These factors, summarized in table 5.1, are conveniently grouped into four categories: *patient factors*, *event factors*, *system factors*, and *therapy factors*. Patient factors are unique to the individual in question; they include prior heart disease, weight, smoking, and genetic factors. Event factors are associated with the cardiac arrest itself and include cardiac rhythm, the presence or absence of witnesses to the victim's collapse, and the presence or absence of bystander CPR. System factors include the time between the victim's collapse and the initiation of CPR and defibrillation, the type and size of the EMS system, the number of responders, the level of experience of the EMS personnel, the presence or absence of dispatcher-assisted telephone CPR, the quality of the system's medical direction, the system's organizational culture, the quality of training, and the presence or absence of CPR training and public access defibrillation in the community. Therapy factors involve the actual treatments used, including pharmacotherapy, hypothermia, and endotracheal intubation, as well as the quality of hospital care. The first two groups—patient and event factors—may be extremely important but are not influenced much by individual or community decisions. In this regard, they could be called "fate factors." The latter two groups—system and therapy factors—can be directly influenced by individual and community decisions. These could be called "choice factors."

Table 5.1 also indicates the strength of each factor's association with survival. Some factors, such as socioeconomic status, are weakly associated with survival; others, such as the amount of time that passes between the victim's collapse and the moment of defibrillation, are strongly associated with survival. In some instances, the strength of a factor's association with survival is unknown, or the science is weak.

Table 5.1. Factors associated with surviving cardiac arrest

Factor	Strength of Association
Patient Factors	
Age	+
Sex	0
Race	++
Comorbidity	+++
Diet	unknown
Obesity	unknown
Medications	+
Socioeconomic status	++
Genetic determinants	unknown
Event Factors	
Type of heart rhythm	+++
Presence of witness	+++
Location of collapse	++
Time of day when collapse occurs	0
Bystander CPR	+++
Cause of cardiac arrest	++
Use of on-scene AED	++
Emesis	+
Symptoms before collapse	unknown
Collapse before arrival of EMS	++
Agonal breathing	+++
Activities preceding collapse	unknown
Environmental factors	0
Position after collapse	unknown
Decision to begin resuscitation	unknown
System Factors	
Time to CPR	+++
Quality of CPR	++
Time to defibrillation	+++
Quality of defibrillation	unknown
Interaction of CPR and defibrillation	+++
Type of EMS system	++
System size	unknown
Number of responders	unknown
Ratio of paramedics to population	unknown
Dispatcher-assisted telephone CPR	+++

Factor	Strength of Association
Quality of EMS care	unknown
Quality of medical direction	unknown
Ongoing medical QI	unknown
Organizational structure and culture	unknown
Administrative support	unknown
Quality of training	unknown
Community CPR training	++
Public access defibrillation	++
Therapy Factors	
Pharmacotherapy	unknown
Defibrillator-guided therapy	+
Impedance threshold device	0
CPR adjuncts	0
Chest-compression-only CPR	+
Airway management	+
Hypothermia	++
Quality of hospital care	unknown

0   no or minimal association

+   weak association

++   moderate association

+++   strong association

Why even list such a factor if the science is so weak? Because the very fact that some data exist suggests possible avenues for future scientific inquiry, even though a current judgment about the factor's association with survival may be based on animal studies or observational studies or may simply be inferred from the association's plausibility. The influence of genetics is a good example of such a factor. Few data exist at present to support our attaching much importance to genetic factors as explanatory in resuscitation, but such an association may be discovered in the future, when genetic information may conceivably come to guide immediate or postresuscitation therapy.

The following discussion emphasizes the direct effects that these factors have on the likelihood of the victim's successful resuscitation. In some instances, the nature of the particular factor may increase or decrease the odds of the individual's having a cardiac arrest in the first place but may have no effect on the likelihood of his or her successful resuscitation. As an example, the consumption of fish oils may decrease the odds of someone's suffering a cardiac arrest but may have no influence at all on the outcome once the arrest has occurred. The goal here is to give a brief summary of the existing knowledge about the confirmed or putative factors directly related to the outcome following a cardiac arrest. Many of the factors discussed here have little or no direct bearing on how a system might be able to improve its management of cardiac arrest, and so greater attention is given to those factors that are directly relevant to the practices of EMS providers and managers.

Patient Factors

The patient factors include the victim's age, sex, race, comorbidity, diet, obesity, medications, socioeconomic status, and genetic determinants. Some of these factors are obviously beyond the individual's control, whereas others can be influenced by his or her personal behavior. This section summarizes what is known about each of the patient factors and about the relative importance of each one to survival outcomes.

Age (Weak Association with Survival)

One might assume that age would be a very strong predictor of survival, but in fact age is only weakly associated with survival. In 2000, Swor and his colleagues reported on 2,600 cardiac arrests in Royal Oak, Michigan, a suburb of Detroit. They found decreased survival with advancing age. Starting with patients between the ages of forty and forty-nine, and increasing by ten-year increments the ages of the patients they studied, they found, for each of these age groups in ascending order, that the likelihood of survival was 10 percent, 10 percent, 8.1 percent, 7.1 percent, and 3.3 percent, respectively (the latter group consisting of patients between the ages of eighty and eighty-nine). There were even survivors among patients ninety and older.[8] Similarly, a report from King County by Kim and her colleagues found reasonable survival rates among patients in their eighties and nineties.[9]

Sex (No Association with Survival)

Men are more likely than women to have heart disease and are therefore more likely than women to suffer cardiac arrest, but sex is not a predictor of survival. Women and men at comparable ages have equal probabilities of survival.

Race (Moderate Association with Survival)

Several studies have shown that African Americans have both a higher incidence of cardiac arrest and poorer survival rates than Caucasian Americans. For example, a 1993 study from Chicago found a higher incidence of cardiac arrest in African Americans, and dismal survival rates overall—0.8 percent of African Americans survived, compared to 2.6 percent of Caucasian Americans.[10] Contrary findings were reported by Chu and his colleagues in a 1998 study from Royal Oak, Michigan, where there was no association of race with survival.[11] An investigation from Seattle demonstrated racial differences in resuscitation after cardiac arrest in which ventricular fibrillation had occurred.[12] When demographic and clinical factors were controlled for, people of European ancestry were found to be twice as likely as people of African ancestry to survive cardiac arrest with VF. The reasons for this discrepancy are not readily apparent.

Comorbidity (Strong Association with Survival)

Comorbidity (underlying disease) is the totality of chronic or acute illnesses that are present at the time of cardiac arrest but that are not direct causes of the arrest. For example, a person who has a cardiac arrest caused by ischemic heart disease may also have emphysema, diabetes, and dementia. The latter three diseases are comorbid conditions. Comorbidity is definitely inversely correlated with survival.[13] It is not surprising that a person with comorbid conditions would do less well than an otherwise healthy person. The best study demonstrating this relationship was one published in 1996 by Hallstrom and his colleagues, who looked at the comorbidity of 282 victims of out-of-hospital cardiac arrest.[14] The victims' comorbidity was determined from interviews that were conducted with the people who had called 911, or with other witnesses of these cardiac arrests, approximately seven weeks after they occurred. There was a strong association—the greater the victim's comorbidity, the lower the likelihood of his or her survival. Before this study was published, it had been assumed that comorbidity did decrease the likelihood of survival, but this was the first study to quantify the effect of underlying disease. Hallstrom and his colleagues concluded that comorbidity is a factor that is often overlooked in studies of cardiac arrest. I agree. Comorbidity probably explains why some resuscitations are not successful even when VF is present and therapy is provided quickly. Comorbidity is so powerful as an explanation for unsuccessful resuscitations that it undoubtedly establishes the maximum rate of resuscitation and survival for cardiac arrest in any given community—that is, the rate of resuscitation and survival that is possible in ideal conditions. As I will argue later on, the maximum rate of resuscitation and survival for VF is around 50 percent. This figure is admittedly an estimate, and is based on community survival rates that include all people who have suffered VF—the relatively healthy as well as the severely ill.[15]

The challenge in measuring the effect of comorbidity is in obtaining clinical information about victims' underlying disease. Most EMS systems do not collect information about comorbidity in a systematic way. Furthermore, it is very difficult to obtain this information from hospital records, or from patients' families in the event of death.

Few EMS centers have the resources to gather such complete clinical particulars. It is possible, however, for one kind of information routinely collected by EMTs and paramedics to stand in for comorbidity data—the list of all the medications that have been prescribed for the victim. The more meds, the more comorbidity.

Diet (Unknown Association with Survival)

In 1995 David Siscovick, a cardiovascular epidemiologist at the University of Washington, coauthored a report stating that a diet high in fish oils and omega-3 fatty acids protects against cardiac arrest.[16] This association of fish oils with reduced risk of sudden cardiac death has been demonstrated repeatedly. It is felt that the omega-3 fatty acids stabilize the cell membranes in the heart and therefore lower the risk of an arrhythmia such as VF. Dietary factors may offer a partial explanation for the differences in rates of sudden death in different countries. In Japan, for example, where there are high national rates of ingesting fish, the rates of sudden death are lower than in the United States. Many other authors have also touted certain diets as cardioprotective. The Mediterranean diet, for example, which is high in monosaturated oils, such as olive oil, has been promoted for this benefit, but good comparison data are hard to come by. That is one reason why it is a challenge to study and compare cross-cultural dietary practices. Though diets high in omega-3 fatty acids are shown to protect against the onset of VF, there is no evidence that diet per se is associated with increased likelihood of successful resuscitation. Furthermore, fish oils do not reduce atherosclerosis or nonfatal myocardial infarction.

Obesity (Unknown Association with Survival)

The connection between obesity and the likelihood of surviving cardiac arrest has not been well studied. In 2006, Becker and his colleagues presented a study on the body mass index (BMI) of seventy-six patients in Chicago who had suffered cardiac arrest. The morbidly obese patients (BMI >40) proved less likely to survive, but it was noted that this group of patients had received shallower chest compressions than those administered to patients with normal body mass index. Presumably, CPR is more difficult to perform for obese patients, and this may partly or wholly explain their worse outcomes.[17] An earlier study, this one by White and his colleagues, showed no relationship between body weight and successful defibrillation.[18]

Medications (Weak Association with Survival)

As noted earlier, a patient's comorbidity can be extrapolated from his or her prescribed medications, and this comorbidity in turn decreases the probability of successful resuscitation after cardiac arrest. Likewise, the patient's medications may become another cofactor along with his or her underlying conditions.

There are virtually no studies demonstrating that patients taking specific medications are more difficult to resuscitate, with one exception—diuretics are commonly prescribed for patients with congestive heart failure, and some diuretics cause depletion of potassium. If this depletion is severe enough, it can both lead to cardiac arrest and make successful resuscitation much more difficult.

It is also conceivable that some medications may improve the likelihood of resuscitation. Patients who are taking beta-blockers, for example, may be less likely to refibrillate after an initial defibrillation and may therefore have better chances of survival. In the absence of data, however, this is a purely speculative proposition.

Occasionally there is publicity in the media about a drug that has been recalled because of some newly discovered side effect. For example, certain drugs may actually have the potential to increase the likelihood of cardiac arrest. Thus when Vioxx was found to present an increased risk of myocardial infarction, that discovery led to new warnings about the medication (as well as to a number of lawsuits),[19] and recently a popular drug for diabetes was also found to increase the risk of cardiac events. Usually such a risk, unless it is major, is difficult to detect through routine therapeutic use of a medication. Most of these adverse associations are discovered during large drug trials, and a trial may be stopped prematurely when an increased risk of cardiac arrest is noted. As an example, the Cardiac Arrhythmia Suppression Trial (CAST) was stopped when it was found that one anti-arrhythmic medication actually led to more of the cardiac arrhythmias that the drug was intended to suppress.[20]

Socioeconomic Status (Moderate Association with Survival)

Several studies have demonstrated a relationship between socioeconomic status and incidence of cardiac arrest. One 1995 study from Portland, Oregon, showed that people from low-median-income census tracts had higher rates of cardiac arrest than did people from high-median-income tracts, though the authors found no relationship between median income and survival.[21] A more detailed two-year study, published in 2006 and also using data from Portland, found that lower median income, greater poverty, lower median home value, and lower educational attainment were strongly associated with higher incidence of sudden cardiac arrest, but this study did not report on the relationship of these factors to the likelihood of survival.[22]

Other studies, however, have found a relationship between socioeconomic factors and survival: the lower the socioeconomic class, the lower the rate of survival. In a 1993 study, Hallstrom and his colleagues found that higher rates of survival after cardiac arrest were associated with higher assessed home value in Seattle: for every $50,000 increase in home valuation there was a 1.6-fold increase in the rate of survival.[23] And in 2005 Clarke, Schellenbaum, and Rea, using median household income as the measure of socioeconomic status, found in King County that higher income was associated with greater likelihood of survival.[24]

It is not evident why a wealthy person should be more likely than a poor person to survive cardiac arrest. Perhaps better health care and more successfully controlled comorbid conditions before the cardiac arrest may be factors. In other words, there may be a relationship between comorbidity and socioeconomic factors when it comes to surviving cardiac arrest. If that is the case, and I suspect that it is, then it may be difficult to sort out exactly what this relationship may be. And, to further cloud the picture, an earlier study from several communities in Michigan found no association between median household income and survival after cardiac arrest.[25]

Genetic Determinants (Unknown Association with Survival)

A recent report in the *New York Times* described the discovery of a genetic factor that increases the risk of heart disease up to 60 percent in people of European descent.[26] Though this finding is not related to the likelihood of resuscitation after cardiac arrest, the discovery of this genetic factor certainly brings with it great potential for identifying people who are at risk of developing ischemic heart disease. Thus early interventions, like control of blood cholesterol and blood pressure, may be able to reduce the likelihood of cardiac arrest in the first place.

While it is clear that genetic factors are linked to heart disease and to cardiac arrest, the question here is whether genetic factors influence the outcome once a cardiac arrest has occurred. It is known that genetic factors determine one's responsiveness to particular medications. Theoretically, the potent pharmacotherapy used in resuscitations could be individually tailored on the basis of the particular patient's genetic susceptibility. Similarly, there may be genetic determinants involved in a patient's responsiveness to defibrillatory shocks or hypothermia. Such relationships are plausible, but very little is known about them at this time, and we are probably years away from understanding the genetic determinants of resuscitation.

Event Factors

Event factors are those associated with the cardiac arrest itself: the type of heart rhythm; the presence or absence of a witness to the collapse; the location of the collapse; the time of day when the collapse occurs; the availability of bystander-initiated CPR; the cause of the cardiac arrest; the use of an on-scene AED; the presence of emesis; the presence or absence of symptoms before the collapse; the timing of the collapse in relation to the arrival of EMS personnel; the presence or absence of agonal

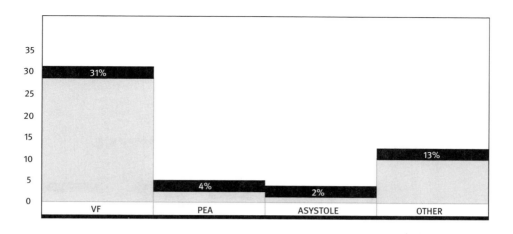

5.1 Percentages of patients surviving cardiac arrest, by rhythm, King County, Washington, 2005–2011.

breathing; the patient's activities and other possible triggers preceding the collapse; environmental conditions; the victim's position after the collapse; and circumstances surrounding the decision to begin resuscitation.

Type of Heart Rhythm (Strong Association with Survival)

The type of heart rhythm found in the patient is an extremely strong predictor of whether or not a resuscitation attempt will succeed (see fig. 5.1). A patient found in ventricular fibrillation has the best chance of survival. Patients whose hearts exhibit other rhythms, such as pulseless electrical activity and asystole, have almost no chance of survival.[27]

Presence or Absence of a Witness to the Collapse (Strong Association with Survival)

The presence of a witness—someone at the scene who sees or hears the patient collapse—is another extremely strong predictor of the patient's survival. Figure 5.2 shows how the presence or absence of a witness is related to survival for patients exhibiting the rhythms of ventricular fibrillation, pulseless electrical activity, and asystole. When we walk into a room and see someone who has collapsed, there is of course no way for us to tell just by looking whether the person collapsed mere seconds ago or a whole hour ago. It is likely, however, that many, perhaps all, patients who have collapsed without a witness, but have still gone on to survive, were able to do so because they collapsed just minutes or even seconds before they were discovered. Patients who collapse in the presence of a witness and who are found in ventricular fibrillation have the best chances for successful resuscitation.[28]

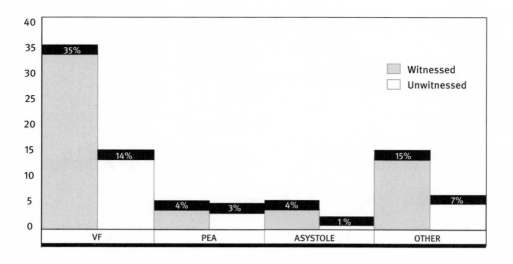

5.2 Percentages, by rhythm that caused witnessed and unwitnessed collapse, of patients surviving cardiac arrest, King County, Washington, 2000–2011.

Location of the Collapse (Moderate Association with Survival)

As in real estate, so in cardiac arrest—location, location, location. And here, I mean not just the community where a cardiac arrest occurs—as we've seen, you are forty-six times more likely to survive in some communities than in others—but the precise place where the collapse occurs within a given community. Patients who collapse in public locations are more likely to survive than those who collapse at home. And patients who collapse in public locations in the presence of witnesses, and who are found to be in ventricular fibrillation, survive 56 percent of the time, whereas patients who collapse at home, with witnesses, survive only 41 percent of the time. This difference in survival rates is partly explained by the fact that there are more likely to be people able to perform CPR in public locations (see fig. 5.3). It is also possible that people who are out and about in public are less likely to have significant comorbidity than are people who may be confined to home because of illness. Nevertheless, patients in nursing homes who suffer cardiac arrest and ventricular fibrillation in the presence of witnesses have the lowest likelihood of survival—17 percent—undoubtedly because of their higher comorbidity by comparison with people who do not require care in a nursing home.

Time of Day When the Collapse Occurs (No Association with Survival)

The time of day when the collapse occurs has no relation to the likelihood of the patient's survival. Furthermore, neither the month nor the day of the week has any relation to the outcome for the patient. Some studies do show a relationship between

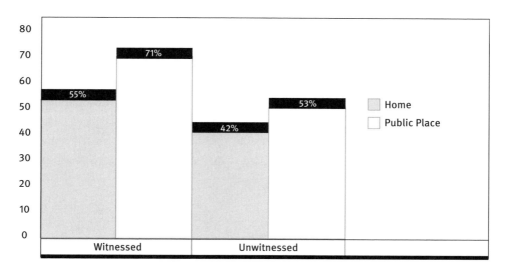

5.3 Percentages of bystander CPR, at home and in public, for witnessed and unwitnessed cardiac arrests due to heart disease, King County, 2000–2011.

time of day and the cardiac event itself; for example, more myocardial infarctions appear to occur in the early-morning hours. But once the cardiac arrest has occurred, the patient's survival is unrelated to the time of day, the day of the week, or the month when the arrest occurred.

Availability of Bystander-Initiated CPR (Strong Association with Survival)

There is a large literature on the benefit of bystander CPR. Though not all studies agree, the vast majority do show an approximate doubling in the likelihood of the patient's survival if bystanders begin CPR before the arrival of EMS personnel.[29] It is usually easy to ascertain whether bystander CPR did or did not occur before EMS personnel arrived, but it is often difficult to measure precisely when it began. King County's cardiac arrest registry uses information from the incident form and the dispatch tape recordings in attempting to reconstruct the timing of bystander CPR. Admittedly, this is a labor-intensive process. Communities that have fewer registry resources can estimate the time that elapsed between the patient's collapse and the initiation of bystander CPR by using half the response time of the first unit that arrived on the scene (that is, half the time between the call to 911 and the arrival of EMS personnel on the scene).

Cause of the Cardiac Arrest (Moderate Association with Survival)

The association between a patient's survival and the cause of his or her cardiac arrest is one that is hard to quantify, but I believe it to be a real one nevertheless. The patient with a cardiomyopathy is less likely to be found in ventricular fibrillation than is one whose cardiac arrest is associated with ischemic heart disease. As a result, the patient whose cardiac arrest is the result of a cardiomyopathy is less likely to survive. The patient with a primary arrhythmia usually exhibits VF and may be easier to resuscitate than is a patient who has suffered an ischemic-associated cardiac arrest. Sometimes the patient who has suffered an ischemic-associated arrest may have had a large myocardial infarction, and it may be impossible to resuscitate this patient. Thus the cause of the patient's cardiac arrest is related to the likely success of an attempted resuscitation.

Use of an On-Scene AED (Moderate Association with Survival)

An on-scene automated external defibrillator can quickly provide defibrillatory shocks. It would certainly be fortunate if a person collapsed at a location where there was an AED. The situation would be analogous, in some ways, to one in which a bystander at the scene of a collapse knew how to perform CPR. Many other conditions would have to be met, of course. Someone would have to recognize that the collapse had occurred, the victim would have to be in VF, a bystander would have to remember the presence and the location of the AED, and the AED would have to be properly attached to the patient and then properly operated. Despite all these challenges, the provision of AEDs in public locations does have the potential to improve outcomes, as demonstrated by a large public access defibrillation (PAD) trial.[30]

Presence of Emesis (Weak Association with Survival)

It is assumed that when emesis (vomiting) is associated with cardiac arrest, the likelihood of successful resuscitation is decreased because of the airway's obstruction and the aspiration of the stomach's contents into the airway and lungs. One study that compared the outcomes of cardiac arrest on the basis of the presence or absence of emesis found a negative association between survival and emesis; in other words, if the patient vomited before or during the resuscitation, there was a lower likelihood of survival.[31]

Patient's Symptoms Before the Collapse (Unknown Association with Survival)

When a patient, before collapsing, experiences symptoms like chest pain or difficulty breathing, the symptoms suggest ischemia or cardiomyopathy as the likely cause of the event. By contrast, a cardiac arrest that occurs without symptoms is probably the result of a primary arrhythmia—namely, VF. As already discussed, the cause of the event can be related to its outcome; therefore, it is likely that the presence or absence of symptoms is also related to outcomes. The relationship between symptoms and outcomes is complicated, however, by the question of whether the collapse occurred before or after the arrival of EMS personnel. Patients who experience symptoms may collapse either before or after EMS personnel arrive, whereas those with no symptoms invariably collapse before the arrival of EMS personnel.

Timing of the Collapse in Relation to the Arrival of EMS Personnel (Moderate Association with Survival)

Someone who suffers a cardiac arrest after the arrival of EMS personnel has a higher likelihood of survival than someone whose cardiac arrest occurs before EMS personnel arrive on the scene. This is logical, since EMS personnel, once they arrive, can provide CPR and defibrillation almost instantly. It would be reasonable to suppose that the survival rate for such patients should approach 100 percent, but their actual rate of survival is approximately 60 percent. This rate, so much lower than what might be expected, is probably explained by the fact that patients who collapse after the arrival of EMS personnel have serious and ongoing symptoms, hence the reason for the 911 call. These are the types of symptoms likely to indicate acute coronary syndrome or the worsening of a cardiomyopathy. The underlying condition may have progressed to the point of fatality, so that even instant care may not be sufficient. For example, the person may be suffering a myocardial infarction so massive that the outcome will be death, regardless of how soon help arrives.

Patients who collapse before the arrival of EMS personnel are a heterogeneous group and include those with no symptoms at all as well as those who have symptoms but who delay the call to 911 long enough for the collapse to occur. In both cases, because of the delay in treatment, there is a lower likelihood of survival among this group of patients than among those who collapse after EMS personnel arrive.

Presence or Absence of Agonal Breathing (Strong Association with Survival)

Agonal breathing—the abnormal breaths that occur immediately after cardiac arrest and last up to several minutes—is an underappreciated phenomenon. Most programs that train citizens in CPR make no mention of it, and many emergency dispatchers are not specially trained to recognize it. This is regrettable, since a dispatcher who hears that a victim's breathing is abnormal may mistakenly conclude that the victim is not in cardiac arrest and may therefore fail to offer CPR instructions over the phone. But the presence of agonal breathing is strongly associated with survival because it is a surrogate for a brief period of cardiac arrest: agonal breathing occurs only during the first few minutes of a cardiac arrest, so its presence suggests that the arrest has just occurred.

In a study from King County, Clark and her colleagues reported agonal breathing in approximately 40 percent of all cardiac arrests; survival in the group of patients with agonal breathing was 27 percent, compared to 9 percent when agonal breathing was not present.[32] The presence of agonal breathing was also strongly associated with the underlying heart rhythm—56 percent of patients in VF had agonal breathing, compared to 34 percent for patients whose hearts had other rhythms. When cardiac arrests were witnessed, patients had agonal breathing 55 percent of the time, compared to 16 percent of the time for patients whose cardiac arrests occurred without witnesses.[33]

Patient's Activities and Other Possible Triggers Preceding the Collapse (Unknown Association with Survival)

As noted in chapter 4, vigorous exercise transiently increases the risk of sudden death,[34] but there is no evidence that exercisers who suffer cardiac arrest are more or less likely to be resuscitated than are nonexercisers. To make a useful comparison, of course, one would have to control for comorbidity in the two groups—presumably, exercisers have less comorbidity.

It is possible that other activities and possible triggers—such as sex, smoking, caffeine or alcohol consumption, emotional stress, anger, or even high-fat foods—are associated with VF. While these associations are plausible, there are no good data to clinch them. The question for us, however, is this: Once cardiac arrest has occurred, does either the presence or the absence of any of these presumed triggers alter the likelihood of resuscitation? Conceivably, some of these activities and other possible triggers could impede resuscitation. For example, if the patient had been smoking, the nicotine in his or her system could make the heart more resistant to defibrillation.

Would EMS personnel provide different types of therapy if they knew that the patient had just been smoking or exercising or had been in a knock-down argument? Probably not, though it is possible that an immediate trigger might be neutralized by some therapeutic factor. Still, the science on this matter is simply too meager for us to draw firm conclusions.

Environmental Conditions (No Association with Survival)

Several studies have found an association between environmental conditions and cardiac events. For example, a 2007 study from the University of Washington reported that long-term exposure to air pollution had led to an increase in cardiovascular events in women.[35] Another study found an association between air pollution and EMS calls for complaints of chest pain.[36] Environmental factors like these may play a role in triggering cardiac arrests, but I suspect that they have little or no relevance to the likelihood of resuscitation.

Victim's Position after the Collapse (Unknown Association with Survival)

The position of the victim after his or her collapse may play a role in the outcome, in two ways. First, the victim's position may delay the start of bystander CPR. For example, the victim may be wedged between the toilet and the bathtub, or crumpled on a stairway, or too heavy to move to the floor, or positioned in one of countless other ways that preclude rapid initiation of CPR.[37] Second, the victim may collapse with his or her head flexed so that the airway is obstructed. In this situation, a bystander attempting to perform CPR may not understand the importance of straightening the victim's head and neck and may have a difficult time providing mouth-to-mouth ventilation. Moreover, if the victim collapses with a flexed neck, there may be no opportunity for air to move back and forth during agonal respirations. Although this kind of abnormal respiration does not allow the victim to breathe normally, it can still provide a limited amount of ventilation, but a flexed neck will prevent even this kind of suboptimal breathing.

Circumstances Surrounding the Decision to Begin Resuscitation (Unknown Association with Survival)

There are no rules that can tell a rescuer whether a person in cardiac arrest has a good chance, a poor chance, or no chance of successful resuscitation. And even though EMTs and paramedics are trained to start resuscitation whenever there is a chance of success, there are clearly situations in which resuscitation should not be attempted. Therefore, when EMTs and paramedics arrive at the scene, they must make a split-second decision to begin or not to begin resuscitation.

The basis for a decision not to begin resuscitation varies from system to system, and it may even vary among EMS personnel within a single agency. For example, I once had occasion to review the "do not attempt resuscitation" medical protocols for each of the counties in Washington State, and I was struck by the variation in these protocols. Most of the counties required a paramedic to contact the medical control doctor, but some counties allowed the paramedic at the scene to make the decision about whether or not to begin resuscitation. In some counties, it was permissible not to resuscitate only if there were findings of absolute incompatibility with life (for example, decapitation or rigor mortis). Other counties allowed more subjective signs, such as cool temperature or lividity, as a basis for withholding resuscitation. And similar variation in standards undoubtedly exists throughout the country. Whatever these decisions are based on, they can affect the denominator of attempted resuscitation and thus have an influence on survival rates.[38]

System Factors

System factors are those associated with the organization, practices, and delivery of EMS care in a community. They include the time between the collapse and the start of CPR; the quality of the CPR; the time between the collapse and the start of defibrillation; the quality of the defibrillation; the interaction between CPR and defibrillation; the type of EMS system; the size of the EMS system; the number of responders; the ratio of paramedics to total members of the community; the use of dispatcher-assisted telephone CPR; the quality of EMS care; the quality of medical direction; the existence of an ongoing program for medical quality improvement; the organizational structure and culture of the emergency medical system; the level and nature of administrative support; the quality of EMS training; the existence of a community program for training citizens in CPR; and the existence of a community program for encouraging public access defibrillation.

Time Between the Collapse and the Start of CPR (Strong Association with Survival)

The amount of time that passes between the moment of collapse and the initiation of CPR is one of the strongest predictors of survival (see fig. 5.4). Note, however, that the rate of survival is relatively constant for everyone with respect to the first four min-

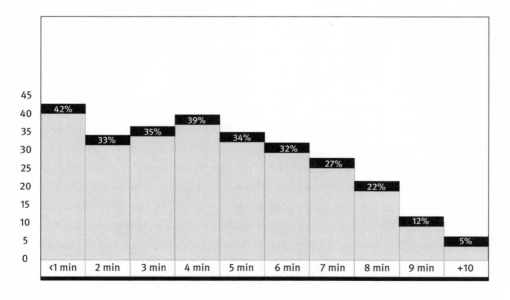

5.4 Percentages, by time between collapse and start of CPR, of patients who survived cardiac arrest with witnessed ventricular fibrillation due to heart disease, King County, Washington, 1990–2007.

utes. The flatness of this part of the curve, in the early minutes of the cardiac arrest, probably reflects the fact that the body still has oxygenated blood. Once this oxygen is used up—probably after four minutes—the fall in the survival rate begins, and it continues relentlessly, dropping by approximately 5 percent for every minute that goes by. This differential rate of survival—high for the first four minutes, then rapidly dropping—is explained in the three-phase model of cardiac arrest that has been proposed by Weisfeldt and Becker.[39]

The first phase, as already mentioned, lasts approximately four minutes and is called the "electrical" phase. Defibrillatory shocks are all that is needed during this phase, and CPR is of lesser importance. The second phase is called the "circulatory" phase. CPR is very important during this phase, since it restores oxygenated blood to the brain and other organs. The circulatory phase probably begins after four minutes and lasts until ten or twelve minutes into the cardiac arrest. The third phase is called the "metabolic" phase. Therapy, or at least the kind based on our current science, is not effective during this phase, because cellular damage has occurred beyond the point where modern science can help, although hypothermia may still be of benefit during the metabolic phase.

Quality of CPR (Moderate Association with Survival)

The quality of CPR, probably because it is difficult to measure in clinical situations, has been an underappreciated factor and is only now beginning to emerge as an important aspect of successful resuscitation. It is only natural, of course, to assume that the quality of CPR is important, and several studies from the mid-1990s seem to confirm this assumption.[40] Nevertheless, the quality of CPR is actually a very difficult factor to study. For one thing, there are few or no cameras at the scene of a cardiac arrest. For another, minimal-quality CPR could turn out to be as good or almost as good as letter-perfect CPR.

Despite these challenges, Aufderheide and his colleagues, in Milwaukee, were able to offer an indirect demonstration of a negative relationship between outcome and quality of CPR.[41] In this study, an observer monitored the number of ventilations provided by EMTs to thirteen victims of cardiac arrest. The key finding was that EMTs compressed the chest too quickly and gave too many ventilations; there were no survivors among the thirteen people whose cardiac arrests were observed. The same researchers then studied pigs in a model of cardiac arrest to determine the effects of too much ventilation. They demonstrated that overventilation led to a fall in blood pressure, which was due to an excess of air in the chest that prevented adequate return of blood to the heart. Thus they showed that poor-quality CPR—in this case, too much ventilation—can decrease the likelihood of successful resuscitation.

Another group of researchers has demonstrated that incomplete chest recoil during CPR worsens hemodynamics.[42] This study used piglets, but the findings were fairly convincing: leaning on the chest during CPR, and not allowing the chest to fully expand on the upstroke, led to worse systolic blood pressure and worse coronary perfusion pressure while substantially reducing myocardial blood flow.

In the matter of determining the quality of CPR and its association with successful resuscitation, technology may yet come to the rescue. Current defibrillators already offer the ability to assess the quality of CPR during an actual resuscitation and to verbally coach the rescuer, giving instructions to slow down or speed up compressions, deliver compressions that are deeper or not so deep, and give fewer or more ventilations. These newer defibrillators also record the quality of the CPR so it can be reviewed by a medical director. Future defibrillators may be able to do all that in addition to determining the volume of ventilations. Other devices, some currently available only in hospital settings, may one day play a role in assessing the quality of prehospital CPR. For example, echocardiography may be able to determine the quantity of forward blood flow associated with CPR and even determine whether there is any mechanical impediment to adequate blood flow.[43]

Time Between the Collapse and the Start of Defibrillation (Strong Association with Survival)

The amount of time that passes between the moment of collapse and the start of defibrillation is arguably the single most important predictor of survival. As seen in figure 5.5, this relationship is striking. With each minute that defibrillation is delayed, the

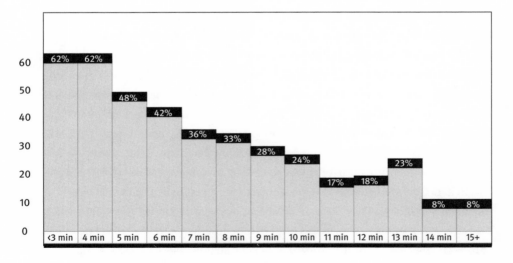

5.5 Percentages, by time between collapse and first defibrillatory shock, of patients who survived cardiac arrest with witnessed ventricular fibrillation due to heart disease, King County, Washington, 1990–2007.

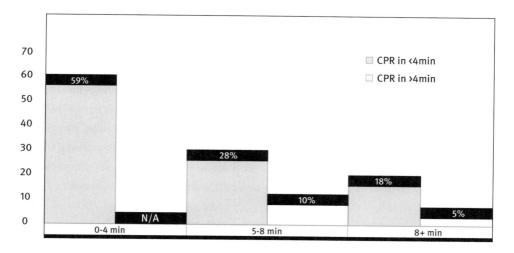

5.6 Percentages of patients who survive VF cardiac arrest in King County, Washington, from collapse to start of CPR and from collapse to first defibrillatory shock.

likelihood of survival falls by 5 percent. Note, however, that the survival rate does not fall for the first four minutes. This phenomenon probably reflects the same one we saw when we looked at the time between the collapse and the start of CPR. The body continues to be well oxygenated for the first four minutes after cardiac arrest, and defibrillation is as effective as CPR during the electrical phase of the arrest.

The benefit of defibrillation can also be modified by other factors, the most important of which is CPR—early delivery of CPR appears to extend the period during which defibrillation is effective. In this regard, CPR slows the dying process. When defibrillation is given very early, however, it may be all the therapy that is required, though more therapy is likely to be needed as the time increases between the collapse and the first defibrillatory shock. This additional therapy may include further shocks, intravenous medications like epinephrine and lidocaine, or other rhythm stabilizers like amiodorone or beta-blockers.

In the case of both CPR and defibrillation, we have seen the numbers that demonstrate the importance of the intervals between the victim's collapse and the initiation of these therapies, and the numbers are additive. Clearly, the best scenario is one in which both intervals are short, and the worst scenario is one in which both are long. Figure 5.6 shows the relationship between each of these two intervals and the victim's survival.[44]

Quality of Defibrillation (Unknown Association with Survival)

In much the same way that the quality of CPR is being appreciated as an important factor in successful resuscitation, there is some evidence to suggest that the quality of defibrillation is also important. Here, the word "quality" refers to the actual mechanics of attaching and operating the defibrillator.

One group of researchers looked at where on the patient's chest the defibrillator's electrode pads were placed.[45] The subjects of their study were patients in the process of having defibrillators implanted, and as part of the study procedure, VF was induced in the patients in order to test the implantable defibrillators. The researchers found that placement location affected the measurement of VF amplitude—in other words, if the pads were not correctly placed, it was possible to reach the false conclusion that VF was not present when in fact it was. This provocative study suggests that training in proper placement of electrode pads may also be an important factor in survival.

Interaction Between CPR and Defibrillation (Strong Association with Survival)

It used to be taught in cardiac arrest protocols that the most important principle of defibrillation was to deliver shocks quickly and repeatedly. The mantra was "Shock fast, and shock often." But this old mantra has been replaced with a new one: "Shock wisely."

Data from animal studies have suggested an important interaction between CPR and defibrillation; in other words, the sequence and timing of the two are emerging as important factors in resuscitation. These studies have revealed that when CPR is delayed or stopped, the left ventricle is quickly drained of blood. If a shock is given to a heart drained of blood, there is no coronary artery perfusion pressure (this is the pressure that fills the coronary artery), and if the coronary artery is empty of blood, a shock will not be successful.[46]

Rea and his colleagues in King County, observing that the old protocols were causing long periods without CPR, changed their EMS system's cardiac arrest protocol for VF in such a way as to minimize the time that the victim was left without CPR. The delivery of multiple shocks—up to three in a row, called "stacked shocks"—was eliminated, as was the practice of stopping for a pulse check after each shock. The new protocol required one shock, followed immediately by two minutes of CPR and then by a reassessment of the heart rhythm. The goal was to provide as much CPR as possible between single shocks. The results were dramatic. The survival rate for witnessed VF, which had been 33 percent under the old protocol, rose to 46 percent ($p < .05$) under the new one.[47] In fact, this new protocol was adopted by the American Heart Association at its 2005 conference on international guidelines. Thus the entire nation is now using this protocol, and it is hoped that survival rates will improve nationally.

Still to be settled is the question of whether CPR should always precede the first defibrillatory shock. For example, if there is no bystander who can perform CPR, and if the fire department is first on the scene, should the EMTs start CPR first, or should they defibrillate immediately? Back in the early 1970s, it was dogma that CPR should precede defibrillation, to "prime the pump" and rid the heart of lactic acid. By the 1980s, a growing body of information was suggesting that the time between the victim's collapse and the first shock was the best predictor of outcome, and so a defibrillatory shock became the priority, and it was to be given as rapidly as possible. But two recent studies, one from Seattle and the other from Oslo, posed the question of whether it might instead be advisable to deliver CPR for several minutes before defibrillation. Both studies concluded that when EMS personnel provided CPR before defibrillation (for ninety seconds in Seattle, and for three minutes in Oslo), survival rates were higher than when the patient received a shock as quickly as possible.[48] Nevertheless, neither of these studies used a scientific methodology that was able to offer definitive proof—the Seattle study used a before-and-after design, and the Oslo study demonstrated a benefit from immediate CPR in only a small subset of patients. To add further weight to arguments for quick defibrillation, a third study, this one from Perth, Australia, randomized immediate defibrillation versus defibrillation after ninety seconds of CPR among a group of 256 patients and found no difference in survival rates between the two groups.[49] Thus it remains unclear what the better approach is—immediate shock, or three minutes of CPR before any shock is given. A large and ongoing North American clinical trial is studying this very issue as one aspect of the Resuscitation Outcomes Consortium (ROC), which appendix 4 discusses in greater detail.

It may well turn out that both approaches are correct—immediate shock for witnessed VF or VF of short duration, and CPR before shock for VF of longer duration. But while the debate rages, defibrillators are advancing to the point where the debate may well become irrelevant. As mentioned elsewhere (see the discussion of CPR quality, earlier in this section, as well as the discussion of defibrillator-guided therapy in the section titled "Therapy Factors"), a new generation of defibrillators capable of guiding therapy is beginning to emerge. These defibrillators will be able to interpret information within the VF signal and advise either immediate shock or a period of CPR and/or medication before the shock. Despite the appeal of such devices, however, they have yet to be proved effective in prehospital use with human subjects.

Type of EMS System (Moderate Association with Survival)

EMS systems can be characterized in many ways. There are private systems, public systems, fire department–based systems, health department–based systems, police department–based systems, single-tier systems, and tiered-response systems.

Despite this great variety of systems, there are no studies that compare administrative structures to outcomes for cardiac arrest, and only a single study indirectly compares single-tier systems to tiered-response systems. In 1990, my colleagues and I compared twenty-nine EMS systems reporting survival rates for cardiac arrest and noted a strong relationship between type of system and rate of survival: systems that utilized paramedics as a single tier reported an average survival rate of 17 percent for ventricular fibrillation, compared to an average survival rate of 29 percent for systems that utilized a tiered response of EMTs capable of defibrillation, along with paramedics.[50] Presumably, this difference in survival rates was due to the ability or inability to deliver certain therapies (such as defibrillation) in a timely fashion. One must take such a study with a giant grain of salt, however. Since there were probably many factors and variables affecting the communities that we studied (whether they were rural or urban, for example, in addition to their differences in terms of response times, the ages of the victims, and differences in comorbidity), any kind of direct comparison must be very qualified. The only definitive way to compare systems would be to start with identical communities and randomly assign the type of system. But such a study would be impossible.

Tiered-response systems vary in terms of number of responders. A common approach utilizes an aid unit as the first-in vehicle, staffed with two (sometimes three) EMTs. The second-in unit is a paramedic unit, staffed with two paramedics (or one EMT and a paramedic). In this system, both vehicles are capable of transporting the patient to the hospital. But there are many variations on this theme. Some communities may send a fire engine as the first-in vehicle (that is, a vehicle incapable of transporting the patient), with a paramedic unit as the second unit. Other communities may send three vehicles to a cardiac arrest—an engine company, an EMT unit, and a paramedic unit.

In 1999, the Ontario Prehospital Advanced Life Support (OPALS) study measured the benefit of adding a paramedic program to an existing program of EMT defibrillation, but it failed to demonstrate any benefit from adding paramedic services.[51] The paramedics' experience (or relative lack thereof) and specific protocols may explain this negative finding. In King County, however, contrary to the OPALS findings, we dramatically improved survival rates for cardiac arrest by adding paramedics to existing EMT services.[52] This change led to a survival rate of 28 percent for cardiac arrest involving VF, compared to 15 percent when only basic EMTs provided care. When our study began, in 1976, basic EMTs were not authorized to defibrillate. It was clear that basic EMT services alone, with no authorization to defibrillate, saved considerably fewer lives than did paramedic services when a cardiac arrest involved ventricular fibrillation.[53] In King County it is clear that, over a thirty-year period, the progressive addition of higher-level skills and services has increased survival rates for VF. Basic EMT services, without the authorization to defibrillate, achieved the lowest survival rates. The use of EMTs trained to defibrillate (as all EMTs now are), but without paramedics, achieved intermediate survival rates for VF. And the tiered-response system, with defibrillation-capable EMTs providing first-in care and paramedics providing second-in care, has achieved the highest survival rates.

Is there an optimal size for an EMS program? There is indirect evidence of lower survival rates in small rural communities and mega-urban communities than in midsize communities. This discrepancy may reflect the logistics of getting EMTs and paramedics quickly to the scene; such factors as housing density and traffic congestion come into play in very large cities.

There may also be an optimal size when it comes to what is called "sphere of authority," a managerial term used in connection with the ratio of supervisors to field personnel. Fire departments, based as they are on a military model, are generally able to create adequate supervisory staffing. In a large community, however, medical direction becomes more problematic. Can a single medical director know and supervise hundreds of personnel?

In King County we have one county medical director and six medical directors of paramedic programs, serving a total population of almost 2 million, and each base-station hospital has a physician on duty in the emergency department who provides line control to the paramedics. None of the seven medical directors works full-time as medical director; all have other responsibilities. If we exclude the emergency room physicians and add up the part-time hours of the seven medical directors, we can say that we have a total of two full-time-equivalent medical directors supervising 250 paramedics in a community of fewer than 2 million people. For us, this arrangement works well—one full-time equivalent medical director per 125 paramedics and approximately 1 million people. Nevertheless, there are no data to suggest what the optimal size of an EMS system would be.

Number of Responders (Unknown Association with Survival)

A cardiac resuscitation should unfold like a choreographed dance, with each individual performing assigned tasks. Some researchers speculate that a critical mass of EMS providers leads to better outcomes for cardiac arrest. The concept of a critical mass means that each skilled task can be carried out by a preassigned individual, without the chaos of multitasking. For example, in a tiered-response system, the first-arriving EMTs perform CPR and provide one or more initial defibrillatory shocks (a third EMT, if present, takes charge of the AED). When the paramedics arrive, the lead—generally the paramedic not driving the vehicle—immediately takes charge. He or she starts the patient's peripheral or central line and orders the medications. Meanwhile, the other paramedic, upon arrival, places the patient's endotracheal tube and draws up the medications. It seems logical to assume that a situation involving a sufficient number of personnel will achieve better outcomes than one that is understaffed, but there are no data to shed light on this matter.

In Seattle and King County, usually three vehicles are sent to the scene if the dispatcher thinks a cardiac arrest has occurred. The first-in unit may be a fire engine (generally staffed with three EMT firefighters and dispatched because it is the closest vehicle), and the second vehicle is an EMT unit. This arrangement allows CPR (and defibrillation) to begin as quickly as possible while the third vehicle—the paramedic unit—is still on the way. The luxury of having many personnel allows for efficient division of labor.

Ratio of Paramedics to Total Members of the Community (Unknown Association with Survival)

In any given community, the number of paramedics per capita is related to the type of EMS system. Some communities utilize a firefighter paramedic system in which paramedics respond to every 911 call. There are variations on this approach, with private paramedics or a combined team of EMTs and paramedics responding instead of firefighters to every EMS call. In communities with systems like these, there are many paramedics, and so there is a high paramedic-to-population ratio. Other communities utilize a tiered-response system (described earlier, in the discussion of types of EMS systems) in which firefighter EMTs respond to all calls and paramedics respond only to calls for which their advanced skills are needed. In these communities, there are fewer paramedics, and so there is a low paramedic-to-population ratio.

One author has speculated that when there are too many paramedics in a community, their opportunities to use critical skills are diluted, and ultimately the performance of the EMS system suffers.[54] This is an intriguing concept, but there have been no studies to establish any relationship between a high paramedic-to-population ratio and lower performance of an EMS system.

Use of Dispatcher-Assisted Telephone CPR (Strong Association with Survival)

Dispatcher-assisted telephone CPR presents both the opportunity to instantly instruct someone who has never had a CPR class as well as the chance to help someone who simply needs to be reminded about what to do. I am a strong believer in the benefits of telephone-assisted CPR. In King County, our dispatcher-assisted telephone CPR program has led to a 50 percent increase in the incidence of bystander CPR, which now occurs in over half of all cardiac arrests in our community. Probably one-third of all bystander CPR is due solely to the existence and efforts of our telephone-assisted program.

Theoretically, 100 percent of cardiac arrests could involve telephone-assisted CPR. In practice, however, that would be impossible. Many calls to 911 are third-party relays, as when the caller is a security guard in the lobby of a building and the person in cardiac arrest is on the eighth floor. Moreover, the victim may collapse too far from a phone, or the caller may be too frail to perform CPR, or it may be impossible to lay the victim flat on the floor.

In any case, it cannot be proved that telephone-assisted CPR saves lives, since a resuscitation event includes many interventions, and it is often impossible to tease out the influence of each separate factor. Nevertheless, Rea and his colleagues, in a large community study, demonstrated a strong association between telephone-assisted CPR and increased survival.[55] Clearly, the amount of time that passes between the victim's collapse and the initiation of CPR is a determinant of survival. Therefore, it follows logically that telephone-assisted CPR is a means of bringing about more bystander CPR. The only valid question here is whether the quality of telephone-assisted CPR is as good as it would have been if the bystander performing it had been taught CPR in a traditional classroom setting. From simulations using mannequins, however, it appears that the quality is comparable.

Quality of EMS Care (Unknown Association with Survival)

There have been almost no studies on the quality of EMS care (as used here, "EMS care" means all the prehospital components of an EMS system, including dispatching and the services of EMTs and paramedics). The dearth of such studies is not due to lack of interest but to the fact that, in practice, it is nearly impossible to agree on how quality should be measured.

One surrogate for quality is experience, but here too there are almost no data. A study from England showed that victims' chances of surviving cardiac arrest were greater when the attending EMTs had four years of experience, and when the attending paramedics had one year of experience, than when these responders had less experience.[56] It seems intuitively correct, moreover, that experience should matter, especially with respect to such skill-based activities as defibrillation, intubation, and administration of intravenous medications. The data supporting a positive relationship between EMTs' and paramedics' experience and patients' survival are slim, but it would still perhaps be useful for agencies to pair newly trained EMTs and paramedics with more experienced partners for some period of time.

Another possible surrogate for quality is the degree of attrition in an EMS agency, since low attrition is directly related to experience. For example, one survey from 2006, conducted by the *Journal of Emergency Medical Services* (*JEMS*), found that fire departments had a low annual attrition rate of 6 percent, compared to 17 percent for private ambulance agencies.[57] Still another factor that may be related to quality is the salaries paid to EMS personnel. The survey just cited also found that the average salary of a fire department–based EMT was $37,500, compared to $23,000 for an EMT employed by a private ambulance agency.[58] Another study found that the paramedics employed by one community's fire department received $42,000 annually, compared to $32,000 for the paramedics working for a private ambulance agency.[59] I do not know whether EMTs and paramedics working for fire departments deliver higher-quality care than do those who work for private ambulance agencies. No one knows, since such data do not exist. All I am doing here is pointing out the large salary differences and wondering whether salary is related to quality of care.

Quality of Medical Direction (Unknown Association with Survival)

There are no studies that measure the quality of an EMS system's medical direction and relate it to outcomes of cardiac arrest. The main challenge here is how to define what quality consists of in terms of medical direction. Without such a definition, it is impossible to discern high-quality medical direction from mediocre or even poor direction. Does high-quality medical direction necessitate the director's full-time involvement? Does it consist of his or her personal review of critical EMS calls? Does it require his or her supervision of the cardiac arrest registry? Does it call for frequent visits from the medical director to paramedic stations? Does it depend on the medical director's riding along on calls? The matter of defining what quality means in the area of medical direction is not unlike the challenge of defining what high-quality performance means in any other service profession, whether we are measuring the police department, the fire department, or a municipal utility. I personally believe that both the quality and the amount of medical supervision in an EMS system are directly related to the overall quality of that system. But this is an assertion that I cannot prove.

Existence of an Ongoing Program for Medical Quality Improvement (Unknown Association with Survival)

As is the case with many other factors discussed here, there are no studies directly linking higher rates of survival for cardiac arrest in a particular community with the existence of an ongoing program for medical quality improvement (QI). Nevertheless, most of the communities cited in chapter 1 as having the highest survival rates for cardiac arrest involving ventricular fibrillation also have active programs for surveillance of cardiac arrest and for medical QI. This fact suggests that ongoing medical QI is part and parcel of a high-quality program.

The medical director of an EMS program uses medical QI to measure skill in the performance of particular tasks and to identify educational needs. An ongoing program for surveillance of cardiac arrests, for example, and an ongoing program for monitoring telephone-assisted CPR would constitute, in essence, medical QI. When an EMS system has an ongoing program for medical QI, that program serves as concrete recognition by the medical director and the administrative director that the system must monitor itself continuously and strive to do better.

Just as character helps to define an individual, culture can define an organization. The perfect EMS culture would include the facets of professionalism, uncompromising standards, high expectations, and a relentless drive to improve. All these facets are summarized in the phrase "culture of excellence."

Many medical directors, dispatchers, EMTs, and paramedics are proud of their systems, and of the hard and valuable work they do. But organizational pride is not the same thing as organizational culture. An organization's culture is a quality that permeates and percolates throughout the organizational system. In the case of an EMS system, it begins at the top with the medical director and the administrative director, and it is instilled in every other member of the system. Members who don't fit into the culture may be ostracized in subtle or not so subtle ways, and they often leave. Thus a culture has a tendency to perpetuate itself. This is a good thing when the culture is one of excellence, but it is not so good when the culture is negative.

Most EMS systems are based in fire departments. By their very nature, fire departments are quasi-military organizations. Even the ranks—chief, battalion chief, captain, lieutenant—are based on those found in the military. But the fact that an organization has a quasi-military structure does not mean that the organization itself is autocratic or dictatorial. A good organization, whether it is a fire department or a Fortune 500 company, encourages internal communications, values the experience of workers, and instills the group with a sense of mission.

One assumes that a well-run organization, and one with high expectations of excellence, would perform better than an organization lacking these qualities. Nevertheless, although there is a large literature on management, organizations, and culture, I am not aware of any literature that relates the organization and culture of an EMS system to rates of survival for cardiac arrest.

Level and Nature of Administrative Support (Unknown Association with Survival)

The term "administrative support" refers to the staffing and budgetary resources devoted to such matters as a cardiac arrest registry, a medical QI program, and data infrastructure. As is true for quality of medical care, there are no data relating the factor of administrative support to outcomes of cardiac arrest. Clearly, if a community is to measure its performance, it will require the resources to do so, though I cannot define what the level of resources should be. In King County, for example, there are several employees dedicated to maintaining the registry and the QI program, and at least three full-time staff members are assigned to the overall database of EMS incidents. Even more important, however, than the particular level of the resources directed to administrative support is the full backing of the top administrator, whether he or she is the fire chief or the EMS director. Without this backing, no amount of staff effort will lead to success in measuring the system's performance.

Quality of EMS Training (Unknown Association with Survival)

Few would argue that the quality of the training for dispatchers, EMTs, and paramedics is anything but a crucial element of a successful EMS program. The challenge is how quality in training should be defined. There are no studies measuring relationships between the quality of training and the outcomes of cardiac arrest. One can certainly measure the number of hours required for certification and recertification, and the types of training provided—didactic instruction versus hands-on mastery of practical skills, or completion of an online curriculum versus face-to-face teaching. By comparison with national standards, the dispatchers, EMTs, and paramedics in Seattle and King County are required to meet extremely high standards and requirements for training and continuing education; more hours of paramedic education are required in Washington State, and in Seattle and King County in particular, than anywhere else in the country. I suppose it would be possible to rank or score EMS systems on the basis of required training hours or other performance measures. But the challenge is to isolate training as a factor and associate it with survival. And because quality of training is associated with other factors (such as organizational culture, quality of medical direction, and level of administrative support), it is difficult to tease out the independent contribution of training.

Existence of a Community Program for Training Citizens in CPR (Moderate Association With Survival)

In 1972, Seattle's Medic Two program pioneered the concept of training citizens in CPR. It was recognized early on that the sooner CPR begins after a cardiac arrest, the better the outcome for the victim. The concept is a simple one: if you can train enough citizens in CPR, then the odds of having a CPR-trained person at the scene of a collapse will increase. The large number of CPR-trained citizens in Seattle and King County accounts for the consistently high rate of bystander CPR in Seattle. Before the dispatcher-assisted telephone CPR program began, in 1983, an average of about 30 to 40 percent of cardiac arrests included bystander CPR. With the creation of the program, this rate has climbed to over 50 percent.[60]

The American Heart Association endorses dispatcher-assisted telephone CPR, and many if not most dispatch centers offer this assistance. Nevertheless, without a dedicated staff to monitor and review calls and provide constructive feedback to dispatchers, such a program can easily become one of unmet expectations. I make this point because there are several proprietary telephone CPR programs that exist as components of comprehensive computer-aided dispatch programs. These proprietary programs have been neither evaluated nor validated. My concern is with whether they convey the key steps of CPR quickly enough, and with whether the exact wording of their instructions leads to the expected performance. It seems more than reasonable to require each of these proprietary programs to publish indicators of its performance for several key steps. For example, how quickly did dispatchers recognize the presence of cardiac arrest? What was the average time that elapsed between the moment when the dispatcher picked up the 911 call and the moment when the first ventilations and first compressions were given? In what percentage of 911 calls were instructions offered by dispatchers? What were the false positive rates for delivering telephone CPR instructions? When every second counts, it is important that telephone instructions be as efficient and effective as possible. The beginning of this chapter described the Utstein Criteria for reporting cardiac arrest survival. It would be helpful if there were comparable Utstein recommendations for reporting a dispatch center's telephone CPR performance.

Existence of a Community Program for Encouraging Public Access Defibrillation (Moderate Association with Survival)

The PAD trial demonstrated that automated external defibrillators in public locations can improve survival rates for cardiac arrest.[61] That large randomized trial proved that an AED at the scene can save valuable time between the victim's collapse and the start of defibrillation, and this time savings translates directly into higher survival rates. In Seattle and King County, there is an active program to encourage and register AEDs in the community. Each AED supplied to a public location is listed with the local dispatch center so that dispatchers can remind callers that an AED is on the premises.[62]

Although public AEDs do offer the opportunity to shave the time between collapse and defibrillation, one still has to put the potential benefits in perspective. For one thing, only 15 percent of all cardiac arrests occur in public locations. For another, a cardiac arrest is more likely to occur in some public locations than in others. Most cardiac arrests in public places occur in airports, jails, health clubs, and shopping malls, and so these are the most logical sites where AEDs should be placed, and where staff should be trained to use them.

Cardiac arrests that occur in public places are far more likely to be witnessed and to involve ventricular fibrillation, and so the benefits of public access defibrillation outweigh the fact that cardiac arrests in public locations are relatively uncommon. An active community program encouraging public access defibrillation can make a significant contribution to a community's VF survival rate.

Therapy Factors

Therapy factors are those associated with the types and quality of therapy provided in the event of cardiac arrest. This group of factors includes the use of pharmacotherapy at the scene, the use of defibrillator-guided therapy, the use of impedance threshold devices, the use of CPR adjuncts, the use of chest-compression-only CPR, the quality of airway management, the use of hypothermia, and the quality of hospital care.[63]

Use of Pharmacotherapy at the Scene (Unknown Association with Survival)

It has always been assumed that pharmacological therapy delivered to a patient in cardiac arrest, or shortly after the return of spontaneous circulation, will improve the outcome, but there are surprisingly few data to support this assumption. The main drugs administered during a resuscitation are cardiac stimulants, including epinephrine and vasopressin; anti-arrhythmics, which are meant to stabilize the heart rhythm and include lidocaine, amiodarone, beta-blockers, and, rarely, procainamide; pressors, which are meant to increase the blood pressure, and among the most common of which are norepinephrine and dopamine; rate increasers, such as atropine; and a few other miscellaneous medications, such as sodium bicarbonate, which is meant to neutralize acidic blood.

Although a few of these medications, such as amiodarone and lidocaine, have been compared to each other, none of them have been rigorously evaluated or studied in randomized clinical trials and compared to placebos. The lack of definitive information about these drugs is partly explained by the fact that most of them have been around for a long time, having entered the pharmacotherapeutic armamentarium long before rigorous randomized clinical trials were mandatory. In nonrandomized trials or in case series, they seemed to help, and consequently they crept into the standard of care through the back door. Now they are difficult to study precisely because they are thought of as reflecting the standard of care.

One pharmacological workhorse, epinephrine, which has been used in the management of intractable VF as well as in that of asystole and PEA since resuscitation standards were first put forth, was recently evaluated in a large clinical trial in Singapore. The researchers, using a before-and-after study design, looked at one year of resuscitation efforts that did not use epinephrine and then compared the survival rates to those associated with a year of efforts that did add epinephrine to the resuscitation protocols. They found that epinephrine was not associated with any significant increase in survival.[64]

Use of Defibrillator-Guided Therapy (Weak Association with Survival)

When you and I look at the pattern of VF, we see a bunch of squiggles. But a new generation of defibrillators can interpret this information and predict the likelihood that the next shock will be successful. This interpretive and predictive capability in turn can guide a rescuer through the timing and appropriate energy level of defibrillatory shocks and advise him or her on whether further CPR is required.

For example, some automated external defibrillators (this is the type of device mostly used by EMTs) can determine whether or not to advise a shock on the basis of how probable it is that the shock will be successful. The probability threshold can even be set in the device by the program or medical director. Manual defibrillators (this is the type of device mostly used by paramedics) are in development that can display the probability of successful defibrillation on the monitor. Since the device can calculate this probability in real time, it can display it as a percentage from 0 to 100. If the percentage is low, the rescuer will devote attention to CPR, and/or to administering medication, and wait to defibrillate until the displayed percentage is higher than 50.

Defibrillator-guided therapy, still in its infancy, offers great promise for seeing how CPR and therapy can alter the VF waveform, and it may help in the development of protocols for cardiac arrest. It is even conceivable that defibrillator-guided therapy can one day also make use of physiological information, such as the patient's blood lactate levels or acid-base values, to recommend specific pharmacological therapy as well as appropriate doses. Nevertheless, because this technology remains mostly a promise at this point, it cannot be said to have more than a weak association with survival.

Use of Impedance Threshold Devices (No Association with Survival)

An impedance threshold device, or ITD, is a clever little mechanism that works well in animals and offers some promise of improving circulation during CPR, and therefore of improving survival rates for cardiac arrest.[65] The device, about the size of a plum, works by impeding the passive return of air into the lungs that comes with chest decompression (the upstroke of CPR). This impedance in turn allows more blood to fill the major vessels in the chest and thereby improves blood flow with the next downward stroke of CPR.

An ITD is easy to use during a cardiac arrest. It takes literally only seconds to apply. An EMT simply places it between the face mask and the bag-valve mask. A paramedic places it between the end of the intubation tube and the bag-valve mask.

I am always a little skeptical – actually, quite massively skeptical – about the ability of any device (other than a defibrillator) to improve outcomes during cardiac arrest. The Resuscitation Outcomes Consortium Trial of the ITD was published in 2011 in the *New England Journal of Medicine*.[66] In this trial, 4,345 patients in cardiac arrest were randomized to receive a working ITD or a sham ITD. There was no difference is survival. At this time there appears to be no role for an ITD in cardiac arrest.

Use of CPR Adjuncts (No Association with Survival)

Many CPR adjuncts have been proposed over the past several decades. These include compressed-air piston devices, used to perform chest compression; plunger devices, used to achieve active compression and active decompression of the chest; and compression straps, used to compress the chest automatically.[67] All are meant to reduce the labor of performing CPR and to improve cardiac output. While many of them appear promising in animal studies, none seems particularly suitable for use with humans.

Use of Chest-Compression-Only CPR—Hands-Only CPR (Weak Association with Survival)

In most U.S. communities, rates of bystander CPR are very low. As a result, many EMS leaders have argued for a radical change in public CPR training and in telephone CPR instructions. These leaders urge the elimination of the mouth-to-mouth component of CPR and argue that chest compression alone is sufficient therapy for the initial stages of cardiac arrest. Several EMS medical directors have decided to make chest-compression-only CPR an element of their dispatch centers' telephone instructions.[68] The American Heart Association issued a Science Advisory in April 2008 endorsing chest-compression-only CPR for cases of witnessed sudden collapse in adults.[69] The AHA calls this technique "Hands-Only CPR" and urges that all bystanders not formally trained in CPR "provide high-quality chest compression by pushing hard and fast in the center of the chest, minimizing interruptions." Bystanders previously trained in CPR may choose to perform hands-only CPR or standard CPR. In effect the AHA is saying these two methods are equivalent. Furthermore, the AHA states that CPR-trained individuals who are not confident in their ability to perform mouth-to-mouth ventilation should provide hands-only CPR.

Several arguments have been offered in favor of chest-compression-only CPR. One of them addresses the perception that citizens in general are unwilling to perform mouth-to-mouth ventilation but would be more willing to administer chest-compression-only CPR. Let me, at least on the basis of my own experience, dispel this perception right away. In twenty-five years of monitoring telephone CPR in King County, I have not seen this alleged reluctance to be a problem, primarily because most CPR occurs in the home. Even for cardiac arrests that have occurred in public locations, however, I am unaware of any instances in which full CPR was inhibited by the prospect of contact with a stranger's mouth. I do readily acknowledge, however, that rates of bystander CPR are lower in other communities than they are in King County, so it is certainly conceivable that performance of mouth-to-mouth ventilation may be an inhibiting factor.

A second argument against the need for mouth-to-mouth ventilation holds that the blood is still fully oxygenated at the moment of cardiac arrest, and so the only need is to perform chest compression. This may be true for the first several minutes, but the saturation of oxygen in the blood falls very rapidly thereafter and can be replenished only with artificial respiration (mouth-to-mouth ventilation). But few if any systems, anywhere in the world, can get EMS personnel to the scene of a cardiac arrest within three or four minutes of the victim's collapse, and Peter Safar, one of the first proponents of modern CPR, would be spinning in his grave if he knew that researchers today are advocating the elimination of the "P" from CPR. Safar's elegant experiments in the 1950s convincingly demonstrated that chest compression alone is not sufficient to maintain oxygenated blood.[70]

Yet a third argument is that chest compressions are easier for ordinary citizens to perform, and that mouth-to-mouth ventilation is especially difficult for dispatchers to teach over the telephone. But compression-only CPR's ease of performance is irrelevant if it remains an ineffective therapy. Furthermore, the mouth-to-mouth instructions for telephone CPR can help sort out real cardiac arrests from false positives. Mouth-to-mouth ventilation is an irritant, and someone who is not in cardiac arrest is likely to push the would-be rescuer away. Better an annoying puff in the mouth than a cracked rib.

Is there any scientific evidence to support the benefit of chest-compression-only CPR? Perhaps. There has been one prospective randomized study comparing dispatcher-assisted chest-compression-only CPR with standard dispatcher-assisted CPR.[71] This twelve-year study, which took place in Seattle, found no difference between the two kinds of dispatcher-assisted instructions in terms of survival rates. It should be pointed out, however, that in Seattle the average response time for EMTs— that is, the time between their being dispatched and their arrival at the scene of a cardiac arrest—is three and a half minutes, one of the fastest response times in the country. This quick response time probably precluded opportunities to observe the advantages, if any, of mouth-to-mouth ventilation over chest-compression-only CPR. In other words, both methods may be equally effective in a community where the average response time is very short. In 2007, an observational study from Japan showed that chest compression alone was better than standard CPR, but this was not a randomized trial, and it did not involve telephone instructions, nor did it contain any explanation of why twice as many bystanders chose to perform chest-compression-only CPR rather than standard CPR.[72] Two international randomized trials are now in progress, and they should resolve the issue, at least as far as dispatch centers are concerned.[73] But controversy will continue over how best to train the public.[74]

There may be a middle ground. It may turn out that chest-compression-only CPR would be the best option for a witnessed cardiac arrest, especially in a community with rapid EMS response times, whereas standard CPR might be the preferred option for an unwitnessed cardiac arrest, or for an arrest that occurred in a community where response times were slow. Thus the dispatcher, once having determined whether or not the collapse was witnessed, could give the appropriate instructions.

Such a conditional approach to therapy, if it can be developed, will be able to take account of how long the victim is likely to have been in cardiac arrest and of how much bystander CPR can be provided before professionals arrive to take over. Moreover, the dispatcher's instructions can be determined in part by the average response time in the community, since the dispatch center will have this information. Therefore, it may be possible to customize dispatchers' CPR instructions to specific sets of circumstances.

Quality of Airway Management (Weak Association with Survival)

It seems intuitive that good airway management should improve a patient's odds of surviving cardiac arrest. Indeed, a study of cardiac arrest patients in King County by Shy and his colleagues demonstrated that patients who were quickly intubated had higher survival rates—46 percent of patients in the quick-intubation group survived, compared to 23 percent in the slow-intubation group.[75] This was a retrospective observational study, and it hardly constitutes proof of a causal link between the quality of airway management and the likelihood of the patient's survival, but it does suggest that our intuition concerning this relationship may be correct.[76]

Use of Hypothermia (Moderate Association with Survival)

The idea of hypothermia has been around for decades. It seems logical to assume that cooling the body and the brain would slow metabolism and afford more time for healing—and, as mentioned earlier, the postulated third phase of cardiac arrest, the so-called metabolic phase, may respond to hypothermia.

In 2002, two different randomized trials demonstrated that cardiac arrest patients treated with hypothermia had better outcomes.[77] The publication of these findings generated much excitement. Some would even say that this was the best evidence of hypothermia's therapeutic benefit to come along in many years. Endorsements by the American Heart Association and the International Liaison Committee on Resuscitation followed in 2005 and, in effect, made hypothermia the new standard of hospital care.

Some programs began pushing the envelope even further and exploring whether hypothermia could be initiated in the prehospital setting. For example, a 2005 pilot study in Seattle showed that two liters of cooled IV fluids could be administered by paramedics to begin the cooling process even before the patient arrived at the emergency room.[78]

The benefits of hypothermia are still being explored. Will it benefit all rhythms, or only VF? How effectively can it be started in the prehospital setting? Are there pharmacological adjuncts to hypothermia? Should hypothermia be induced quickly or slowly? Though the degree (pun intended) of hypothermia's benefit has yet to be determined, it appears to offer a new therapeutic option, and thus an option for improving outcomes in some cardiac arrests.

In King County, eight hospitals receive the vast majority of resuscitated patients. If the quality of their care in hospitals varied, we would expect to see differences in survival rates among the resuscitated patients admitted to these eight hospitals, but no such differences exist. The rates of discharge for these resuscitated patients are virtually identical among all the hospitals. Therefore, the quality of hospital care, at least in King County, can be considered a constant factor, which is not surprising, since post-resuscitation care is fairly well standardized.

Nevertheless, a study from Sweden has found contrary results.[79] Among 3,853 patients taken to twenty-one hospitals, the rates of survival—with the patient's survival defined as his or her still being alive one month after cardiac arrest—varied from 14 percent to 42 percent. Another study, this one from neighboring Norway, demonstrated that a hospital's predefined postresuscitation protocol improved survival rates by comparison with those of historical controls.[80] There have been too few other studies to enable me to draw a definitive conclusion here. Could these differences in survival rates have been due to different protocols, or to variations in the quality of hospital care? Clearly, although the quality of hospital care has an unknown association with survival, it is a potentially important factor.

CARDIAC ARREST: A FORMULA FOR SURVIVAL

This chapter has identified fifty known or speculative factors associated with surviving cardiac arrest, and there are probably more. It should be clear that these factors are not independent of one another. For example, a bystander who initiates CPR makes the time between the victim's collapse and the start of CPR shorter than it would be if the start of CPR had to wait for EMTs to arrive. Similarly, the existence of a program for dispatcher-assisted telephone CPR means that more bystanders will perform CPR, just as a public access defibrillation program may allow earlier defibrillation in some cardiac arrests, and so on. But whatever the means of shortening the time between the victim's collapse and the start of CPR, regardless of whether CPR is performed by trained bystanders or by novices with the help of dispatchers, rapid delivery of CPR remains a critical factor in the victim's chances for survival.

If we had perfect understanding of all fifty of these factors and their respective influences on survival, and if we perfectly understood whatever factors are yet to be identified, we could construct a formula giving the exact likelihood that any particular patient would survive a cardiac arrest. This kind of global formula would be of academic interest, and it could help us understand any variances within it (that is, discrepancies between predicted and actual instances of survival), thereby allowing us to discover and explore additional predictive factors. A global formula could also help family members understand why a loved one did not survive cardiac arrest.

In terms of an EMS system's performance, however, a more meaningful formula would be one that focused on those factors that can be readily changed or influenced by community decisions. In this list of fifty factors, those that I have called "patient factors" and "event factors" are set in stone. They are largely determined by fate or circumstances and are not easily altered by the programmatic structure of an EMS system or by therapeutic decisions made at the scene of the cardiac arrest. It is not possible to alter such patient factors as gender, for instance, and little if anything can be done at the time of the arrest to offset the victim's body mass index or comorbid factors. Similarly, no one really has any control over such event factors as the victim's heart rhythm at the time of the arrest or the presence of witnesses. But that is not the case with what I have called "system factors" and "therapy factors." These two groups of factors are directly determined by the type of EMS system and by the multitude of decisions made by administrators, medical directors, and personnel at the scene.

A survival formula focused on system and therapy factors would allow a community to instantly visualize where it succeeds and where it falls short. Such a formula would contain all the known system and therapy factors that determine the likelihood of surviving ventricular fibrillation. The list of these factors is actually rather a short one: (1) the time between the patient's collapse and the initiation of CPR, (2) the time between the patient's collapse and the first defibrillatory shock, (3) the interaction of CPR and defibrillation, (4) the provision of timely and skilled care by paramedics, and (5) the institution of hypothermia for patients who achieve a pulse and blood pressure but do not wake up. The effects of these five factors are the direct determinants of survival. All the other factors exert contributory influences in that they lead indirectly to improved chances of survival.

In offering the following formula for calculating, on the basis of system and therapy factors, the probability of surviving cardiac arrest with ventricular fibrillation in a particular community, I have arbitrarily set 50 percent as the highest likely survival rate. This is not an absolute ceiling, of course; as better therapy and methods of delivery are derived, the rate may be set higher. At this time, however, the best systems in the United States—in Seattle–King County, Washington, and in Rochester, Minnesota—are reporting a survival rate of 46 percent for witnessed ventricular fibrillation. Admittedly, this formula is a model and a generalization. It is based on a moderate amount of science combined with fair amounts of conjecture and estimate. Even if the formula is inexact, however, its thrust should be clear. With these qualifications in mind, here is how the formula might look:

Likelihood of surviving witnessed VF (maximum survival rate: 50 percent) = average time between collapse and start of CPR (15 percent for four minutes, 10 percent for five minutes, 5 percent for six minutes)

+ average time between collapse and first defibrillatory shock (20 percent for six minutes, 15 percent for seven minutes, 10 percent for eight minutes, 5 percent for nine minutes)

+ 5 percent for carefully monitored interaction of CPR and defibrillation, minimizing the time without CPR

+ 5 percent for timely delivery of skilled care by paramedics

+ 5 percent if the EMS system has a record of starting hypothermia within two hours of the patient's collapse in more than 50 percent of cases

Note that the model is based not on how long it takes the dispatcher to pick up the call to 911, or on how long it takes the first-in unit to reach the scene, but on the interval between the patient's collapse and the start of CPR and between the collapse and the start of defibrillation. When bystanders initiate CPR, the time between the collapse and the start of CPR is arbitrarily designated as 50 percent of the interval between the pickup of the 911 call and the first-in unit's arrival at the address. According to this formula, then, King County would score 20 percent on the first factor (time between collapse and start of CPR), 15 percent on the second (time between collapse and start of defibrillation), 5 percent on the third (interaction of CPR and defibrillation),[81] 5 percent on the fourth (timely and skilled care from paramedics), and 0 per-

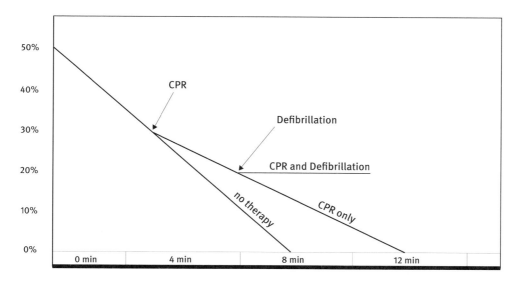

5.7 Influence of particular therapies and times on patient's chance of survival, expressed as a percentage.

cent on the fifth (provision of hypothermia),[82] for a total survival probability of 45 percent—spot on with the current survival rate.

It deserves repeating that this formula is more a model than a precise survival calculator. It includes several arbitrarily assigned values (I like to think of them as educated estimates). For example, although the value of 5 percent is assigned to the interaction between CPR and defibrillation, to timely and skilled care from paramedics, and to the EMS system's record of initiating hypothermia, these are not factors that can be precisely quantified at this time. I must emphasize that this formula has not been validated, and that it is based only on observational data. Moreover, it may not apply to all communities. Nevertheless, it offers a good approximation of the system factors and therapy factors that determine survival, and of what it takes for an EMS system to achieve a high score.

The formula can also be graphically represented. It is crucial to appreciate that cardiac arrest is an event with an extremely rapid course, one measured in minutes. From the moment of collapse, the clock of resuscitation starts to tick. By eight minutes, if there has been no therapy, the potential for resuscitation falls to zero (see fig. 5.7).[83] Rapid provision of CPR alters the potential for survival by slowing the dying process. If CPR begins at four minutes, the process is slowed, but survival will still fall to zero, since CPR by itself will not achieve a life-sustaining cardiac rhythm. Let's

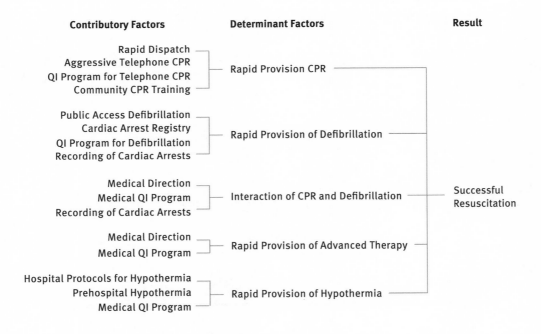

5.8 Contributory and determinant factors leading to improved survival rates for cardiac arrest.

assume that defibrillation is delivered at six minutes. Since defibrillation is definitive therapy for VF, the maximum probability of survival is defined by when this therapy is delivered. In the theoretical illustration offered by figure 5.7, a survival probability of 20 percent can be attained if CPR begins at four minutes and defibrillation is provided at six minutes. This probability can be boosted even higher if there is good interaction of CPR and defibrillation, with timely arrival of care from paramedics.[84] Yet another way to improve the overall probability of survival is to institute hypothermia at an early point. Each of the three latter factors may increase the patient's chances of survival by another 5 percent.

The formula is also useful in identifying areas that need improvement. In addressing this challenge, it is helpful to remember that many of the system and therapy factors are contributory and exercise direct influence on the determinant factors (see fig. 5.8). It is common sense that to solve a big problem, you have to break it down into its component (or contributory) parts—improve the parts, and the big problem will take care of itself.[85] A task viewed in this way becomes more manageable. For example, if a fire chief were ordered to shave two minutes off the time between collapse and the start of defibrillation and one minute off the time between collapse and the start of CPR, that order might appear overwhelming at first, but if four or five contributory factors could be identified, the task would go from seeming impossible to being merely difficult. To carry it out, the fire chief might consider any of a number of actions, such as instituting a rapid-dispatch program to ensure a quick response by the first-in unit (and therefore a quick time to CPR), or using digital voice recordings of resuscitations to reconstruct the sequence of events and identify possible correctable delays in therapy, or creating an aggressive dispatcher-assisted telephone CPR program to increase the rate of bystander CPR (and therefore shorten the average time between the collapse and the start of CPR), or bringing in strong medical leadership to supervise proper adherence to protocols, or establishing a target time of sixty seconds between the arrival of the first-in unit at the patient's side and the delivery of the first shock. Thus the secret of success lies in making improvements in the contributory factors, which in turn will bring about improvements in the determinant factors.

SIX

Location, Location, Location

Best Places to Have a Cardiac Arrest

The fire chief and the medical director from the City of D. spent the first day meeting with the Seattle Medic One battalion chief, visiting the alarm center, and riding all afternoon and into the evening with two paramedics. The second day they visited the quality improvement office to understand the data collection system and then had lunch with the Medic One medical director. Eventually the discussion came around to the issue of what makes the Seattle system work so well. The D. fire chief asked directly, "What is the secret of Seattle's success?" The Seattle medical director was not surprised by the question. Almost every visitor to the Medic One program asked it. The visitors imperceptibly leaned forward anticipating the response . . .

If you are going to have a cardiac arrest, one of the best places to have it is Seattle. So said *60 Minutes* on a national TV broadcast in 1974. The claim was not just media hype —it happened to be accurate, and it remains accurate to this day. Seattle and the surrounding King County community, along with Rochester, Minnesota, have the nation's highest survival rates for cardiac arrest. The latest data from King County and Rochester indicate that 46 percent of patients who collapse with ventricular fibrillation in the presence of witnesses walk out of the hospital alive. The survival rate in Seattle, at 45 percent, is virtually identical.[1] So if you're going to have a cardiac arrest, where should you try *not* to be? The obvious choices would be Los Angeles, New York, Chicago, and Detroit, cities with the nation's lowest published survival rates for cardiac arrest involving ventricular fibrillation—7 percent, 5 percent, 3 percent, and 1 percent, respectively.

What accounts for these drastically different survival rates? To begin to answer this question, this chapter closely examines the communities with the highest survival rates—Seattle, King County, and Rochester. What are the elements of success in these communities? Do their EMS systems have a secret ingredient that is missing from the systems in other communities? Can successful systems like the ones in these communities be exported to other cities?

THE SEATTLE AND KING COUNTY EMS SYSTEMS: HISTORY, FOUNDATION, DESIGN, AND STRUCTURE

What are the elements of an EMS system's success? What is it that makes Seattle one of the best places to have a cardiac arrest? I posed these questions to two individuals who are eminently qualified to answer it—Leonard Cobb (we met him in chapter 2), the cofounder of Seattle's paramedic program, and Michael Copass, the program's director of training for thirty-three years and its current medical director.

History: Two Leaders, One Vision

Leonard Cobb and Michael Copass have different, contrasting leadership styles, but in one area they are in total agreement—they refuse to accept anything less than full commitment to helping patients.

Cobb and Copass, Copass and Cobb—these two complex, dedicated men made Seattle's Medic One program what it is. It is difficult to speak of one without the other, since they are both so intimately tied to the program. And their strengths and personalities are perfectly complementary—Cobb is the professor, the thoughtful investigator who wants to know what works and how to make things better, and Copass is the enforcer, the one who gives orders and demands nothing less than 100 percent loyalty and effort.

I've known Leonard Cobb since 1971, when I arrived in Seattle for an internship and residency in internal medicine.[2] Cobb—he was "Dr. Cobb" to me at the time—was the attending physician on one of my first rotations, at Harborview Medical Center's coronary care unit. I vividly recall seeing several patients who had been resuscitated after out-of-hospital cardiac arrest, and I remember Cobb explaining the workings of the Medic One system and the role that paramedics played in resuscitation. At the time, I assumed that every hospital had a number of such patients; only later did I learn how unusual Harborview was.

As for Michael Copass, his gruff demeanor is legendary. I have heard him described many times, and some of those descriptions were less than kind, but my favorite saying about him is this one: "He'll make you feel like you're going to run out of ass before he runs out of teeth." But beneath his harsh exterior shines a soft and caring soul.

I met Copass a few months after I met Cobb, while I was on a rotation in Harborview's emergency department. Copass, then Medic One's training director, often had interns or residents ride on the night shift with student paramedics and evaluate their work. I volunteered to do this and enjoyed every minute of it. The students were a great group, eager to learn and highly motivated to do well. I got to see emergency medicine as it unfolded in people's homes and on the streets of Seattle. And it was a boyhood dream come true for me to be speeding along with the fire department's medic unit as the lights flashed and the sirens wailed.

As director of training, Copass taught every single paramedic in the Medic One program, and he left an indelible mark on every one of them, not only in terms of knowledge and skills but also, and just as profoundly, in terms of the attitude and code of behavior befitting a health care professional. Copass demanded that every patient in every situation be treated with respect and dignity; he would accept nothing less. Once when I was meeting with Copass in his office, a student paramedic knocked at the door and sheepishly entered to say that he had followed up on a problematic situation by contacting the patient in question and explaining a medication error.

Copass glared at the student. "You almost killed that little old lady," he snapped. "Don't you ever, *ever* make a mistake like that again!"

The student left, no doubt grateful that anything at all remained of his behind. After the door closed, Copass turned to me and winked.

"He's really a good student," he said.

Maybe I've read too much into that wink, but what it showed me is that Copass's "Billy Goat Gruff" behavior is mostly an act. It's an effective one, though. That student was retained in the paramedic program, and I doubt that he will make any more medication errors for the rest of his career.

Despite his fearsome reputation, Copass is a humble person, and he places great stock in others' humility as well. He distrusts bravado and ostentatious displays of celebration; his motto could very well be "When you get to the end zone, act like you've been there before." He says of paramedics, "They are dealing with disease, terrible disease. They need to realize that practicing medicine is not a winning game. It's a holding game, and it's hard work. They have to be willing to do an enormous amount of work for an occasional splendorous moment."

Foundation: The Medical Model and the Importance of Medical Control

When I asked Cobb and Copass what makes the programs in Seattle and King County work so well, they both unhesitatingly gave the same answer: "Medical control."[3] From the system's earliest beginnings, Cobb has viewed its paramedics as extensions of physicians, serving as their eyes, ears, and hands out in the community. Though physically separated from physicians, the paramedics are connected to them by radio and telephone. Thus the paramedics—and this is a key concept—are not practicing medicine; the physicians are the ones practicing medicine, and they authorize paramedics to administer medications and perform other medical procedures on their behalf.

Cobb feels very strongly that the medical model of the Seattle and King County programs is a major key to their success, just as he believes that the paramedics' accountability to authorizing physicians makes for excellent care. Virtually every EMS system everywhere in the country has a medical director, of course. But, as Cobb might say, there are medical directors and there are medical directors. That might sound like a glib remark, but it hints at the core of the Seattle and King County systems. The medical director is fully in charge of all medical care and holds everyone in the system accountable—dispatchers, EMTs, paramedics, and everyone else delivering care to patients. The medical director reviews every medical incident report, and if something is lacking or less than perfect, the person responsible for the shortcoming is going to hear about it.[4]

Copass's views are very similar to Cobb's. Like Cobb, he sees the role of the medical director as paramount. "A doctor and the people he supervises have personal responsibility for every patient," Copass says. "There is no margin for error." For Copass, shared responsibility is most effective when it is accompanied by the element of face-to-face accountability, without administrative layering. Paramedics are directly accountable to the medical director—they know him, and he knows them.[5]

When, nearly four decades ago, Cobb and Gordon Vickery, then the fire chief, established Medic One, there was no conflict between them over who would run what. (The precise delineation of responsibilities within the system, especially the role of the fire department and its paramedics, is described in the following section, "Design: One System, Six Programs.") Cobb was the physician in charge, and Vickery was the fire chief in charge. According to Cobb, the EMS systems in most other cities do not follow this unequivocally medical model, one in which the paramedic is totally responsible to a supervising physician for care delivered to patients. Cobb himself does not hire or fire paramedics, but if a paramedic fails to meet medical expectations, he or she is removed from the paramedic role. The fire chief is the one who carries out the paramedic's removal, but the recommendation for this action comes from the medical director.[6]

Though Cobb and Vickery were mutually supportive, that level of harmony was not always present between Cobb and subsequent fire chiefs. There have been eight chiefs over the course of the program's existence, and two of them attempted drastic revisions to the program. Those two fire chiefs had good intentions, but they had come from communities where other EMS models were in use, and their visions of paramedic care would have destroyed the carefully considered design of the Seattle–King County system. Fortunately, neither of those fire chiefs stayed long in the job, and each left before the EMS system had been irreparably altered. Where the Medic One program is concerned, however, complementarity between medical control and administrative direction is key—the fire chief and the medical director need each other.

Cobb's view of the primacy of medical control is essentially a very logical one— since resuscitation is a medical procedure, it should be run by physicians. Cobb would never presume to tell a fire chief how run the fire department, nor would he advise a police chief on how to ensure public safety, so he expects to run his medical program without interference by nonphysicians. This is not to say, however, that he thinks he should be wholly unaccountable. The fire and police chiefs report to the mayor or the city council, and Cobb is accountable both to the chair of the University of Washington's Department of Medicine and to the dean of the School of Medicine. Thus the Seattle–King County EMS model, with its strong academic connections, makes its medical director accountable to other physicians while helping to insulate medical control and medical practice from politics.

Two other points about the EMS system's medical model deserve mention.

The first point is that the model, from its inception, called not just for a strong medical director but also for line physicians who would give direct orders to the paramedics. It was apparent from the beginning that Cobb could not carry a radio with him around the clock. Therefore, line control was delegated to the resident on duty in Harborview Medical Center's emergency department. This resident, designated the Medic One doctor, was to carry a pager and a radio at all times while on duty. That way, when paramedics needed permission to deliver some form of therapy or to carry out another procedure, or when they needed advice in a challenging medical situation, they could call or radio in to the Medic One doctor. Thus medical control could be maintained at all times.[7] The rule was that paramedics would contact the Medic One doctor every time they went out on a call. This arrangement left the Medic One doctor in charge of directing care but also reinforced the concept that paramedics were part of the chain of emergency care, a chain stretching from the field all the way into the hospital. As Cobb puts it, "The skills are important, but there is an important attitudinal aspect. The paramedics need to be regarded by doctors, hospitals, and nurses as essential to patient care, with an important role. Doctors and nurses in the receiving hospital need to respect and trust the care in the field."

The second point to be made about the system's medical model is that the program was designed to use very few written protocols (also known as "standing orders"). Some paramedic programs have many detailed medical protocols by which the medical director preauthorizes paramedics to administer therapy and perform medical procedures. These multiple protocols and standing orders can reach book length. In Seattle, however, the preauthorization protocols apply only to cardiac arrest and major trauma. In both situations, paramedics are preauthorized to carry out a limited number of procedures and therapies. For example, they can intubate, defibrillate, give initial drugs for cardiac arrest, and start large-bore IVs in major trauma. Clearly, these are procedures that must be performed right away, without the delays that might be entailed in reaching the Medic One doctor. After that, though, there is the opportunity for the Medic One doctor, and therefore medical control, to play an active part in every therapeutic decision. It was partly because Cobb and Copass wanted to preserve the central role of the Medic One doctor that they resisted the idea of standing orders from the start, but they also believed that the care of critically ill patients was too complex to be entrusted to a cookbook-style approach (in this and other matters, Seattle is not a protocol-driven community).

In the final analysis, the power of the system's medical model lies in the attitude it fosters. Cobb sums it up this way: "Medical accountability somehow strengthens the concept of your being there for the patient and never giving up. It is a job with a mission."

Design: One System, Six Programs

7:45:23 A.M.	"911. Police, fire or medical?"
7:45:35 A.M.	*Call transferred to Seattle Fire Department's alarm center.*
7:45:38 A.M.	"What is the problem?" *Dispatcher determines possible cardiac arrest.*
7:46:10 A.M.	*Aid 25 and Medic One dispatched to address.*
7:46:25 A.M.	*Dispatcher asks caller if she would like to perform CPR, begins instructions.*
7:49:49 A.M.	*Aid 25 arrives at address.*
7:50:37 A.M.	*Two EMTs from Aid 25 reach patient's side. One takes over CPR while the other attaches AED.*
7:51:29 A.M.	*First shock is delivered.*
7:53:44 A.M.	*Medic One arrives at address*
7:54:15 A.M.	*Two paramedics from Medic One reach patient's side, instruct EMTs to continue CPR as they take charge of resuscitation. Two more shocks delivered. Patient intubated and IV started.*
8:05:18 A.M.	*Patient achieves regular rhythm, pulse detected.*
8:07:13 A.M.	*Paramedics phone Medic One doctor, describe what happened, request permission to take patient to Harborview Medical Center.*

There are six paramedic programs in King County, and the 255 paramedics in Seattle and King County staff a total of twenty-three full-time and two part-time paramedic units. The Seattle program, serving the entire city, is operated by the Seattle Fire Department and provides the system's EMT and paramedic tiers. The remainder of the King County program is made up of five paramedic programs—in the communities of Shoreline, Redmond, Bellevue, Vashon Island, and south King County—the latter program is known as King County Medic One. Like the Seattle program, the Shoreline,

Redmond, Bellevue, and Vashon Island programs are run by fire departments and serve their respective cities as well as surrounding communities. The King County Medic One paramedic program, which serves fifteen cities and communities in the southern portion of King County, is the only one of the six programs that is not run by a fire department. Instead, it is administered by the health department. (The annual report for the King County EMS system is at: www.kingcounty.gov/healthservices/health/ems.)

Seattle and King County have tiered-response EMS systems. When a call comes in to 911, an emergency dispatcher determines the nature of the medical problem. If it is a minor problem, an aid unit is dispatched to the scene from the fire department. The aid unit is staffed with two firefighter EMTs who, like all the system's EMTs, are trained to use an automated external defibrillator. If the dispatcher determines the problem to be major—for example, if the victim has chest pain and difficulty breathing or is unresponsive and seems to be in cardiac arrest—the responders will include both the fire department's aid unit and a paramedic unit staffed with two paramedics (sometimes an engine company with three EMTs is sent if it happens to be closer to the scene). In any case, because there are more aid units and engine companies than paramedic units, the aid units and engine companies almost invariably—95 percent of the time—are the first to arrive.[8]

Since EMTs arrive before paramedics, they are the ones who start therapy for cardiac arrest, by beginning CPR (or continuing CPR, if a bystander has initiated it) and delivering one or more defibrillatory shocks. If the call turns out not to be serious, the EMTs can also relay a "code green" message to any paramedics who are en route, just as they can request the presence of paramedics if the call turns out to be more serious than the dispatcher realized.

In Seattle and King County, paramedics are always the ones who transport critically ill patients to the hospital (the group of patients considered to be critically ill includes all those who have been resuscitated). A stable patient who is not critically ill may be transported to the hospital by firefighter EMTs in their aid unit, or a private ambulance may be used, especially when the fire station is far from a hospital.

Structure: Three Crucial Elements

If, as Leonard Cobb and Michael Copass have said, medical control is the foundation of the Seattle and King County EMS systems, then the structure is composed of three crucial elements: response, training, and medical quality improvement.

Response

As soon as the heart stops, life begins to slip away like sand through an hourglass, and the patient has ten minutes at most before, figuratively speaking, the sand runs out completely. The EMS response systems in Seattle and King County are designed to get care to the patient within critical time intervals.

There are two such critical windows of time. The first is the interval between the patient's collapse and the initiation of CPR, and the second is the interval between the patient's collapse and the first defibrillatory shock.

Where the first of these critical intervals is concerned, once the patient's heart goes into ventricular fibrillation, there will be irreversible damage to the brain, the heart, and other organs within four to six minutes unless CPR is started. Therefore, CPR must begin within this time frame. This urgent need can be met in three ways—a bystander who is already trained in CPR can begin giving ventilations, the 911 dispatcher can give the bystander CPR instructions over the phone, or an aid unit staffed with firefighter EMTs can be quickly dispatched to the scene. Seattle and King County are fortunate to have fire stations peppered throughout the community, so the average response time to any address is four minutes. Furthermore, the community is composed mostly of single-family dwellings (in Seattle, large apartment buildings and high-rise condominiums are still in the minority, being phenomena of very recent years), so once the fire department arrives at the scene, EMTs don't need much more time to reach the patient.

As for the second critical interval—the time between the patient's collapse and the start of defibrillation—the sooner the first shock is given, the better. After ten minutes, defibrillation is seldom successful, but CPR, if started promptly, can extend that critical window of time by several minutes. When the Medic One program began, only paramedics were trained and authorized to defibrillate, but since the development of automated external defibrillators, in the 1980s, EMTs have been allowed to deliver the first shock, before paramedics arrive. Thus the Seattle system, on average, can deliver the first shock within seven minutes of a witnessed collapse—one minute for the caller to reach 911, one minute for the aid unit to be dispatched, four minutes for the unit to reach the address, and one minute for EMTs to attach the AED and deliver the first shock. And even though EMTs can now deliver defibrillatory shocks, the role of paramedics has scarcely been marginalized. They conduct the vital and highly skilled interventions of performing endotracheal intubation, gaining intravenous access, and administering such medications as epinephrine and rhythm-stabilizing drugs.

Training

EMTs are certified at the state and national levels. The National Registry of Emergency Medical Technicians (NREMT), established in 1970, offers certification at the basic, intermediate, and paramedic levels. NREMT exams are used in twenty-four states and territories as the sole basis for certification at one or more levels, and fifteen additional states and territories accept NREMT exams as equivalent to their own state or territorial examinations.

The curriculum for EMTs is standardized by the U.S. Department of Transportation (DOT). Basic EMT certification currently requires 110 hours of training. Basic EMTs are trained to assess the nature and severity of a medical or traumatic problem, initiate CPR, deliver oxygen with nasal prongs or a bag-valve mask, and use an AED. They are not trained to start an IV, use advanced airway-control measures, or administer medications. Intermediate EMTs are authorized in most states to start an IV, use advanced airway-control measures, and administer selected medications. Intermediate EMTs are often used in rural areas, where paramedics may be unavailable or may take a long time to respond.

The DOT published a recommended minimum curriculum for paramedics in 1998, but the training of paramedics is only partially standardized at the national level. While the DOT curriculum does not mandate a specified number of hours, it does state that the "average" program with "average" students will achieve "average" results with about 1,000 to 1,200 hours of training, and it recommends that one-half the training consist of classroom instruction, with one-quarter devoted to clinical experience and the remainder devoted to field experience in the form of an internship. But some training programs for paramedics have additional certification requirements. Seattle's Medic One training program, for example, is one of the most extensive in the nation, offering more than 2,800 hours of classroom, clinical, and mentored experience—almost three times more than the low-end DOT recommendation. Paramedics in Seattle and King County are also subject to very stringent requirements for continuing education, which they must fulfill in order to maintain their certification. Annually, every paramedic must complete fifty hours of classroom or other didactic training, perform a minimum of twelve intubations, and start a minimum of fifty IVs. Every two years they must pass a recertifying examination.

Medical Quality Improvement

In an era of budget constriction, it may be tempting to think that quality improvement (QI) should be the first area of retrenchment. But eliminating QI would be a big mistake. Without QI, a system will stagnate, and it cannot improve. Seattle and King County devote considerable resources to medical quality improvement (some organizations use the term "quality assurance"), at the level of the individual and at the level of the system.

At the level of the individual, the most concrete example of medical QI is the review of run reports by the medical director of the programs. Nothing gets a paramedic's attention like a "see me" scribbled by the medical director on a run report. The "see me" may be there for a minor infraction, such as lack of proper documentation, or it may be there for a major mistake, such as a missed diagnosis.

Tom Rea is medical director for the King County Medic One Program serving the southern portion of the county. This area is larger than Seattle and has a population of 800,000, compared to Seattle's 600,000. Rea supervises seventy-five paramedics who staff seven paramedic units. He reviews all resuscitations, intubations, and central-line placements and provides feedback, both positive and negative, to the paramedics involved in these procedures. For paramedics in training, he conducts a very detailed review of each case, such as the one that follows:

Medical Quality Improvement Review, November 7, 2008

    To: Paramedic James A.

    From: Tom Rea, M.D.

    Date of event: 11/05/08

    Patient: Marilyn M. (62-year-old female, sudden collapse—VF arrest)

    You have marked both VF and pulseless electrical activity for the initial rhythm. My impression is that the fire department arrived on scene, determined cardiac arrest, and delivered a shock based on the initial rhythm assessment. So my take is that the initial rhythm is VF. Please clarify.

    It is interesting that she did not have prior established heart disease or even risk factors other than obesity. I am confused about when you recorded a 12-lead. The time on the 12-lead is 14:31, but you have the patient in VF at that point. Your care plan does not indicate when the 12-lead was performed.

    The ECG demonstrates an acute infarction and is the probable cause of her arrest—VF secondary to acute MI. You could also wonder if she had a primary CNS [central nervous system] event, given the HA [headache] and the relative bradycardia [abnormally slow heart rate], but I think this is quite unlikely.

    In reviewing the flow sheet, I agree with proceeding to magnesium, especially since she takes a tricyclic antidepressant, according to her med profile. Pressor drips are reasonable when she regains an organized rhythm, though they should be used to supplement CPR and potentially a fluid challenge.

    Based on my review of the incident report and airway report, care was very good in this case. At King County Medic One, the goal is to resuscitate each and every VF patient, even though in reality we know that this will not be possible. However, you should develop the expectation and attitude that a patient who presents with VF as an initial rhythm will make it to the hospital alive.

At the level of the system, the most concrete example of medical QI is the effort to collect systemwide information on selected conditions, such as cardiac arrest.[9] Since 1975, dozens of research colleagues, associates, and assistants have studied the circumstances and outcomes of every cardiac arrest in our community. Every case has involved a patient who suffered out-of-hospital cardiac arrest due to underlying cardiac disease, and for whom EMS personnel were called to the scene and continued or initiated CPR. In each case, the etiology of the arrest was determined from a review of the run report, the death certificate, or hospital discharge records. This effort was and remains a collaborative undertaking between the EMS division of Public Health–Seattle and King County and the University of Washington.

The QI system in King County has been funded in part by federal and foundation grants, and in part by tax levies.[10] Other communities may wonder how they can afford such an extensive QI system, especially in view of rising costs and decreased revenues. But perhaps the question should be turned around: How can a community afford *not* to make this expenditure?

OTHER TYPES OF EMS SYSTEMS

The fire department–based, tiered-response system used in Seattle and King County is not the only model of EMS. For example, a community may use responders from its police and fire departments but may also place paramedics within a third public agency, which may be run by the city or by a private company under contract with the city. In the past, New York City combined this public agency model with a single-tier system (the city has since integrated its EMS personnel into its fire department), and Kansas City contracts with a private company to provide paramedic-level care.

Regardless of the model being used, an EMS system may have a single tier (such a system is also called a "single-layered system") or, as in Seattle and King County, it may have multiple tiers (sometimes this kind of system is called a "multilayered system" or a "tiered-response system"). An EMS system may be run outright by the police, or, as in Rochester, Minnesota, the police may help provide the first-in response. It is also possible for a community to use a mixed system, with the fire department providing EMTs as the first tier and another agency providing paramedic-level care as the second tier.

To add even more complexity to this heterogeneous picture, a community may have a single-tier system that uses a blend of EMTs and paramedics. For example, Washington County, adjacent to Portland, Oregon, uses an engine company of four firefighters to respond to every medical emergency call, and at least two of these firefighters are paramedics, though accidents of scheduling may mean that the responding crew includes as many as three or four paramedics. This kind of system is also called a "fire-medic system"—paramedics (the "fire-medics") who are members of a firefighter crew respond as a single tier to every EMS call. Private ambulance companies also play an important role in this type of system. They are dispatched simultaneously with the fire-medics and collaborate with them at the scene. They also transport patients to the hospital, thus freeing the fire-medics to respond to the next 911 call. This blend of public and private providers working in partnership is an increasingly common model for EMS care in many communities.

Other communities use private ambulance companies to provide paramedic-level care, either in a single-tier system or in collaboration with a fire department that provides EMT care. Still others have hospital-based EMS systems, or systems in which emergency medical services are provided by a health department, as in the southern portions of King County. The latter two models are relatively uncommon, however.

Every year, the *Journal of Emergency Medical Services* (*JEMS*) surveys EMS programs in the 200 largest cities of the United States.[11] The cities surveyed have ranged from New York (population 8 million) to Vallejo, California (population 117,500). The 2006 survey revealed that the most common EMS model in that year was fire department–based (35 percent), with the private ambulance model (34 percent)

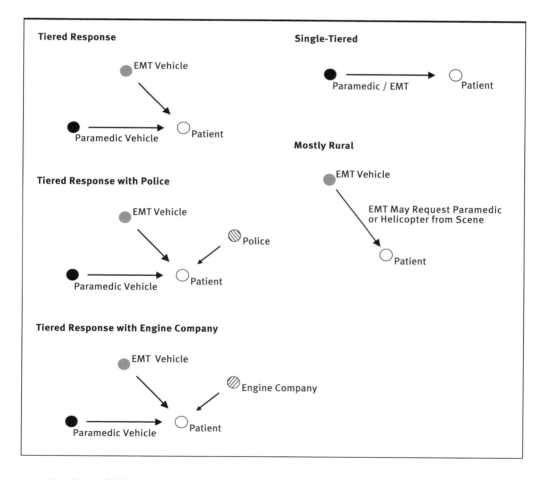

6.1 Types of EMS systems.

close behind. Less common were the public agency model (14 percent), the hospital-based model (5 percent), and the public utility model (5 percent); one community reported a police-based system. To add to this multitude of models, there were also three public-private partnerships. Almost all the systems used a combination of EMTs and paramedics, though there did appear to be a trend in larger cities to use paramedics as the only responders. Every community's EMS system had a designated medical director, but in 44 percent of the systems the medical director devoted fewer than ten hours a week to that role. There were full-time medical directors in 23 percent of the communities.[12] The survey offers a snapshot of EMS in America, though it is a snapshot taken through a blurred lens, since many prominent systems were not surveyed.[13]

In sum, there is no such thing as a uniform national model of EMS care, and systems vary considerably from community to community. Cities use a blend of private ambulance companies, fire departments, hospitals, health departments, police departments, and public agencies (see fig. 6.1), and they may be administered at the city, the county, or sometimes the regional level. Staff may include EMTs, paramedics, and sometimes police (often trained as first responders) in various proportions, or a system may use only paramedics or only EMTs. In rural systems, volunteer EMTs and even volunteer paramedics play a large role.

The funding of EMS systems is just as complex as their administrative arrangements. Some systems, especially those run by private companies operating under contract with cities, not only charge patients for paramedic care but also charge separately for transport. Or a city, under its contract with a private entity, may pay for paramedic care while allowing an ambulance company to charge patients for transport. A public EMS service, whether based in a fire department or using a third public agency, may employ a mix of funding.[14] Often the initial care is provided at no cost to the patient, but a transport fee is charged.[15] It is the rare system that provides both initial care and transport by paramedics at no cost to the patient.[16]

THE ROCHESTER MODEL

Rochester, Minnesota, a city of 97,000, is much smaller than the Seattle–King County area but has equally impressive survival statistics for cardiac arrest. Like Seattle, Rochester has a tiered-response system, but police instead of firefighter EMTs provide the first-in response for most cardiac arrests.[17] Actually, however, Rochester could be considered a triple-response system, since police and firefighters deliver CPR and defibrillation with AEDs, and hospital-based paramedics provide advanced care.[18]

Rochester's incorporation of police into its EMS system allows for quick defibrillation. When the city's public safety communications center is alerted to a possible cardiac arrest, police and fire vehicles are dispatched simultaneously, and the call is transferred, usually within ten to fifteen seconds, to the Mayo Clinic's emergency communications center at St. Mary's Hospital, which dispatches a paramedic-staffed vehicle from the Gold Cross Ambulance Service.[19] Since three different vehicles are dispatched—one from the police department, one from the fire department, and one from the hospital—any one of the three, according to its location, may be the first to arrive at the scene. About 50 percent of the time, the police or fire department arrives first; the rest of the time, the paramedic vehicle is the first one in. The average interval between the call to the dispatch center and the delivery of the first shock is just over six minutes. This is a very fast response time, and it undoubtedly explains Rochester's high survival rate.

Roger White is the medical director of Rochester's EMS system. In 1990, when he began as medical director of the city's police department, the police were already responding to medical emergencies and providing CPR to victims of cardiac arrest. Paramedics employed by the Gold Cross Ambulance Service provided advanced care, including defibrillation. At the time, the fire department played little or no role in providing emergency care. When White noticed how often police arrived before paramedics—several minutes earlier, in many cases—he realized that there was an opportunity for police to provide a quick defibrillatory shock. As a result, he proposed a two-year trial of training police officers and equipping them with AEDs, to determine whether they could improve survival rates for cardiac arrest. The trial was a success, and Rochester's experimental police AED program became a permanent one, the first of its kind in the United States.

From the very beginning, the police had been supportive of expanding their role, probably because of their long-standing history of providing basic first aid, which they had been doing since the 1940s. In their new role, they were even instructed to leave the scene of a minor traffic infraction if a call about a cardiac arrest came in. Today, every police vehicle in Rochester is tracked with GPS technology, and when a cardiac call comes in, the closest police vehicle is dispatched to the scene.[20]

This particular use of police has not worked in every community. Miami, Louisville, and Cincinnati have had mixed success, and there has hardly been a stampede of police chiefs demanding police AED programs; on the contrary, a recent survey of law enforcement officers found that attitudes toward police use of AEDs were considerably negative.[21] White thinks that the unique success of Rochester's police AED program is due to the department's long history and established culture of providing basic first aid and CPR, but that imposing such a culture on a police department that lacked a comparable history would be an uphill battle, especially if it were a large and busy department.[22] He has met with many police chiefs, and they give him a variety of responses: "We have altogether too much to do already." "The unions will never allow it." "We'll never get the support we need."

Despite such cultural barriers, White is hopeful that the police AED model can be successfully transplanted to other communities. White firmly believes that a police AED program must have strong medical control, and in this he echoes precisely the views of Leonard Cobb and Michael Copass. He is aware of some police AED programs that have little or no medical control, and he can barely hide his contempt—such programs may trumpet an occasional success, he says, but without medical control they cannot sustain or improve their performance.

After every cardiac arrest to which police, firefighter, or paramedic crews have responded, White himself reviews the ECG recording, and he personally gives feedback to the responding crews. He tries to do so within a day or two of the event. If a crew member cannot make it to White's office, he pays a visit to the police or fire station or to St. Mary's Hospital and reviews the tape there. This type of dedication is infectious, and it makes every police officer, firefighter, and paramedic want to try just a little harder on the next call.

White is a full-time faculty member at the Mayo Clinic College of Medicine, and this academic connection enhances his credibility in the role of medical director. As an academician, he also has a responsibility to share and publish his findings, and he thinks that this mission is one that the field personnel also view as important, since it helps them feel that they are participating in a larger effort—what is learned in Rochester may help people in other communities, too.

MORE PERSPECTIVES ON EMS SYSTEMS

Researchers

Tom Rea

We've seen what Leonard Cobb, Michael Copass, and Roger White believe—medical control should be the foundation of an EMS system. The structure that is then built on the foundation consists of a tiered-response system, training and continuing education, and medical QI. Tom Rea believes that organizational culture is another key component of the structure.

The term "culture," as used by Rea, refers not to historical traditions, such as the long-standing provision of basic first aid by the Rochester police department, but rather to attitudes and expectations within the organization. The program's culture can do much to create a high standard of practice and instill pride and motivation. There is relatively little turnover among paramedics in Seattle and King County, where being a paramedic is a career-long endeavor, unlike in some other parts of the country. Moreover, most paramedics come from within the ranks of firefighter EMTs—the introduction of "fresh blood" is uncommon. On occasion, however, a paramedic does come into the system after having worked elsewhere, and he or she invariably notes striking differences in culture. For example, the new paramedic may hear more senior paramedics say things that throw these cultural differences into relief: "We've got three minutes to turn this critical patient around—let's get going" or "This patient is in VF, and if we don't resuscitate her, we've failed." As Rea sees it, a culture that reinforces expectations for good outcomes is a culture that perpetuates itself. As he puts it, "Paramedics are optimistic and determined, and they bring to every cardiac a mindset that they will succeed."

Graham Nichol

Graham Nichol is director of the Center for Prehospital Emergency Care at the University of Washington. He is an endowed professor of medicine and works closely with Cobb, Copass, and Rea (and with me, for that matter). Nichol arrived at the university in 2006 from Ontario, Canada, and is currently codirector of the coordinating center for the Resuscitation Outcomes Consortium (ROC) trial. I mention these credentials because they give Nichol a unique perspective from which to evaluate an EMS system.

Nichol has strong opinions about why some communities succeed in managing cardiac arrest and others fail. He thinks that one underappreciated factor is the number of providers at the scene of a cardiac arrest. In Seattle and King County, there are at least four providers—two EMTs and two paramedics—and typically there are six or more. For Nichol, a successful resuscitation effort is like a finely choreographed ballet, with all participants knowing their parts. In fact he uses the term "choreographed" when he describes his impressions of riding with paramedics, and he contrasts these impressions with those that he formed in situations where only two or three EMS personnel were on the scene, moving around in a comparatively chaotic way. For Nichol, other underappreciated factors include the type of providers and the ratio of providers to the overall population. In Seattle and King County, 255 paramedics and 3,500 firefighter EMTs serve a total population of 2 million, whereas in communities of similar size there may be 1,000 paramedics. According to Nichol, the more paramedics there are, the fewer opportunities they have to use and maintain their proficiency in critical skills.[23]

Through his position with the ROC, Nichol has had the chance to observe at first hand the differences in survival rates among the participating communities, and he notes that there is a sevenfold difference.[24] He calls this a "dirty little secret," one that would lead to action, he claims, if people knew about it. The solution, Nichol thinks, is to make cardiac arrest a reportable disease—only mandatory reporting, he says, can focus the spotlight of public awareness on this intolerable situation. But he also thinks that there's a psychological explanation for why there is so little awareness of this discrepancy in survival rates. "People simply don't want to talk about cardiac arrest," he says. "It is too unpleasant a topic." Avoidance is a powerful force.

Peter Kudenchuk

Many factors explain a particular community's success or failure in managing cardiac arrest. Peter Kudenchuk, professor of cardiology at the University of Washington, characterizes these factors as "hard" and "soft." The hard factors are those with good scientific support, and the soft ones are those that are difficult to quantify. Kudenchuk thinks that one vital factor, leaning toward the soft end of the spectrum, is voice recording of cardiac arrests. Some EMS programs use AEDs and manual defibrillators that have built-in digital voice recorders, which simultaneously record the patient's ECG rhythms and all the words spoken during the resuscitation. Playing a recording back is a wonderful way to reconstruct the events of a resuscitation—the listener is almost in the patient's home, listening to barking dogs and slamming doors—and to facilitate meaningful quality improvement. Kudenchuk once did a study that showed very poor correlation between clinical information taken from written incident reports and information obtained from voice recordings of the same patients' resuscitation attempts. This finding was not a surprise, since an incident report is reconstructed after the event, sometimes after the end of a busy shift, when it can be difficult to recall exact timing and details, whereas a digital recorder passively and accurately registers everything. Kudenchuk believes that any community serious about improving its survival rates must institute the use of voice recordings and use them to identify the EMS program's strong and weak elements. EMTs and paramedics can be expected to resist voice recordings at first, but their resistance should dissipate when they realize that the recordings will be used for the system's improvement rather than for disciplinary purposes. And people tend to want to do their best when they know that their efforts are being recorded.

As a researcher and principal investigator for the Seattle and King County sites in the ROC trial, Kudenchuk has the opportunity to see at first hand the quality of the cardiac arrest registries maintained by the other participating communities (the ROC has ten clinical centers that encompass eleven different geographical areas in the United States and Canada). All the sites are challenged by this monumental endeavor, some more than others; Kudenchuk acknowledges the "tedium and grunt work," as he calls it, involved in maintaining a registry and keeping it accurate. In his experience of surveying these registries, usually the raw data supplied from the field are missing key components and often require clarification. For example, two boxes that are mutually exclusive, such as "witnessed collapse" and "unwitnessed collapse," may both be checked on an incident report, so someone has to reach the EMT or paramedic and clarify the matter. It is thankless work, and yet ultimately it is the most important kind of activity a system can undertake if improvement is a major goal. And after good medical QI data have been obtained, there must be a direct connection between a program's QI efforts and the program's other operations. In many instances, however, there is a disconnect, as if the organization had suffered a stroke—the body (the program) knows what it has to do (because the QI data have identified the changes that are needed), but the muscles (the various operations within the program) do not respond (because they refuse to acknowledge the importance of the QI information). This is another reason why the position of medical director is such an important one —the medical director is the logical person to lead the QI efforts, and the logical person to use QI information for operational improvements.

Al Hallstrom

Al Hallstrom, professor of biostatistics at the University of Washington, is an international expert on prehospital emergency medical research and has worked closely with researchers from Seattle and King County. As director of the Clinical Trials Center at the University of Washington, he has also coordinated many multisite national trials. Until recently he was the head of the coordinating center for the ROC trial.

I have known Hallstrom for more than thirty years, and he has provided invaluable assistance as coinvestigator and statistical consultant for many clinical studies. Hallstrom is well aware of the challenges involved in explaining the differences in survival rates among communities. He thinks that medical control of the EMS program may be a key factor, but he admits the difficulty of isolating its effect. He once joked that the best experiment would be to ship Leonard Cobb and Michael Copass off for several years to some community with a low survival rate and see if its rate began to improve.

Hallstrom has been in the business long enough to realize the limits of resuscitation. He concurs with my speculation that the maximum community survival rate for witnessed ventricular fibrillation is approximately 50 percent. The remaining 50 percent of patients—people with severe comorbidity or a large myocardial infarction or severe pump failure as the cause of arrest—cannot be resuscitated, no matter what therapy is provided. This explains why some patients die even though they have everything going for them in terms of rapid initiation of CPR and defibrillation; they simply do not have heart muscle that is normal enough to respond to therapy. For the 50 percent who do have a chance, the major challenge is to provide therapy quickly enough, but it isn't at all clear what that therapy should be. Hallstrom thinks that 90 percent of the resuscitation guidelines are based on little or no science, but once something enters the guidelines, it is nearly impossible to get it out. The most unequivocally beneficial therapy is to defibrillate someone whose arrest occurred within the past four minutes, but for anyone whose arrest occurred more than five minutes ago, the best therapy or sequence of therapies is unclear—and it is these cases, of course, that account for the vast majority of attempted resuscitations. Hallstrom sees this as the biggest challenge in resuscitation research. Though we are on the cusp of "smart" defibrillators that will be able to guide therapy, Hallstrom plans to withhold judgment until the data are in. "Perhaps they will help," he says of these next-generation devices, "and perhaps not."

Michael Sayre

Michael Sayre has credentials as a medical director as well as a researcher. From 1992 to 2000 he was medical director of the Cincinnati EMS program and is currently associate professor of emergency medicine at Ohio State University.

Sayre was a leading investigator for the AutoPulse Assisted Prehospital International Resuscitation (ASPIRE) trial.[25] This prospective, randomized trial, using common protocols and data collection methods, took place from 2002 to 2004 in Ohio (Columbus), Pennsylvania (the suburbs of Pittsburgh), Washington State (Seattle), and the Canadian provinces of Alberta (Calgary) and British Columbia (Vancouver) and studied the effect in these five communities of using a chest-squeezing device designed to improve blood pressure during CPR. The trial showed no benefit from use of the device, but because data had been collected in a common manner, it was possible to compare characteristics of the five communities.

When the research was published, the average response time of the first-in EMS vehicle was reported to be approximately one minute less for Seattle than for the other sites, whereas the average response time of the first-in paramedic vehicle was reported to be approximately half a minute longer for Seattle. The time between the patient's collapse and the first shock was approximately ten minutes for all the sites. But even though these times were reasonably similar, the survival rates were quite different. In Seattle, the survival rate was 18.3 percent (the study included cardiac arrest due to all rhythms, so the survival rate was lower than for VF alone), and in the other communities the overall survival rate was 5.6 percent.

We might reasonably ask why there was this threefold difference, when the times were so similar. But were they? In Seattle, the first-in unit arrived a minute faster, on average, than in the other communities, and analysis did show that the response time of the first-in vehicle was strongly and positively correlated with survival, so this fact may explain some of the difference in survival rates. But in the cases studied, there was no effort to determine the actual, precise time of the patient's collapse. When it comes to positing relationships between time and outcomes, the only relevant events are those that involve a witnessed collapse, and the most meaningful time intervals are the estimated times between the actual collapse and the initiation of CPR and defibrillation. Reporting the response times of EMS vehicles gives only a partial picture of the key time intervals. This is a poor metric on which to base comparisons between and among communities, since vehicle response times alone cannot fully explain differences in survival rates.

Sayre thinks that the difference in survival rates between Seattle and the other four communities is explained by the Seattle paramedics' higher level of skills, and that these skills are due to the fact that Seattle has fewer paramedics performing more procedures. There are 600 paramedics in Columbus, for example, versus 60 in Seattle, yet the populations are 750,000 and 600,000, respectively. The EMS system in Columbus is an all-paramedic system. When a cardiac arrest call comes into the alarm center, two vehicles are dispatched—the first-in fire engine has one paramedic and three EMTs, and the second-in paramedic vehicle has two paramedics. In addition, a supervisor paramedic often responds, so there are typically four paramedics and three EMTs managing any one cardiac arrest. The strong possibility that paramedics' skill levels were a critical factor in determining these difference in survival rates has led Sayre to lobby vigorously for change in the Columbus system and to urge that it use fewer paramedics. The firefighters' union in Columbus is open to discussing this idea, and if, as a result of these changes, Columbus improves its survival rate, there will be at least indirect evidence to support the contention that paramedics' skills are a factor in determining survival rates.[26]

Paramedics

Tod Levesh and Aaron Tyerman

In March 2007, Tod Levesh and Aaron Tyerman, both King County paramedics, were returning to Seattle with their families after a joint vacation and were waiting to board their flight. With only fifteen minutes left until boarding, they noticed a small crowd and two police officers hovering over a man who was lying on the floor. The officers were trying to rouse the man by kicking his feet—no response. He turned out to be forty-one years old and in cardiac arrest.

No one was doing CPR, so Levesh and Tyerman identified themselves to the police. Levesh secured the patient's airway while Tyerman started chest compressions. The police brought an AED, and the two King County paramedics applied it to the patient's chest and delivered one shock.

Then local paramedics arrived and took over CPR, using the incorrect ratio of two ventilations to fifteen chest compressions (the correct ratio is two ventilations to thirty chest compressions). Again the King County paramedics offered to help, and help they did—the local paramedics did not know how to operate the defibrillator properly, so Levesh showed them how to read the patient's heart rhythm off the AED cable. The local paramedics were also unable to place a peripheral IV in the patient's arm, despite repeated attempts, so Levesh placed a 16-gauge IV line into the man's external jugular. Tyerman heard one of the local paramedics exclaim, "Whoa! That was cool!"

Meanwhile, another local paramedic—"shaking like she had advanced Parkinson's," Tyerman later recalled—managed to intubate the patient on the second try.

The patient refibrillated and received a second shock (the local paramedics had wanted to use the wrong energy level but were steered to the proper setting), which in turn led to slow pulseless electrical activity. Levesh and Tyerman reminded the paramedics to try atropine, a medication used to speed the heart up.

Tyerman then asked one of the paramedics for a Doppler (a type of radar device) so he could see whether there was a faint blood pressure.

"What's a Doppler?" the paramedic asked.

Now other rescue personnel arrived, and Levesh and Tyerman were relieved of their duties. As they were boarding their plane with their families, they learned that the resuscitation had been "called" (stopped), and that the patient had been taken to a hospital to be declared dead. One of the rescuers told them, "We ceased efforts. He was still in PEA, but after we gave the epi and atropine, that was all we could do in our protocol."

The two King County paramedics were dumbfounded. During the long flight back to Seattle, they could not stop wondering how a witnessed case of VF in a forty-one-year-old man had not had a successful outcome. As Levesh later remarked to me, "I would have gotten him alive to the hospital." This was said not as a boast but as a simple matter of fact.

It is unusual for two teams of paramedics from two different cities to be working side by side on the same patient, and that is what makes this event so telling. A simple comparison of the difference in skill levels between the King County paramedics and the local paramedics can explain some of the differences that we see in the survival rates of various communities. This anecdote presents only one side of the events that occurred, and it is, after all, just that—an anecdote. But it certainly is revealing.

I mean no disrespect toward the EMS personnel in the other city. I know that they did the best they could. But the theme of paramedics' skills, for which the paramedics-to-population is a presumed surrogate, has come up repeatedly. How does one measure paramedic quality? I don't have a ready answer, but I do think that the quality of paramedics' skills is directly related to survival rates for cardiac arrest. The point of my relating this incident is to demonstrate how likely it is that training and expectations of success—difficult things to quantify—will be determinant factors in a successful resuscitation.

Mike Helbock

Mike Helbock wanted to be a paramedic, and he knew that the best route was to first become a firefighter, so he got himself hired by a small department north of King County and worked there from 1977 to 1982. At that time, the community he served did not have paramedics. Patients in cardiac arrest were thrown into the back of an aid unit and rushed to the hospital.

"You wouldn't believe the chaos," Helbock told me, "the driver racing to the hospital with four guys in the back of the aid unit, two guys doing CPR and two guys holding the two doing CPR so they wouldn't smash into the side of the van as we careened around corners—every time we arrived in the hospital, the staff would take over CPR, do it for a few minutes, and then declare the patient dead. We never saved anyone."

In 1982, Helbock was hired by the Bellevue Fire Department, and within nine months he had entered the paramedic training class. He has now been a paramedic for more than twenty years and is currently the training director for King County EMS. When I asked him why Seattle and King County succeed in managing cardiac arrest whereas other communities do not, his answer largely echoed Leonard Cobb's. He believes that strong medical control was and is the distinguishing feature of the Seattle and King County programs.

As a paramedic student training in Seattle, he had observed that the medical chain of command was very short indeed. It went directly from the medical director to the paramedics. This arrangement was totally new to him. As a firefighter, his experience had been that there were plenty of hierarchical layers—lieutenants, battalion chiefs, deputy chiefs, chiefs. Among firefighters, everything is done by protocol; the chain of command is deep and always adhered to. Paramedics, by contrast, have very few protocols. They must think for themselves, and quickly. As Helbock puts it, "Protocols are great when things are black and white, but in medicine everything is gray, and you must use your judgment with every patient. The more difficult the resuscitation, the more we are challenged, and the more we shine."

Medical control has to be built on trust. You have to train a paramedic to the skill level of a specialist and then trust him or her to do the job. Endotracheal intubation offers a perfect example of this principle. Many programs allow paramedics to place endotracheal tubes, a complex and potentially dangerous skill, but few programs allow paramedics to administer intravenous succinylcholine to paralyze the patient before intubation, as is allowed in Seattle and King County.[27] Other communities are more cautious, and the result in these communities is a lower success rate for endotracheal intubations. In some communities, in fact, the success rate is so low that thought is even being given to dropping this procedure and using a procedure for airway protection that is less secure but easier to perform. But published data from Seattle show that the city's paramedics have a success rate of 98 percent for endotracheal intubation.[28]

"If succinylcholine is the gold standard in the emergency department," Helbock observes, "why should we settle for anything less in the streets?"

Why, indeed?

Fire Chiefs
Mario Trevino[29]

Mario Trevino used to be a battalion chief in Seattle and the fire chief in Las Vegas and San Francisco and is now the fire chief in Bellevue, Washington. Some might say that Trevino, in his three and a half decades of service, has experienced the worst and the best that fire department–based EMS has to offer.

Trevino was hired in San Francisco in June 2001. He had arrived from Las Vegas, and this was the first time in the San Francisco Fire Department's 145-year history that an outsider had been hired as chief. The mayor had brought him in specifically to complete a merger between the fire department and emergency medical services, which had previously been under the health department. This merger, which had been urged since 1998, was meeting a great deal of resistance from firefighters. But to call it resistance is perhaps too mild—the firefighters' union was vehemently opposed to the merger, and this opposition had been taking the form of verbal and even physical assaults.

Trevino, who came to be well aware of the history surrounding the issue, estimated that it would take five years to complete the merger and achieve its universal acceptance. He set out on his merger plan by canceling the current discussion process (the fire commissioners had established a round-table discussion group) and starting afresh with an implementation team of representatives from the firefighters' union, the paramedics' union, and fire department administrators. He chaired the team himself.

The team made progress, and paramedics began to work in conjunction with firefighters. The goal was to start putting paramedics on fire engines in the periphery of the city and then, over a two-year period, work toward the downtown core. Things seemed to be going well enough, but then the plan hit the wall of the downtown firehouses, where opposition to the paramedics was fierce.

Some of the paramedics had been hired from outside the system, but some had cross-trained from within the ranks of the San Francisco Fire Department itself. It made no difference—all the paramedics were ostracized. They had to eat separately from the firefighters, were harassed by firefighters, and were sometimes called vulgar names while on duty—hardly the picture of harmonious collaboration.

Trevino contrasts the reception of the paramedics in San Francisco to what he had seen while he was a battalion chief in Seattle.

"In Seattle," he says, "the paramedics are considered an elite group. In San Francisco, they were viewed as second-class citizens. Many dropped out of the program, and many others simply quit the department."

Trevino left San Francisco and returned to the Northwest in early 2004. Since his departure, things in San Francisco have reportedly devolved to resemble the old system except that paramedics continue to be employed by the fire department instead of the department of health; the hoped-for integration of EMS into the fire department has not been fully achieved. But Trevino now belongs to an EMS world that is 180 degrees different from what he saw in San Francisco. In Bellevue, and throughout Seattle and King County, paramedics are highly respected, and they smoothly work side by side with firefighter EMTs. All of the paramedics, except those in the south county program, are also cross-trained as firefighters.

Trevino has seen the power of organizational culture to make or break a program —it was culture that prevented San Francisco from developing a world-class EMS system, and it is culture that facilitates Bellevue's success. Trevino's firsthand experience should give pause to anyone who thinks than an EMS system can be turned around on a dime. Fresh ideas and innovation are much to be desired, but the wheels of inertia and the baggage of history are strong countervailing forces.

A. D. Vickery

A. D. Vickery has been with the Seattle Fire Department for more than forty years. As assistant chief of operations, he is currently responsible for all emergency medical services and fire-suppression activities.

If anyone has seen it all, it is Vickery. He is the son of Gordon Vickery (the former fire chief and co-founder of the Seattle Medic One program) and he was in the second class of Seattle paramedics to be certified in 1971. He served as a paramedic for twelve years. A. D. Vickery's participation in many national organizations and his service on EMS, fire, safety, and homeland security task forces have given him a broad and unique perspective.

Vickery thinks that Seattle's success with cardiac arrest is due to a fortuitous combination of community support, medical oversight, and a fire department–based EMS system that is able to deliver CPR and defibrillation quickly. Community support is demonstrated by citizens' massive willingness to be trained in CPR as well as by their knowledge about how to recognize cardiac arrest and when to call 911. Medical oversight is evidenced by the EMS system's tight medical control as well as by its constant investigation into how survival rates can be improved. And the fire department–based EMS system is flexible enough to respond to new information and has been able to reconfigure itself as necessary to achieve success. For example, when the Seattle Medic One program began, there was only one paramedic rig stationed at Harborview Medical Center, and the survival rates for cardiac arrest were good but not stellar. But as every cardiac arrest was studied, it became evident within two years that the interval between the patient's collapse and the initiation of CPR was a critical determinant of a successful outcome. This knowledge led to a major reconfiguration of the system. Now the first of the fire department's vehicles to be dispatched became the one that was closest to the scene of the cardiac arrest, even if that vehicle was a fire engine. CPR training for citizens began, and paramedic vehicles were now scattered throughout the city so that paramedics with defibrillators could reach patients more quickly. Suddenly survival rates for VF increased, climbing into the range of 30 percent and higher. As Vickery puts it, "Success is not a red rig running down the street. Success is a community, a fire department, and a medical director working together to construct the best system possible."

Vickery notes that visitors to Seattle's paramedic program have come from all over the world—from Australia, New Zealand, Great Britain, Singapore, Japan, China, Sweden, France, and Norway—but in the last decade, visitors have come from only one or two American cities. I have noticed the same thing.

"Can other communities emulate the Seattle cardiac arrest experience?" Vickery asks rhetorically. "Can they reproduce our system? Probably not, but at least they could improve things."

Vickery thinks that most EMS programs in the United States are closed systems with little maneuverability. There are exceptions, of course. New York City, to take one example, did manage to incorporate its EMS program into the fire department. San Francisco has not had the same success, but at least that city recognizes the need for change.

Vickery's is not entirely pessimistic, however. He thinks that federal performance standards for EMS systems hold promise. The National Fire Protection Association, for example, has already issued EMS standards, and almost everyone would agree that performance standards have the potential to improve EMS care.[30] Indeed, it is hard to imagine how they could make things worse. The challenge is how to implement them in the face of national indifference, and Vickery articulates this situation well.

"It amazes me that there is no national focus on prehospital care," he says. "Critical emergencies start in the field, and yet we as a society ignore that component. EMS is part of health care, but we are so focused on hospital care that we forget about what happens before the patient enters the emergency department."

EMTs

Terry Sinclair

Terry Sinclair wears two hats. He is a full-time coordinator for the training section of the King County EMS and a half-time lieutenant at Eastside Fire and Rescue, a department east of Seattle. He is a twenty-one-year veteran of the department, having started as a volunteer in 1987, and received his EMT training shortly after joining the department.

With his experience in training and in the field, Sinclair has a unique perspective, one that has been enriched by his dozens of visits to fire departments throughout the United States. He thinks that two things in particular—attitude and training—set the Seattle and King County EMS systems apart from systems in other communities.

When Sinclair talks about attitude, he means one that embraces high expectations and high standards. He thinks that this attitude is shared by all ranks in his

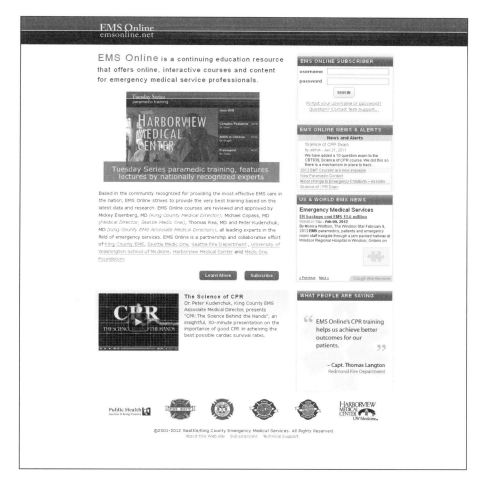

6.2 Home page of EMS Online (EMSonline.net).

department, from the chief on down, and that it permeates the system, leading everyone to want to do better; substandard performance, whether that means failure to maintain a piece of equipment or failure to adhere to a protocol, is simply not tolerated. And training, Sinclair says, is the means of attaining high standards.

In all his visits to other departments, Sinclair has not seen one whose training requirements are as high as those in his own department. "It's one thing to put out an EMT," he says, "but it's another thing to continuously enhance and improve that EMT's skills." Not only does every EMT in the system participate in EMS Online (www.emsonline.net, an Internet-based continuing education program), there is also constant review of practical skills in addition to drills in medical procedures (see fig. 6.2). Every run report is read and critiqued by a paramedic QI coordinator, and these critiques are reinforced with written feedback and monthly meetings.

I asked Sinclair whether his department's resuscitation can be improved. He reflected a moment, and then he said, "Of course it can. We have to make sure CPR is done letter-perfect. That's the key to making us even better. If we are to save more lives, it will be because of the details." When I asked him what it will take for other systems to improve, he answered without hesitation. "People at the top with different attitudes," he replied, "the chiefs, the mayor, the councils." For Sinclair, the culture of excellence has to start at the top, and he himself is the embodiment of high expectations and high standards.

Dispatchers

Mark Morgan[31]

Valley Communications Center is one of three large dispatch centers in King County. It serves the south and southeast portions of the county, taking 911 calls from a region of 800,000 people and dispatching for fourteen fire departments, the King County Medic One paramedic agency, and the police departments in the area. Mark Morgan, interim director of this center, brings seventeen years of experience to the job. Because of his experience in emergency telecommunications, Morgan also serves as a subject-matter expert for the Loaned Executive Member Assistance Program (LEMAP) of the Washington Association of Sheriffs and Police Chiefs (WASPC) and as a team leader for the Member Advisory Assistance Program (MAAP) of the International Association of Public Safety Communications Officials (APCO). Thus he has the opportunity to visit many centers throughout the state and nation and to perform peer reviews.

Morgan believes that the keys to success in a dispatch center are the same ones that would lead to success in any public service agency—progressive thinking, high expectations, high-quality training, continuing education, ongoing performance evaluation, and quality improvement. He also cites two specific elements that enhance his center's functioning when it comes to dispatching for cardiac arrest. The first is the countywide telephone CPR program, through which dispatchers provide instant CPR instructions over the phone to callers who may not know how to perform CPR or who may need a refresher.[32] A half-time QI person in the King County EMS office reviews digital recordings of every call involving dispatcher-assisted telephone CPR and provides feedback to the individual dispatcher. Most of the time, the feedback is simply "Great job," but sometimes opportunities for improvement are pointed out (QI forms can be found at survivecardiacarrest.org). The second element is the committee that constantly reviews dispatch recordings, and information from the incident reports completed by EMTs and paramedics, to refine and improve dispatch guidelines. This committee functions as an oversight body, constantly endeavoring to create a more efficient and more effective dispatch system. One example of the committee's work is the effort it made to alert dispatchers that a 911 call for a seizure may in fact be a call for a cardiac arrest (when the brain is deprived of oxygen, there may be seizurelike activity for a few seconds).

Morgan also believes that the practice of rapid dispatch (also called "accelerated dispatch") is one that should be adopted by every EMS dispatch center in the nation. The concept is simple. After determining that there is a medical problem, the dispatcher verifies the address and gets the initial unit or units rolling while continuing to gather information from the caller. Once enough information has been obtained for an informed decision, the dispatcher upgrades or downgrades the response, as necessary. This practice adds slightly to the dispatcher's workload, but it can shave a minute or more off the time needed for the first-in unit to reach the patient.

Cleo Subido

Cleo Subido worked for twelve years as a dispatcher and supervisor with the Seattle Police Department Communications Center. She is now program manager for King County Emergency Medical Dispatch Training and QI. Her responsibilities include organizing and presenting the initial forty-hour emergency medical training course for dispatchers as well as the courses designed to fulfill the requirement for eight hours a year of continuing education. Subido has visited many dispatch centers, and she is convinced that three factors—training, continuing education, and QI—make the difference between a center that is good and one that is excellent.

Ten of the initial forty hours of training are devoted to recognizing the signs of cardiac arrest and agonal respirations, as described by callers to 911, and to offering callers CPR instructions over the telephone. The training also includes instruction in how to avoid unnecessary questions that eat up precious time. Subido teaches the King County dispatchers to be very aggressive in offering telephone CPR instructions. She thinks that this assertiveness defines the culture in the dispatch centers, and she reinforces that culture and improves the continuing education courses with feedback that uses information from the QI review of dispatch tapes.

Dispatchers often ask Subido why she spends so much time training them to recognize the need for telephone CPR and deliver CPR instructions over the phone, since most of the calls they pick up don't require them to use those skills. Subido's answer is simple: "Because it's the most important thing you do."

Administrators

Tom Hearne[33]

Tom Hearne is director of the King County EMS Division. His ten years as director, plus his twenty-two years as the EMS associate director and research project director, have given him a wealth of experience in managing the complexities of emergency medical services.

Hearne does not view the EMS system through a medical lens. Trained as a social scientist (he has a Ph.D. in anthropology), he readily acknowledges that some of the factors responsible for the success of the EMS system are difficult to quantify. These are more qualitative factors—"mushy," as he calls them.

Hearne works in a complex world of county government, a world that includes the county health department, several dozen fire departments, dispatch agencies, an advisory board, a trauma council, and the board of health. He readily acknowledges that one of his major roles is keeping the entire regional system together. "My role is to minimize division and separation," he says. "I try to maximize consensus, partnerships, cooperation, and common goals."[34]

Hearne places great value on regionalization, and he thinks that it is one of the key factors explaining the successful programs in Seattle and King County. The term "regionalization," in this case, refers to the fact that thirty-three fire departments, six paramedic programs, and five dispatch agencies are all working under common protocols and standards. The region's paramedics and EMTs can easily cross city borders, since standards and protocols are identical everywhere within the area. The regional standard that all paramedics be trained at Harborview Medical Center ensures the same high level of skill across the entire paramedic group. And regionalization also offers opportunities to realize economies of scale in the program's operations as well as in its financing. For example, considerable time and effort are saved by the use of a single system for data collection and a regional purchasing plan, since individual departments do not have to maintain their own EMS databases and purchasing plans. Moreover, there are few turf issues because all the various agencies buy into the system and its level of oversight.[35]

The regionalization of the EMS system in King County has been successful partly because regionalization has been directed toward improving early access to the patient, early CPR, early defibrillation, and early advanced care—as Hearne puts it, "We polish all four links in the chain of survival."[36] As a result, Hearne is able to devote his division's energy and resources to improving dispatch guidelines, telephone CPR, community CPR training, EMT training, and continuing education as well as to providing and coordinating paramedic services. In King County, which includes Seattle, there are fewer than 2 million citizens. Thus the entire region is small enough for the key players to get to know and trust one another. But would regionalization be as successful in an area with a population of 4 million, or 10 million? Or would it fail under the pressure of the region's sheer size? Is successful regionalization associated with an optimal size for the region's population? Hearne suspects that it is, but this is probably another "mushy" factor that resists being quantified.

The King County EMS Division, in addition to providing the regional coordination for the entire county, directly provides paramedic services to a population of 800,000 in the southern part of the county (King County Medic One), and Hearne thinks that their services are vital to the overall program. The seventy-five paramedics who work in this paramedic program are employees of the health department, but they receive the same training and use the same protocols as the 180 paramedics who staff the five fire department–based programs in Seattle and the remainder of the county. Many of the paramedics working in the south county paramedic program, as well as most of the officers, come from the fire service as does the administrator of the program who used to be a fire chief. As Hearne says, "We're as 'fire service' as we can be without pumping water on the patient." Hearne thinks that the fire department–based model is a very effective one for EMS; firefighters, he says, "understand the importance of service and time. Fire departments know that flashover is the direct result of not getting water on the conflagration fast enough. A failed resuscitation is the result of not getting the defibrillator to the patient fast enough."

Hearne must have been a fire chief in a past life.

PUTTING IT ALL TOGETHER

The views of Cobb, Copass, White, Rea, Nichol, Kudenchuk, Hallstrom, Sayre, Levesh, Helbock, Trevino, Vickery, Sinclair, Morgan, Subido, and Hearne are based on several hundred collective years of directing, evaluating, training, and researching EMS systems. Though each of these informants has a slightly different view and emphasis, together their remarks suggest that the successful management of five key elements appears vital to the creation and perpetuation of a high-quality EMS system. These elements are medical control; administrative control; system configuration; training and continuing education; and ongoing quality improvement, including maintenance of a cardiac arrest registry.

These five key elements are all imbued with and infuse an EMS system's culture. In turn, the system's culture must embrace high expectations and high standards— the system must have, in other words, what some refer to as a "culture of excellence" —and while such expectations and standards must be set from the top, ultimately the entire EMS system must embrace them. As Mario Trevino has made crystal clear, an EMS system can be either enhanced or destroyed by its culture. A culture of excellence nurtures and sustains a superior system that strives to do its very best for every patient, 100 percent of the time.

SEVEN

What Can Your Community Do?

The coffee cup saved Mike J.'s life. Mike's wife, Joan, heard it shatter and went running into the kitchen. She saw the shards on the floor, and her husband was slumped over the table. While shouting Mike's name, Joan reached for the telephone. Within thirty seconds of the cup's hitting the floor, she had dialed 911.

Rapid dispatch sent EMS units within twenty seconds of receiving the call, and within ninety seconds the dispatcher had instructed Joan to get her husband onto the floor and begin CPR.

Fire department EMTs arrived at Mike's side within five minutes of having been dispatched. Fifty-five seconds later, they had attached the AED and delivered a defibrillatory shock.

Paramedics arrived five minutes after the EMTs. They intubated Mike and started an IV line. Mike required two more defibrillatory shocks as well as medications to stabilize his heart rhythm. Then he was transported to the hospital.

By the time he arrived, he was starting to move and trying to grab his airway tube, even though his hands were tied to the gurney. He received an implantable defibrillator and was discharged eight days later.

The medical director and the coordinator of the cardiac arrest registry later reviewed the run report as well as the digital voice tapes and the ECG tapes. The final audit listed the patient's collapse as having been witnessed, the time needed to reach 911 as one minute, the time between the patient's collapse and the start of CPR as two and a half minutes, the time between the collapse and the first shock as seven minutes, and the time between the collapse and the initiation of advanced care as eleven minutes. A summary of the event, including the discharge information, was sent to dispatchers, EMTs, and paramedics who were involved in the case. The medical director wrote a congratulatory note on each copy of the summary.

THE CHAIN OF SURVIVAL

The American Heart Association, describing the sequence of the interventions that are required in a successful resuscitation, talks about the "chain of survival" (fig. 7.1). This is an apt metaphor. The four links in the chain are early access, early CPR, early defibrillation, and early advanced care. Each link in this chain builds on the previous one, and timely delivery of each intervention allows the next intervention to be successful. When all the interventions are delivered quickly, the patient in cardiac arrest has a high likelihood of full recovery.

Just how high is the likelihood of full recovery? As we saw in the previous chapter, Al Hallstrom of the University of Washington thinks that the maximum possible survival rate for witnessed ventricular fibrillation is approximately 50 percent, given the realities of underlying comorbidity. I agree with this figure and I'm sure many other researchers would estimate a similar percentage. Some communities are already close to this theoretical ceiling. In special situations, a survival rate above 50 percent is possible. For example, a study published in 2000 reported that 73 percent of patients who collapsed with VF in gambling casinos survived when a defibrillatory shock was delivered within three minutes of collapse, but the overall survival rate in the casinos was still 50 percent.[1] Settings like casinos, airplanes, and airports provide the opportunity to deliver a shock within minutes of collapse.[2] In most other settings, however, it is unlikely for a defibrillator and a trained user to be so instantly or so quickly available. That is why the other links in the chain of survival—early access, early CPR, and early advanced care—are so important.

It is a cliché, of course, to say that a chain is only as strong as its weakest link, but one reason why clichés become clichés is that they express a truth. In the case of the

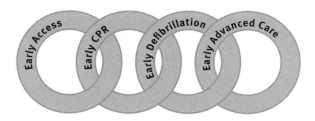

7.1 Chain of survival.

chain of survival, if each intervention occurs rapidly, there is a good chance for the patient's successful resuscitation. A substantial delay in any one intervention, however, means that the patient's death is inevitable, regardless of how efficiently the other interventions can be delivered. The four links in the chain of survival are simplified representations of what is actually a multitude of twenty or more smaller links, each one representing a vital step or action. For the four major interventions to be successful, each of the smaller steps or actions must also be flawlessly carried out.

The following lists give the detailed elements of a resuscitation, more or less in the order in which they appear in an actual emergency. The sequences described here assume a tiered-response system, with EMTs providing the first-in response and paramedics providing the second. All the elements described here are necessary, but none by itself is sufficient. The point of listing them here is to tease apart the complex process of resuscitation and begin to identify the potential weak points along the chain of survival. Some of these elements are not amenable to change, but for those that are, concrete programmatic and individual actions can improve outcomes for patients.

The first link in the chain of survival, *early access*, involves these elements:

1. *Someone (here called a "bystander") sees or hears the victim collapse.*
2. *The bystander recognizes the seriousness of the situation.*
3. *The bystander calls for help and quickly gives all the necessary information to the emergency call receiver or dispatcher.* In most parts of the country, the number to call is 911. I am always amazed when a bystander calls a relative or a doctor instead of 911, though I am also very sympathetic, given the panic and ensuing chaos. The bystander may never before have witnessed a cardiac arrest and may never do so again, so he or she may not do the right thing; it is impossible to be fully prepared for a once-in-a-lifetime event.
4. *The dispatcher quickly identifies the problem and uses rapid dispatch to send the EMT and paramedic units.* As explained in chapter 6, the term "rapid dispatch" refers to the practice of sending the proper unit or units before all the information has been obtained from the caller. For example, if the caller says that her husband has collapsed, this is enough information to get the units rolling. Once the units are on the way, the dispatcher can inquire about the details and then briefly convey them to the responding units. Rapid dispatch can save up to a minute, sometimes more, in the delivery of vital care.

The second link, *early CPR,* involves these elements:

1. *The bystander and/or the dispatcher recognizes the signs of cardiac arrest.*
2. *If the bystander is not trained in CPR, or is trained but needs to be reminded how CPR is performed, the dispatcher quickly offers CPR instructions over the phone.*

A big challenge in recognizing cardiac arrest is recognizing the presence of agonal respirations. Agonal respirations are a sign of recent collapse, and yet their presence often mistakenly leads the caller (and the dispatcher) to believe that the patient is breathing and therefore not in need of CPR.

3. *The caller is able to position the victim on his or her back, preferably on a hard surface, and to perform CPR.* This can be a real challenge, since the victim may have collapsed in an awkward position—say, between the toilet and bathtub. The presence of vomit or blood in the victim's mouth will also inhibit the performance and quality of CPR. The caller must be able to tilt the victim's head in such a way as to open the throat and airway and must be able to form a tight seal around the victim's mouth in order to blow air into the lungs. The caller must also be able to find the correct position for chest compression and must be able to compress the chest a depth of one and a half to two inches at the proper rate and the appropriate number of times. (The correct procedure is to give two ventilations followed by thirty chest compressions. See chapter 5 for a discussion of hands-only CPR. See also learncpr.org.)

4. *The caller is able to continue CPR, without growing fatigued, until EMS personnel arrive.*

5. *EMTs get to the victim's address quickly.*

6. *EMTs quickly reach the victim's side.* Here, the necessary elements are things like having the door unlocked, the elevator available, and the dog locked away. Simple obstructions can cause disastrous delays.

7. *EMTs take over CPR from the bystander or begin CPR if it is not being performed.* The EMTs must ventilate the patient with 100 percent oxygen, preferably using a bag-valve mask. CPR must be continued until just before an AED is used to assess the cardiac rhythm.

The third link, *early defibrillation,* involves these elements:

1. *The first-in unit—EMTs or police first responders—has an AED and is trained in its use.* These personnel must properly attach the electrodes and operate the defibrillator correctly. Ideally, the first shock will be delivered within one minute after the first-in unit arrives at the patient's side.

2. *After delivering the first shock, first responders immediately resume CPR, without waiting for a pulse check.* After two minutes of CPR, the patient's heart rhythm should be reassessed. If a second shock is indicated, it is delivered. If no shock is indicated, the patient's pulse is checked. It is very important to minimize the period of time during which no CPR is being given.

The fourth link, *early advanced care,* involves these elements:

1. *Paramedics arrive quickly.*

2. *Paramedics deliver additional defibrillatory shocks if those already delivered have not been successful.*

3. *Paramedics place and start a peripheral intravenous line.* If a peripheral IV cannot be started, paramedics must start a central or interosseous line.

4. *Paramedics perform endotracheal intubation and ventilate the patient with 100 percent oxygen.*

5. *Paramedics administer emergency medications, such as epinephrine to stimulate the patient's heart, and lidocaine or amiodarone to stabilize the heart's rhythm.*

6. *Paramedics take a 12-lead ECG reading to determine whether an acute myocardial infarction is present.*

7. *Paramedics contact the medical control doctor for consultation, guidance, instructions regarding additional therapy, and plans for transportation.* They then transport the patient to a hospital's emergency room.[3]

MIKE'S RESUSCITATION REVISITED

The cardiac arrest that opened this chapter illustrates the chain of survival and the interdependence of its four links. This event actually took place exactly as described.

1. *Early access:* Mike J.'s wife, Joan, heard the coffee cup shatter, and she ran to her husband within seconds of his collapse. She knew to call 911, and she did so without delay—in less than one minute.

2. *Early CPR:* The dispatcher immediately recognized the critical nature of the call and dispatched aid and medic units simultaneously. She then gave Joan CPR instructions over the telephone. As a result, Mike received two full cycles of CPR within three minutes of his collapse, and CPR continued until the first EMS personnel arrived.

3. *Early defibrillation:* Firefighter EMTs equipped with an automated external defibrillator took over CPR and applied the device to Mike. They gave him the first defibrillatory shock within seven minutes of his collapse. Mike was temporarily defibrillated into a sinus rhythm, and he was in a perfusing rhythm when the paramedics arrived.

4. *Early advanced care:* Five minutes after the arrival of the firefighter EMTs, the paramedics arrived to deliver advanced life support. Mike's heart refibrillated, and the paramedics gave him two more shocks. He also received intravenous medications to stabilize his heart rhythm and prevent further episodes of VF. The medics intubated Mike's airway in order to deliver 100 percent oxygen and protect his airway from aspirated secretions. All this advanced care was started within eleven minutes of Mike's collapse.

Mike would not have lived if any of the links in the chain of survival had been weakened or broken. Nevertheless, his cardiac arrest would have had the same outcome if it had occurred in any community where the actions along the chain of survival had been similarly timely. The secret of a successful resuscitation is not all that mysterious—simply ensure that rapid care is provided along each of the links in the chain of survival. That is easier said than done, however. Few communities can provide all the necessary elements of resuscitation quickly enough. A community may be able to provide one, two, or even three of the necessary elements, but if all four are not provided rapidly enough, that community's overall outcomes will be dismal.

"IT'S THE TIME, STUPID"

James Carville, during Bill Clinton's first presidential campaign, posted a sign at the campaign's headquarters—"It's the economy, stupid"—that was intended as a blunt reminder for Clinton to keep hammering home on a major campaign theme. Similarly, I hope that everyone involved with cardiac resuscitation will post a sign saying "It's the time, stupid" above his or her desk, on the bathroom mirror, or wherever else it can be seen every day. *Two of what we have called "system factors"—the time between the patient's collapse and the initiation of CPR,[4] and the time between the patient's collapse and the first defibrillatory shock—are the most important factors associated with the patient's survival.* Without rapid CPR and defibrillation, nothing else can save the patient. And when a community cannot provide these two interventions quickly, that community's management of cardiac arrest will not be successful.

A COMMUNITY REPORT CARD FOR SUDDEN CARDIAC ARREST

I doubt that many people would move to a city on the basis of on its survival rate for sudden cardiac arrest. Frankly, though, I don't see why that should not be an important consideration, especially if one is contemplating a move to a community where one plans to retire. How often does a senior who is moving to Florida, Arizona, or southern California write to the director of the local EMS agency and ask what the community's VF survival rate is? Not often, I suspect. But if any seniors were to write, here is the letter I think they should send:

> Dear — —,
>
> My husband and I are thinking of retiring to your community in the near future. My husband has coronary artery disease and had a triple bypass four years ago. I needn't go into his medical history except to note that he is at higher risk than most people for sudden cardiac arrest. I am writing to determine the following information about your EMS system. Would you kindly answer the following questions?

What is the average response time for the first responding EMS vehicle, measured from the time a call comes in to your dispatch center to the rescue unit's arrival at the address?

Do you have a single- or tiered-response system?

Does the first responding vehicle have a defibrillator on board and personnel trained to use it?

Does your dispatch center provide telephone CPR instructions?

If "survival" is understood to mean discharge from the hospital, what is your survival rate for cardiac arrest when ventricular fibrillation occurs in the presence of a witness?

If you don't have this information, can you explain to me why you do not?

Thank you for your assistance.

I think that the administrator of the EMS agency would be shocked to receive such a letter. He or she would probably respond as follows:

Dear — —:

Thank you for your letter inquiring about our EMS system. I can assure you that our personnel are highly trained and provide the highest-quality emergency aid and assistance.

To answer your questions, we have a single-tier paramedic-staffed system. All our paramedics are state-certified. All our vehicles have defibrillators, and the paramedics are trained to use them.

We collect response-time data in a way different from the way you requested. I can tell you that our travel time is under ten minutes 75 percent of the time for code red alarms (such as cardiac arrest).

Your inquiry about telephone CPR is difficult to answer because we have given CPR instructions on a case-by-case basis but do not have a formal program.

As for your last question about the survival rate, our program does not routinely collect this information. Our job is to resuscitate the patient and take him or her to the hospital—hopefully, with a pulse and blood pressure. What happens then is up to the doctors.

I hope this answers your questions, and I hope you will consider moving to our community.

Would you be comforted by such a reply? This administrator seems to have missed the point. The letter writer's intention was to find out whether the EMS system kept track of its performance. Unfortunately, this administrator, like 98 percent of other administrators in EMS agencies across the United States, was unable to answer the letter writer's final question: "If 'survival' is understood to mean discharge from the hospital, what is your survival rate for cardiac arrest when ventricular fibrillation occurs in the presence of a witness?" Indeed, there are no national reporting requirements for cardiac arrest.[5] Ideally, however, and at a bare minimum, every community would be reporting and making public two pieces of information: its survival rate for witnessed cardiac arrest involving VF, when "survival" means discharge from a hospital; and the average interval between the first alarm center's receipt of a call and the delivery of the first defibrillatory shock for VF.

A brutal self-assessment is the first step toward improvement. Imagine the world's foremost evaluator of EMS systems paying a visit to your community. What would this expert find? What grade would he or she give your system? How would you stack up against other communities? Admittedly, the report card shown in figure 7.2 is not based on scientific research. There are no studies that rank communities on their survival rates for cardiac arrest, though such studies might be worthwhile. I would be the first to admit that this report card contains subjective criteria. But I think that the criteria do have a basis in common sense, and that they are tinctured with science (for example, there is clear scientific backing for the relationships that have been drawn between intervention times and survival). The report card represents an effort to be as specific as possible, since too much generality would allow every community to score high. For example, every community's EMS system probably has some kind of program for quality improvement, but how many systems have a full-time or even a part-time person dedicated solely to maintaining a cardiac arrest registry? Also, it should be obvious that there is overlap between and among some of the elements in the report card. For example, high rates of bystander CPR are correlated with a shorter average time between the victim's collapse and the initiation of CPR.

All these qualifiers having been noted, let's examine the report card itself, which includes seven categories: medical control, administrative control, dispatch characteristics, system characteristics, training, quality improvement, and community characteristics.[6] The category of medical control includes the most elements, since the medical director is ultimately responsible for the professional behavior of the paramedics. He or she should read every incident report (or at least all critical incidents such as cardiac arrests) and immediately address any problems that are identified. These may be mundane—illegible writing, incomplete data entry, sketchy documentation—or they may involve skill deficits or faulty decision making. For example, the medical director may want to know why a fifty-year-old man with intermittent left-side jaw pain (a possible symptom of angina) was left at home rather than transported to the hospital.[7]

You will undoubtedly find that some of the elements in the report card do not exist in your community's EMS system. When you make this discovery, ask yourself whether

Medical Control

- [ ] At least half-time medical director
- [ ] Medical director supervises no more than 100 paramedics
- [ ] Personaly knows every paramedic
- [ ] Medical director reads every paramedic run report or at a minimum all critical patients
- [ ] Medical director provides feedback directly
- [ ] Medical director measures and corrects skills and professional behavior
- [ ] Medical director appointed by clean, department chair and can only be fired
- [ ] Medical director has an academic appointment (not courtesy appointment)
- [ ] On-line medical control by an emergency department physician or nurse
- [ ] Medical director has authority to decertify or suspend paramedics
- [ ] Medical director has been at position for 5 years or longer (or no more than two years medical directors in past 10 years)

Administrative Control

- [ ] Clear lines of authority for administrative
- [ ] Clearly designates in writing medical direction and medical training to the medical
- [ ] Written agreement with an academic medical center to provide medical control

Dispatch Characteristics

- [ ] Dispatcher assisted telephone CPR program
- [ ] Dispatchers offer CPR instruction in 50% or more of all cardiac arrests
- [ ] Half-time or more person dedicated to reviewing CPR tapes

System Characteristics

- [ ] Tiered response system
- [ ] Average 911 phone pick-up time to onset of CPR less than 4 minutes (3)
- [ ] Avereage 911 phone pick-up time to defibrillatory shock on average 8 minutes
- [ ] Bystander CPR greater than 50% of the time for arrests before arrival
- [ ] Detailed incident report form completed after every event and timely forwarding to administrative agency
- [ ] Rates of paramedic to population to allow skil maintenance : ration of one paramedic per 7500 residents (or fewer)

Training

- [ ] Initial training done in-house
- [ ] Continuing education program for dispatchers, EMTS, and paramedics with mandatory skill requirements
- [ ] Medical director authorizes all medical training

Quality Improvement Program

- [ ] Dedicated staff for cardiac arrest registry. Approximately one FTE person for every million persons in the community.
- [ ] Able to determine the witnessed VF survival rate
- [ ] Available access to hospital discharge information
- [ ] Available access to death certificates
- [ ] Medical program for critical interventons; intubation, central lines
- [ ] Sufficient computer resources and support resources for the medical QI program to succeed

Community Characteristics

- [ ] Tax supported levy or other dedicated source of funding for EMS services
- [ ] Positive attitude toward EMS personnel (good press, lack of lawsuits, drivers pull over in response to sirens, etc)

7.2 Cardiac arrest community report card.

those elements should be included in your system, and how they can be created. Some of these elements represent areas of the system where improvements are easy, and others represent areas where the challenges are considerably greater. Remember, it is not realistic to expect to move overnight from a failing grade to a perfect score. Change is difficult and should be viewed as a continuous process. Scarce resources, cultural impediments, inertia, and complacency are strong inhibitors of change, but change must still be undertaken. EMS personnel are health professionals. As such, they have a duty to their patients to be uncompromising about doing everything possible on their patients' behalf. If the EMS system is failing, then EMS personnel are failing their patients.

Before you can change your EMS system, however, you will need to evaluate it as it is today. The best way to take a snapshot of your system's performance on cardiac arrest is to study ten or twenty or fifty arrests, using data from dispatch centers, EMS providers, and hospitals (assuming that all these entities are willing to provide such information in the interest of assessing the system's performance on critical indices). For example, you may wish to summarize the number of witnessed cardiac arrests in your community, the number of cardiac arrests that involved ventricular fibrillation, the number that involved bystander CPR, and the number in which dispatcher-assisted telephone CPR played a role. You may also want to determine average times between the patient's collapse and CPR, and between collapse and the first defibrillatory shock, and you may want to know how many patients were discharged from the hospital after resuscitation. Then, having completed this audit, you can measure its results against realistic norms and gain an immediate impression of where your system needs to improve.

This chapter has posed the question of what steps a community can take to improve its emergency medical services. The audit that was just proposed is one that is likely to suggest just what those steps should be for a particular system. Be that as it may, I believe that every community should look at how it is providing CPR and defibrillation —the two most critical elements of resuscitation—and rethink both of these components. Every EMS system has its own constellation of history and resources, and it is not realistic to design a new system from scratch. Nevertheless, any community can take at least four concrete steps to speed its delivery of CPR and defibrillation: the institution of an aggressive program of dispatcher-assisted telephone CPR, the adoption of the practice of rapid dispatch, the delivery of defibrillation by police, and the use of public access defibrillation.

EIGHT

A Completed Life

Ruth T. is eighty-five and is on a respirator in the ICU. Two IVs in her arms and one in her neck contain medications to keep her blood pressure up, her heart stable, and her brain from swelling. Her kidneys have failed, and her doctor has talked about dialysis with Ruth's three children, who have flown in from out of town.

Three days ago, at a senior center, Ruth suffered a cardiac arrest and was initially resuscitated by the center's nurse, who used an AED, though further care by EMS personnel was also required.

Ruth's course in the hospital has been stormy, and she has been in a coma since admission. Before the cardiac arrest, her quality of life was already in a tailspin. Her uterine cancer has metastasized to her liver, and the pain, at times sharp, keeps her up half the night. More troublesome to her has been her rheumatoid arthritis—progressive, deforming, and interfering with her everyday activities.

Ruth's doctor has asked her children what their mother would want done if her heart should stop again. The three discuss the matter and can't decide. Apparently Ruth has never spoken with them about her wishes.

HEARTS TOO GOOD TO DIE

One of my research colleagues has definite views about the best way to die. She and I have been studying cardiac arrest for almost thirty years and doing what we can to devise innovative and more effective therapies. Her ironic opinion can be summarized in a few words: "Sudden cardiac arrest—hey, it's a great way to go."

I think many people feel this way. In one respect, my colleague is correct—it is a great way to die. There are no symptoms to deal with (or, if symptoms are present, they are brief), one is spared the indignities of tubes and IVs and the depersonalization of the hospital ICU, there is no gradual loss of mental and physical faculties, and, perhaps most important of all, there is neither pain nor suffering. Her views, of course, don't take into account the lost opportunity for final good-byes and death preparations. This is a separate issue, and one that is irresolvable, since many people, I suspect, would prefer a quick and painless death, but just as many might prefer a slow and painless death over a period of weeks and months, with the opportunity for final partings. Apart from the question of last farewells, however, there actually is a strong case to be made for sudden death, unless—and here comes the punch line—the death is unexpected.

Most of the time, sudden death comes to someone who is living independently at home. The death is completely unexpected. If it had been expected, the person would already have been under observation in the hospital, or with family members. Sudden cardiac arrest is usually death that appears to come before its time—death that occurs too early. Dr. Claude Beck, one of the inventors of defibrillation, summarized this concept nearly fifty years ago, when he defined sudden cardiac arrest as occurring in "hearts too good to die."[1] Beck's phrase captures the essence of sudden cardiac arrest—a heart that is basically fine suddenly fibrillates. If the fibrillation can be reversed, the heart will have years left to beat. Beck lived before our modern era of personal computers, but if he were alive today he might liken a fibrillating heart to a computer that has frozen up because of an errant electrical signal, which can be corrected if the machine is simply rebooted.

Despite, or perhaps because of, the advances in resuscitation, many people today are pondering a fundamental ethical question: Is resuscitation worth it, or does it merely prolong a life already spent? There is much validity to the concept of a completed life. A life lived fully—with satisfying personal accomplishments, education, companionship, fulfilling work, friends, children, grandchildren—need not be artificially prolonged. Then there is the issue of dying with dignity. Spending one's last days and hours of life ignominiously attached to a respirator, an ECG monitor, an arterial pressure monitor, a pulse oximeter, intravenous lines, and a catheter for bladder drainage strikes most people as nightmarish. Added to these indignities are the staggering hospital and doctor bills. Even more awful is the possibility of suffering mental or physical incapacitation and yet being forced, thanks to the miracles of modern medicine, to endure months or even years of a life that is far less than whole and dignified.

Even many of those involved in the quest to reverse sudden death have questioned whether resuscitation is worthwhile. Peter Safar, one of the early founders of modern CPR, asks whether resuscitation is "socially, morally, and economically justified" or whether it is instead "an antievolutionary undertaking." Here is how Safar answers his own question:

Resuscitation applied without judgment and compassion is morally and economically unacceptable. The debilitated, elderly patient or the otherwise
terminally ill patient with incurable disease, particularly the one with irreversible coma or stupor, should be permitted to die without the imposition
of costly and often dehumanizing efforts. [And yet those who die] from
potentially reversible conditions imposed by the arbitrary mischances of
Nature, before they have had time to live full lives, should receive the benefits of emergency resuscitation . . . if there is a chance that life with human
mentation can possibly be restored.[2]

Safar's statement highlights two key concepts involved in the question of resuscitation from sudden death—the death's reversibility and its prematurity. Most men and
women in their fifties, sixties, and seventies, and many in their eighties and even in
their nineties, are hardly willing to call their lives biologically or psychologically completed. Sudden and unexpected death typically occurs in "hearts too good to die" and
in people with uncompleted lives. Sudden death from ventricular fibrillation can be
reversed if the VF is treated in a timely fashion, and the fact that sudden death is often
premature is what justifies communities' massive investments in resources devoted to
emergency medical services and resuscitation.

Of course, we also deal with the opposite situation—not all resuscitations are
attempted on behalf of hearts too good to die. Richard Cummins, professor of medicine
at the University of Washington, refers to the dilemma of resuscitation targeting
"hearts too sick to live."[3] A team of EMTs and paramedics at the scene of a cardiac
arrest cannot instantly determine who should be resuscitated and who should be quietly allowed to die. Emergency medical personnel are trained to swoop down with a
full-court press on everyone they encounter in cardiac arrest. Occasionally it is obvious that resuscitation would be futile and perhaps cruel; perhaps a person with
advanced terminal cancer should not be resuscitated. But when paramedics arrive at
the scene, it is not usually clear to them what the underlying situation is. Their only
option is to resuscitate. And when they do, sometimes a heart too sick to live is brought
back to life. The person whose life has been saved may already have extensive prior
brain damage from underlying disease but must now face a long and expensive hospitalization. This is hardly what anyone would think of as a successful resuscitation.

Even when a heart is too good to die, a difficult or delayed resuscitation may leave
residual and irreversible brain damage due to oxygen deprivation. Mercifully, this kind
of brain damage, if it is severe enough, usually leads to death within days of the
patient's admission to the hospital. But not always. Sometimes the damage, though
severe, turns out to be still compatible with life, and as a result an enormous burden
is placed on the patient, the family, and society.

It would be ideal to begin every resuscitation with the belief that success will be total and that the patient will fully recover. And this is generally what happens when care is provided rapidly. But when care to a good heart is delayed, or simply when care is provided to a sick heart, the outcome after resuscitation may not be optimal. There is a reality to resuscitation that cannot be ignored—it has a bright side and dark side. The bright side is bright indeed. People with lives still very much worth living are brought back from the abyss of death. Two-thirds of survivors of ventricular fibrillation return to their previous lives with little or no impairment from the cardiac arrest.[4] The dark side encompasses a spectrum ranging from shades of gray all the way to black. At the gray end is the fact that one-quarter of survivors have moderate to severe impairment after resuscitation. While these people can usually return home, they often have memory deficits and other cognitive problems.[5] At the black end of the spectrum are the worst outcomes. Approximately 5 percent of cardiac arrest survivors have significant problems after resuscitation and require extended nursing or medical care.

This is the current reality, and we must not deny it. Our challenge is to increase the number of people who make a full recovery. And yet there will always be some survivors with poor outcomes. While a successful resuscitation is going on, or immediately afterward, it is not possible to predict that the patient will or will not fully recover. There are too many unknown and unmeasurable variables—the patient's underlying conditions, the exact intervals between the cardiac arrest and the start of CPR and defibrillation, the rapidity with which full circulation was restored, and so on. And it follows that, without any means of predicting precisely who will fully recover and who will not, there is no possible basis for withholding care or merely going through a "show" resuscitation.[6] On the contrary, once emergency help has been summoned, the patient in cardiac arrest deserves a resuscitation attempt, without exception, unless there is a clear and unambiguous living will that indicates the patient's request not to be resuscitated.[7] With the ability to perform successful resuscitations comes the certainty that some of these efforts will fail, but this is the price that we as a society must pay.

RESUSCITATION AND COMPASSION

Sylvia Feder, a paramedic for South King County Medic One, has repeatedly helped snatch life from the jaws of death for people who went on to live for many years and enjoyed a high quality of life. She would be the first to agree that there can be nothing more gratifying than reviving someone whose life is not yet complete. But Feder has also seen too many attempts to resuscitate people whose lives were already at an end—people with terminal diseases, people whose bodies were wasted and whose minds were numbed by their slow exit from life, people with no further chance to have anything resembling a normal life. Feder believes that it is wrong to attempt to resuscitate someone who has reached the end of life. Death is, after all, life's natural end. Performing such an act violates patients' autonomy (assuming they have chosen not to have resuscitation attempted) and robs them of their dignity. How many of us would choose to have our last moments invaded with endotracheal tubes, monitors, IV lines, oxygen masks, and burly firefighters and paramedics hovering over us and keeping family members away?

Feder and a fellow paramedic, Roger Matheny, decided to take action. With the support of their program's medical director, Jack Murray, they decided to create new guidelines for end-of-life decisions. These new guidelines allow EMTs not to begin a resuscitation when the following conditions are met:

1. The patient is in the end stage of a terminal disease.
2. Family members or caregivers, in the absence of a written DNR order, verbally inform the EMTs that the patient's wish is not to be resuscitated.

Both conditions must be met and if there is any uncertainty or disagreement among family members, the EMTs are to begin resuscitation.

Feder and Matheny describe their guidelines in terms of "withholding resuscitation for compelling reasons," the compelling reasons being that the patient is already terminally ill and that the patient's wishes must be respected. Before these new guidelines were adopted, EMTs in King County—and, for that matter, throughout the rest of the country—were required to initiate resuscitation efforts for almost anyone they found to be in cardiac arrest.[8] And yet, as Feder had seen too many times, families call 911 not necessarily because they want a loved one to be resuscitated but simply because they don't know what else to do. ("How can we be sure he is dead?" "What do we do with his body? Who will come and get it?" "Must Grandpa be taken to a hospital to be declared dead?") That is unfortunate, because the EMS system is incapable of graded responses—its only settings, so to speak, are to be switched all the way on or all the way off; resuscitate first, and ask questions later. And, regrettably, many patients who are near or at the last breath can sometimes respond just enough to pharmacological stimulation to get a pulse back. Then they are transported to a hospital, where indignity upon indignity is piled on. What could have been a peaceful death at home, with family members standing by, ends up becoming a depersonalized and depersonalizing spectacle that unfolds in a sterile environment, often with doctors and nurses looking on and wondering why the patient was brought to the hospital in the first place. Not a pretty scene. Not the way I wish to leave this earth.

Now, with these new guidelines, EMTs are empowered to honor the verbal wishes of patients' family members. Everyone wins—the patient dies with dignity, the family sees that the loved one's wishes are fulfilled, and the EMTs can help the family deal with such end-of-life issues as funeral arrangements instead of attempting a heroic but futile resuscitation. In addition to devising these new guidelines, Feder and Matheny trained hundreds of EMTs in King County in their proper application. For example, "do not resuscitate" does not mean "do not care." Sometimes a dying patient is in pain, or is choking on secretions, and a paramedic can provide needed pain medication or suctioning.

In 2006, after measuring the impact of their guidelines, Feder and Matheny and two colleagues published their findings in the *Annals of Internal Medicine*.[9] (Theirs is probably the only article in that prestigious journal ever to have been coauthored by two paramedics.) They found that since the adoption of the new guidelines, resuscitation had been withheld from 12 percent of patients in cardiac arrest, by comparison with 5 percent in three historical and contemporary control groups. And use of the new guidelines to honor family members' verbal requests had accounted for more than 50 percent of those withheld resuscitations, by comparison with 8 percent of withheld resuscitations in the control groups. Compassionate withholding of resuscitation for compelling reasons is now standard protocol for every fire department and paramedic agency in King County, and this practice is spreading throughout the country.

A BETTER WAY: OPEN DISCUSSION AND COMMUNICATION

But a conundrum remains. When should the reversal of sudden death be attempted? Ultimately, the answer to this question is a very personal one, and each of us must decide for ourselves before a decision is needed, since we cannot make our wishes known once we're in cardiac arrest. Most of us, I believe, if our hearts were basically healthy, would wish to be resuscitated from ventricular fibrillation. But would we wish to be defibrillated if we had an underlying terminal condition like Alzheimer's disease or advanced cancer? In this case, the answer becomes less straightforward. The point is, I cannot know what you want. I cannot tell what value you place on a few extra days or months of life. I cannot tell how you assess your quality of life. And if I have no information about what you want, my obligation is to call 911 and initiate CPR.

My mother died of Alzheimer's. I knew that she did not want to be resuscitated, and I would have known this even if she had not confirmed it with a living will. When she stopped breathing, it would have been cruel to call the paramedics in order to buy her a few more days or weeks of life. My father died of a cardiac arrest. I suspect, though I cannot know, that he was in ventricular fibrillation, but his collapse was unwitnessed, so there was no chance of resuscitation even though paramedics were called to the scene. Would my father have wanted to be resuscitated? He was a vigorous and sharp eighty-two-year-old man, but he also had early prostate cancer as well as fairly bothersome arthritis, and his short-term memory was starting to fail. Though I believe he still had several more good years ahead, I don't know if he wanted to be resuscitated. I simply never asked. The point is moot now, but I wish I had. We should have no inhibition about discussing people's wishes regarding resuscitation. The wisdom of living wills is widely accepted, but these documents are generally relevant only to what happens in hospitals, and there is too little discussion about what happens

Physician Orders for Life-Sustaining Treatment (POLST)

Follow these orders until orders change. These medical orders are based on the patient's **current** medical condition and preferences. Any section not completed does not invalidate the form and implies full treatment for that section. With significant change of condition new orders may need to be written. *Guidance for Health Care Professionals.* http://www.ohsu.edu/polst/programs/documents/Guidebook.pdf.

Patient Last Name:	Patient First Name	Middle Int.
Date of Birth: (mm/dd/yyyy)	Gender: ☐ M ☐ F	Last 4 SSN: ☐☐☐☐
Address: (street / city / state / zip)		

A Check One	**CARDIOPULMONARY RESUSCITATION (CPR):** *Patient has no pulse __and__ is not breathing.*
	☐ **Attempt Resuscitation/CPR**
	☐ **Do Not Attempt Resuscitation/DNR**
	When not in cardiopulmonary arrest, follow orders in **B** and **C**.

B Check One	**MEDICAL INTERVENTIONS:** *If patient has pulse and/__or__ is breathing.*
	☐ **Comfort Measures Only** (__A__llow __N__atural __D__eath). Relieve pain and suffering through the use of any medication by any route, positioning, wound care and other measures. Use oxygen, suction and manual treatment of airway obstruction as needed for comfort. *Patient prefers no transfer to hospital for life-sustaining treatments. Transfer if comfort needs cannot be met in current location.* **Treatment Plan: Maximize comfort through symptom management.**
	☐ **Limited Additional Interventions** In addition to care described in Comfort Measures Only, use medical treatment, antibiotics, IV fluids and cardiac monitor as indicated. No intubation, advanced airway interventions, or mechanical ventilation. May consider less invasive airway support (e.g. CPAP, BiPAP). *Transfer to hospital if indicated. Generally avoid the intensive care unit.* **Treatment Plan: Provide basic medical treatments.**
	☐ **Full Treatment** In addition to care described in Comfort Measures Only and Limited Additional Interventions, use intubation, advanced airway interventions, and mechanical ventilation as indicated. *Transfer to hospital and/or intensive care unit if indicated.* **Treatment Plan: Full treatment including life support measures in the intensive care unit.**
	Additional Orders: _____

C Check One	**ARTIFICIALLY ADMINISTERED NUTRITION:** *Offer food by mouth if feasible.*
	☐ No artificial nutrition by tube. *Additional Orders:*_____
	☐ Defined trial period of artificial nutrition by tube. _____
	☐ Long-term artificial nutrition by tube. _____

D	**DOCUMENTATION OF DISCUSSION:**
	☐ Patient (Patient has capacity) ☐ Health Care Representative or legally recognized surrogate
	☐ Parent of minor ☐ Surrogate for patient with developmental disabilities or significant mental health condition (Note: Special requirements for completion. See reverse side.)
	☐ Court-Appointed Guardian ☐ Other_____

Signature of Patient or Surrogate

Signature: *recommended*	Name (print):	Relationship (write "self" if patient):

This form will be sent to the POLST Registry unless the patient wishes to opt out, if so check opt out box ☐

E	**SIGNATURE OF PHYSICIAN / NP/ PA**
	My signature below indicates to the best of my knowledge that these orders are consistent with the patient's **current** medical condition and preferences.
	Print Signing Physician / NP / PA Name: *required* Signer Phone Number: Signer License Number: *(optional)*
	Physician / NP / PA Signature: *required* Date: *required* Office Use Only

© CENTER FOR ETHICS IN HEALTH CARE, Oregon Health & Science University, 3181 Sam Jackson Park Rd, UHN-86, Portland, OR 97239-3098 (503) 494-3965

8.1 POLST form, Center for Ethics in Health Care, Oregon Science & Health University.

before the hospital comes into the picture. The reality remains that sudden cardiac arrest is the leading cause of death among adults in Western countries. Let your spouse or your friends or your family know what you would want when it comes to resuscitation. I'd rather not decide for you.

The easiest and clearest way of letting your relatives and friends know your wishes is to draw up an advance directive, a legal document that allows you to indicate your wishes about medical care in the event that you are unable to communicate. Advance directives can be obtained from many sources—hospitals, state health departments, office supply stores, Web sites. One popular advance directive can be found at the Web site of the nonprofit group called Aging with Dignity (www.agingwithdignity.org). This organization provides, at minimal cost, a user-friendly advance directive known as *Five Wishes*. This document, developed with grant support from the Robert Wood Johnson Foundation, affords you the opportunity to state your wishes for who you want to make care decisions for you, the kind of medical care you wish to have, how comfortable you wish to be, how you wish to be treated by others, and what you want your loved ones to know about you. The document is now recognized as a valid advance directive by forty states. Another document recognized by many states is the *Physician Orders for Life-Sustaining Treatment (POLST) Paradigm to Improve End-of-Life Care*, available at no cost from www.ohsu.edu/polst. *POLST* is a two-page form that allows you to indicate your wishes regarding CPR, medical interventions, antibiotics, and artificial nutrition (see fig. 8.1). It is signed by you (or your surrogate) and by your physician. The attractive thing about the *POLST* form is that it stays with you, regardless of whether you move from home to the hospital or to a long-term-care facility, and there is no need for you to complete the form all over again every time you move. *POLST* can supplement an advance directive, or it can serve the function of an advance directive in states where the POLST paradigm is accepted.[10] Even if you do not complete an advance directive or *POLST* form, you can at least verbally express your wishes for end-of-life care to family members. This is better than being silent on the subject and leaving family members to guess your desires.

But there is another answer to the question of whether resuscitation is worthwhile. Although it is true that only a very few of the many millions of people in our society will ever actually be resuscitated, we must also acknowledge a greater truth—that the effort of resuscitation is ennobling. The effort to resuscitate reveals much about our society's values, not the least of which is that we have reverence for human life. As Peter Safar so eloquently wrote of resuscitation, "Its moral impact and the commitment it represents may have a much broader influence in a world where life has too often been regarded as cheap." Resuscitation is ultimately a life-affirming act. "Medicine imposes compassion, reason, and decency on a random universe," says Safer. "Thus an increasingly individual-oriented society makes resuscitation evolutionarily positive—it implies a commitment on the side of Life."[11]

NINE

Putting It All Together

The core programs are those that make the chain of survival happen quickly and with high fidelity. Examples are rapid dispatch, dispatcher-assisted CPR, high-performance CPR, and quick defibrillation. But the chain of survival must be embedded in a frame of survival, which supports and nourishes it. This frame is comprised of leadership, training, quality improvement, and a culture of excellence. Put them all together and you have one helluva EMS system.

DR. TOM REA, speaking at
the Resuscitation Academy,
March 12, 2012

Why do some communities succeed in treating cardiac arrest while others fail? It would be convenient if one variable could explain the wide difference in survival rates for cardiac arrest between those U.S. communities that are most successful in treating this major public health problem and those that are least successful. But that would imply an easy fix, or at least a clarity of direction about what needs to change. Regrettably, there is no single variable and no easy fix. Instead, there are multiple variables, each important in itself but insufficient as a single explanation. What we do know is that successful treatment of ventricular fibrillation is associated with an EMS system's ability to deliver care quickly. As we saw in chapter 7, the chain of survival, with its four links—early access, early CPR, early defibrillation, and early advanced care—illustrates the most critical elements of addressing sudden cardiac arrest. Because of the reasonably good scientific evidence showing that hypothermia improves survival,

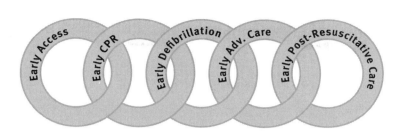

9.1 The chain of survival

I think it appropriate to expand the chain of survival to include post resuscitative care—namely, hypothermia[1] (see fig. 9.1).

Chapter 5 lists fifty factors—patient, event, system, and therapy factors—associated with surviving cardiac arrest (refer to table 5.1). The patient factors and the event factors, although undoubtedly important in determining who will live and who will die, cannot be altered by changes made to an EMS program or to the types of therapy it delivers. They are powerful contributors to survival, but they are factors of fate—of good or bad luck. But the system factors and the therapy factors can all be affected by a community's decisions. The chain of survival describes the key system and therapy factors that insure rapid delivery of care. These include time to CPR, quality of CPR, time to defibrillation, interaction of CPR and defibrillation, dispatcher-assisted CPR (synonymous terms are telephone CPR, dispatcher CPR, and dispatcher-assisted telephone CPR), community CPR training, public access defibrillation, and hypothermia.

QUANTITATIVE FACTORS: THE CHAIN OF SURVIVAL

The system and therapy factors that comprise the links in the chain of survival are quantitative in nature, meaning they have a specific value and can be measured. Some are time related (time to CPR, time to defibrillation); others can be measured by their presence (dispatcher-assisted CPR, community CPR training, community PAD, hypothermia); and two can be scored (quality of CPR can be determined by compressions per minute of CPR and duration of pauses, and the interaction of CPR and defibrillation can be determined by the duration of pauses before and after defibrillation). All can be measured in one way or another.

Does this mean that a community merely has to put these system and therapy factors in place in order to see its rate of survival rise? It would certainly be convenient if this were the key to understanding the disparity in cardiac arrest survival, but, although one can measure these factors, they do not fully explain a system's success or lack thereof. Every community's EMS system already incorporates some if not all of them—at least to some degree—but even these factors, as necessary as they are, are not sufficient. After all, a baseball team can field nine players but still lose every game. What else, then, is needed?

QUALITATIVE FACTORS: THE FRAME OF SURVIVAL

What are needed are the qualitative factors that contribute to a system's success. These factors are far more difficult to measure or score; though lacking in hard numbers, they are just as or more important than the hard metrics. The links in the chain cannot stay connected unless they are embedded in a context of strong medical and administrative leadership, continuous medical QI, a culture of excellence, and stellar training and continuing education for dispatchers, EMTs, and paramedics (see fig. 9.2). These four elements literally frame, surround, and embed the core links of care.

I call this concept the frame of survival. Together, the chain of survival and the frame of survival form a complete and comprehensive system of care. Together, they nurture, sustain, and define a high-quality EMS system. Just as important to the success of a champion baseball team that starts with nine excellent players are sustained practice, superb managing and coaching, continuous review and fine-tuning, and team spirit. In sum, the frame surrounding the chain of survival can be reduced to a single word—accountability. It is accountability, achieved through leadership, quality improvement, training, and excellence, that holds the chain of survival in place and ensures that its links are as strong as they need to be. An EMS system that cannot be accountable to the citizens it serves will at best be mediocre.

The elements comprising the frame are far more difficult to measure than those inside the frame. As opposed to the quantitative chain of survival the frame is purely

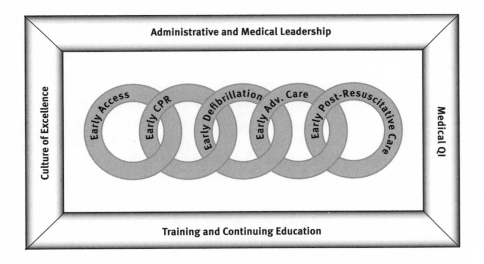

9.2 Frame of survival surrounding the chain of survivall

qualitative. I would be the first to admit that qualitative elements like leadership, culture of excellence, and accountability are "softer" and less scientific than the quantitative tools that directly contribute to the chain of survival. Nevertheless, I believe that qualitative elements are the keys to success in managing cardiac arrest involving VF, and that their relative absence is the reason why some EMS systems fail.[2] It also occurs to me that the frame of survival embodies the characteristics of Drs. Cobb and Copass in Seattle, Drs. Rea and Kudenchuk in King County, Washington, and Dr. White in Rochester, Minnesota. These individuals are natural leaders who can instill in their organizations their vision of high expectations and relentless striving for excellence. They also continuously ask the question, How can the system be improved? Ongoing quality improvement (QI) is the mechanism by which they know where and how to improve. And training and continuing education are the vehicles by which expertise and professionalism are brought to every cardiac arrest.

PUBLIC EXPECTATIONS

Is there a public expectation for high-quality emergency medical services? Before you answer "Of course," consider the evidence. The average citizen of the average city has no idea what his or her community's EMS system's performance is, as measured by survival rates for cardiac arrest. Furthermore, the average citizen has no idea how his or her community's EMS system works, or who provides the services. Are the services contracted? Are they public? Does the EMS program use a tiered-response system? Are the first-in personnel EMTs or paramedics? Who is the medical director? Is there an academic connection? Is there a cardiac arrest registry? Is there assertive dispatcher-assisted CPR? These and countless other questions would never enter the mind of the average citizen. For most people, the local EMS system, whatever it is, seems to work—dial 911, and several minutes later one or more vehicles arrive to whisk the patient off to the hospital. But what if concerned citizens in Detroit realized that virtually no one survives cardiac arrest in the Motor City? What if concerned citizens in New York, Chicago, and Los Angeles realized that very few survive in those cities? What if citizens everywhere understood that most communities, their own included, don't track survival rates for cardiac arrest? How can a problem be fixed if it can't be measured? How will the problem even be revealed?

Nothing will change if the status quo continues to be tolerated. And the status quo in virtually every community is indifference combined with insufficient data—a powerful duo on the side of inaction. If there is to be improvement, one or two or ten or fifty motivated individuals must want the situation to change. The catalyst will probably vary from community to community. It may come from an external group or organization, or it may come from within the EMS system or from the political structure of the community. In some communities, a citizens group or a civic action group may take the lead, or a group of physicians may agitate for change. Coalitions may take shape among the local medical society, the chamber of commerce, health care organizations, chapters of the American Heart Association or the Red Cross, local newspapers or TV stations. Their united voices, especially on behalf of a mission as clearly and widely accepted as improving the community's survival rates for cardiac arrest, can go a long way toward prompting politicians to review the community's EMS services and create an action plan for their improvement.

Community awareness of the incidence of cardiac arrest is an important component of any improvement campaign, but cardiac arrest often falls below the threshold for media attention. After all, cardiac arrest happens to ordinary people, often at home, away from the spotlight. Consider a community of one million residents. In any one year, there will probably be a thousand out-of-hospital cardiac arrests treated by EMS, or about three per day. In response to most of these events, EMS vehicles will rush with lights flashing and sirens wailing to the home of the victim, and EMS personnel will attempt resuscitation. Their efforts are likely to be unsuccessful, however, and the EMS units will quietly drive away. Only later will the victim's neighbors learn of the death. An event that unfolds slowly over time and space doesn't compel media attention in the way that a dramatic explosion or a fatal automobile crash does.

But why should a sudden cardiac arrest be less newsworthy than a fire or an explosion or a car crash or a shooting? Is it the lack of blood? (Recall the old newsroom adage "If it bleeds, it leads.") Is it lack of media access to the scene of the attempted resuscitation? Is it a matter of privacy? Is it because most victims are older? Whatever the reasons why cardiac arrest is not considered newsworthy, I think there is a "hook" to focus media attention. A news media (newspaper, television, or local website) might conduct an investigation to determine the survival rate in its community. The reporter will likely discover how difficult those survival statistics are to find and, assuming they can be determined, how poorly the reporter's own community compares to other communities. That's Part One of the investigative report. Part Two could be what "best practices" the community does or does not have in place. A cardiac arrest registry? Assertive dispatcher-assisted CPR? High-performance CPR? Rapid dispatch? Detailed review of every cardiac arrest? Feedback to EMTs and paramedics? Voice recording of the event? And so on. And Part Three could be a prescription for improvement.

When it comes to impeding change, misperception can be as significant as indifference. For example, people may believe that most attempted resuscitations are successful. This is certainly the impression that the entertainment media give. One study of the cardiac arrests portrayed on television found that only 28 percent were depicted as being due to cardiac causes; most were shown as occurring in children or young adults, and 67 percent of the fictional victims survived to be discharged from the hospital.[3] So, what's the problem, if most resuscitation attempts are successful? This kind of misperception calls for a reality check. Regardless of the type of campaign for change that a community group mounts, a big dose of reality will be needed to contradict the misinformation spawned by the entertainment industry.

It is probable that most people also view cardiac arrest fatalistically—sure, there are all those dramatic saves in the movies and on TV, but for the rest of us cardiac arrest is simply the end. This is certainly true for cardiac arrest associated with asystole and pulseless electrical activity (PEA). What is not appreciated, however, is the good prognosis for ventricular fibrillation. When VF is treated quickly, the prognosis is very favorable. A cardiologist once joked that VF is a benign rhythm, "benign" meaning trivial and easy to treat. Apart from the fact that VF leads to sudden death, he was correct in his characterization—VF is an easily treated condition. If EMS systems began to view VF as a condition with an excellent prognosis, they would both celebrate their successes and investigate every death. Why did the death occur? What could have been done to prevent it?

SERVICE OR LIP SERVICE?

A community's EMS agency, when approached by the media or by a civic organization seeking information or even by an inquisitive citizen, may well be defensive. Officials will often cite figures showing that the agency meets standards for timely response. They may say that the agency has and employs all the latest equipment and trot out sheaves of written protocols and training curricula. But the real question is whether the system saves lives or not. It will be a challenge to determine whether it does, since most EMS systems cannot honestly or definitively answer that question. Here is where an unbiased third party may have something to offer. A medical school or university can provide the names of experts for consultation or the National Association of EMS Physicians might suggest consultants.

Change agents need not come from outside the EMS system. The medical director, paramedics or EMTs, the administrative director, the mayor, the city council—any of these parties, regardless of their official roles, can take the lead to improve the system. For example, the medical director can unilaterally form an advisory group, create a cardiac arrest registry, rewrite the protocols for cardiac arrest, partner with an academic medical center, establish requirements for training and continuing education, obtain follow-up information on patients, and provide feedback to EMTs and paramedics. A simple first step is to ask "Why did this patient with witnessed VF not survive?" Detailed answers are likely to facilitate a local action plan leading to improvement.

Paramedics and EMTs can work to record times and interventions accurately, improve teamwork, train in high-performance CPR, synchronize AEDs with dispatch centers, suggest ways to speed up response times, and collaborate with dispatch centers to institute rapid dispatch. The administrative director and the medical director can work together to revamp the protocols for dispatcher-assisted CPR. The mayor or the city council can mandate a QI program for cardiac arrest, increase the extent of medical control, and synchronize the operations of the dispatch center with those of the EMS agency. There is no limit to what can be accomplished by motivated individuals working within an organization.

Changing an organization's culture is hard work. I would be naive to think that you, the reader of this chapter, could simply shout "Eureka!" and then instantly set about implementing radical changes in your organization. Nevertheless, whatever your role in your EMS system, you can take or contribute to some relatively resource-light actions that are likely to raise your community's survival rate for cardiac arrest—actions whose short-term dividends can encourage and reinforce the will to engage in longer-term, more difficult change efforts.

THE WILL AND THE WAY

In chapter 10, I will provide a game plan with 15 specific steps (10 of which are local and 5 national) to achieve improvements in both the chain and the frame of survival. It takes determination to incorporate these steps into an existing EMS system. Some individual or some group needs to want it to happen. But change can occur, and survival rates for cardiac arrest can improve. Two hundred and fifty years ago, community leaders in Amsterdam decided to improve survival rates for drowning, the sudden death of their time, and they established the world's first rescue society. But resuscitation science was primitive and therapy was not very effective; the leaders of Amsterdam had the will for resuscitation but not the way. The sudden death of our time is cardiac arrest due to heart disease. Science has made great strides, and therapy can be effective. We now have the way; all we need is the will.[4]

TEN

A Plan of Action

Email sent to me:

Dear Dr. Eisenberg: I am a captain in the Cobb City Fire Department and responsible for EMS training and supervision. I plan to visit Seattle next month on my way to a conference in Vancouver, BC, and hope I can visit and ride with your paramedics for a day. I would like to learn all about your program and how it works so I can apply some of what I learn to my own system. And if you have time, I hope we can meet.

Thanks,
Captain David Daniel

My reply:

Dear Captain Daniel: You are welcome to visit. Let me know the date and time you will be available. Though you will undoubtedly learn something about our system, I think a more profitable use of your time would be to attend an upcoming Resuscitation Academy. Better yet, send a small team from your department—maybe you can convince the Chief and Medical Director to join you. The Academy's goal is to provide EMS leaders with the knowledge, skills, and tools to improve cardiac arrest survival in their communities. Though each community and EMS system is unique there are specific programs, which we believe can work in every EMS system and that when put in play will likely improve survival. Check out the next Academy class at resuscitationacademy.org. I hope we will have a chance to meet.

Best,
Mickey

Is it possible to change an EMS system in fundamental ways? Can a community's survival rate for cardiac arrest be dramatically and permanently improved? Is it possible to change not only a system's culture but also its entire structure? I believe that the answer to these questions is an emphatic Yes.

This chapter outlines an action plan to improve community cardiac arrest survival rates. The plan consists of 15 specific steps. The first 10 steps are for local implementation and are grouped by difficulty. There are 4 steps that are relatively easy and do not require much in the way of resources. These may be considered the low-hanging fruit. There are 6 steps that are more difficult and require modest to considerable equipment or resources—the higher-hanging fruit. It is unrealistic to presume that all 10 local steps can be implemented in any given community; an EMS director and medical director have to decide what is doable locally. Last, there are 5 steps requiring implementation at the national level. All the recommended steps are based on the fact that real change requires addressing quantitative as well as qualitative factors. The total picture must entail the chain of survival as well as the frame of survival. The chapter closes with some thoughts on how to implement change.

Table 10.1 An Action Plan of 15 Steps to Improve Survival

Easy steps (the low-hanging fruit)
- Cardiac arrest registry
- Dispatcher-assisted CPR: Training, implementation, and QI
- High-performance CPR: Training, implementation, and QI
- Rapid dispatch

More difficult steps (the higher-hanging fruit)
- Voice record all attempted resuscitation
- Police defibrillation
- Public access defibrillation.
- Local foundation for training and QI
- Hypothermia
- Culture of excellence

National initiatives to improve survival
- National lead agency for prehospital emergency care
- National reporting of cardiac arrest
- National performance standards for cardiac arrest care
- Institute of Resuscitation Research within the National Institutes of Health
- Guidelines for compassionate withholding of resuscitation

Let me offer a disclaimer at the outset. The recommendations put forward in this chapter cannot simply be used as a template and applied to any emergency medical system. Every community has its own constellation of resources, history, culture, and personalities. Indeed, this variety, which makes every EMS system unique, is a strength, offering a crucible for new ideas and new programs, which is why every community can become a source of innovation as well as a testing ground for new ideas. In my role as medical director for King County Emergency Medical Services, I meet every year with all the other county EMS medical directors in Washington State, and I never cease to be amazed by the diverse challenges that my colleagues face. That's one reason why I don't make any suggestions here with the expectation that they must or even can be easily adopted. In fact, I am acutely aware that for some communities implementing even one of the recommendations offered here may prove challenging.

A PLAN OF ACTION: STARTING WITH THE LOW-HANGING FRUIT

The attendees at the Resuscitation Academy, by the end of the two-day training course, are fired up to return home and begin to make changes. It is clear that they are bursting with ideas big and small for their home communities. What should they tackle first? What will give the biggest bang for the buck? We (meaning the faculty) tell them to pick the low-hanging fruit first. Our advice is to reach for the largest, tastiest, juiciest, and closest pear before climbing the tree. Get some success under your belt and keep plugging away, small step by small step, until there is a culture of change allowing one to pick some of the higher-hanging fruit. The steps that can achieve the most are (1) to establish a cardiac arrest registry, (2) to begin a program in high-performance CPR, (3) to begin a program in dispatcher-assisted CPR, and (4) to begin rapid dispatch.

These steps are neither complicated nor costly, but they are not without challenges. Three of them require ongoing QI if they are to reach their potential. High-performance CPR, dispatcher-assisted CPR, and rapid dispatch all require continuous maintenance and nurturing. To do otherwise would be like planting a vineyard and assuming it would do fine without watering and pruning. Programs without constant QI and ongoing training will result at best in mediocre and lackluster performance and at worst in no improvement at all.

Table 10.2 Easy Steps to Improve Cardiac Arrest Survival: The Low-Hanging Fruit

STEP 1. Create a cardiac arrest registry

STEP 2. Implement dispatcher-assisted CPR with ongoing training and QI

STEP 3. Implement high-performance CPR with ongoing training and QI

STEP 4. Implement rapid dispatch

Step 1. Create a Cardiac Arrest Registry

A cardiac arrest registry is the first step to improving survival. It is the essence of measurement. One of the mantras at the Resuscitation Academy is "measure, improve, measure, improve," encapsulating the concept of documenting (measuring) cardiac arrest events and only then implementing changes for improvement. In turn, continued measurement will determine if the improvement has had an effect and will identify further steps. And so on. I venture to say it is the most important mantra of the Academy since it pithily describes the bedrock upon which all programmatic change springs forth.

A registry is a means of taking the entire EMS system's temperature—if cardiac arrest is well managed, it's more than likely that all other conditions will be well managed, too. In this sense, cardiac arrest stands for the whole system. A registry measures more than whether the patient lives or dies but all aspects related to the care. Was bystander CPR performed? Did the dispatcher provide telephone CPR instructions? How good was the EMT CPR? Were there unacceptable pauses in CPR? Did the paramedics intubate successfully? Given enough cardiac arrests, a profile begins to emerge of where the system is succeeding and where it is failing. This information then informs the specific elements that need improvement.

The cardiac arrest registry's efforts must be viewed as a core function, and the registry itself must not be threatened with funding cuts or elimination during lean times. It must have sufficient resources and the full support of the medical and administrative directors. Necessary resources include staff time for gathering information from run reports (electronic or paper), dispatch center reports, AED recordings, hospital records, and, ideally, death certificates. Clearly, a small community will not have the volume of events to justify full-time dedicated staff, but several small communities can join together to establish a registry at the county or regional level.

Investigators from Emory University, with funding from the Centers for Disease Control and Prevention, have established a national cardiac arrest registry—the Cardiac Arrest Registry to Enhance Survival (CARES – mycares.net).[1] The registry is open to EMS systems throughout the nation. As of 2012 there were 50 communities from 17 states participating plus 5 entire statewide EMS programs. The registry entails having the EMS system and local hospitals submit data via a Web-based system. CARES overcomes a major obstacle in most well-intentioned registries, namely obtaining outcome data from hospitals.[2] Did the patient live or die and what was the neurological condition on discharge? The CARES project is based on voluntary participation, and all the participants receive summaries of their own community as well as a national summary.

CARES can be customized for the needs of the local community. CARES also provides templates so communities can review their statistics sliced and diced in any way they

Utstein Survival Report

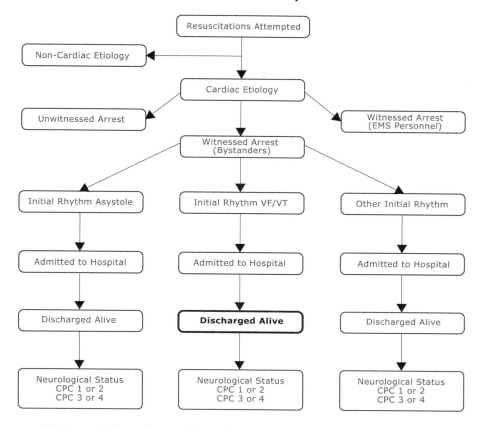

10.1 Utstein survival report for reporting cardiac arrest survival (also known as the Utstein Template). The main metric is "discharged alive" survival from bystander witnessed cases of ventricular fibrillation of cardiac etiology. The survival is expressed as a percentage of all cases meeting this definition (see highlighted box in the figure). When possible the neurological status of the survivors should also be determined from the hospital record. CPC scores of 1 and 2 indicate good to moderately good neurological outcomes and CPR scores of 3 and 4 indicate poor to terrible outcomes.

wish. The main template is the Utstein reporting template (see page 80), which provides the survival (discharged alive) rate for witnessed cases of VF in which the collapse occurs before the arrival of EMS personnel. For agencies participating in CARES, the Utstein template is automatically generated.

To maintain a cardiac arrest registry (whether in CARES or as a free-standing registry) at its basic level, probably a quarter-time person is needed for a community of one million to gather incident data and obtain follow-up information from hospitals. If the tasks associated with maintaining the cardiac arrest registry are combined with those of collecting and managing data for high-performance CPR and the dispatcher-assisted CPR program, there will be enough work for one half-time employee. This estimate assumes that the EMTs and paramedics are assisting in the data collection, such as forwarding run reports[3] and defibrillator downloads, and it also assumes that the dispatch center is providing CAD reports and recordings on CPR calls.[4]

The registry should collect information on all cardiac arrests for which EMS care has been provided, that is, when resuscitation was attempted. The major emphasis, however, should be on cardiac arrests in which VF was the presenting rhythm. For communities with limited resources, restricting the registry to cases of VF or witnessed VF is a reasonable measure. Implicit in the concept of a cardiac arrest registry is the assumption that time intervals will be measured accurately. The most important time intervals are those between the patient's collapse and the start of CPR and between the collapse and the first shock. Admittedly, it is not always possible to know the exact time of collapse. Therefore, the first accurate time is the time the 911 call is answered and this should be the precise moment the EMS clock starts ticking. For cases involving bystander CPR, the initiation of CPR can be arbitrarily defined as having occurred halfway between the time of the call to 911 and the time of the first-in unit's arrival. Ideally, all the system's AEDs will be synchronized automatically or manually to an accurate clock.[5]

It is important to be realistic about what a cardiac arrest registry includes. I think to be fully functional a registry must have the following three elements:

1. *Full capture of all arrests meeting the case definition.* The case definition we use in King County for an event is a cardiac arrest in which EMS personnel initiate or continue CPR. Patients with AED shocks and who do not require EMS CPR are also considered cases. Trauma cases are excluded from the registry unless a case results from a low-speed motor vehicle accident or other trauma in which the cardiac arrest may have preceded the trauma. Patients who are dead on arrival or have a "do not resuscitate" (DNR) order and those who did not receive EMS CPR do not qualify under the "case" definition, but we do include cases in which EMS CPR is started and then stopped after a DNR order is clarified. However, since DNR cases are invariably non-VF cases they do not affect the VF survival rate.

2. *Measurement of critical variables.* Witnessed collapse, collapse before EMS arrival, first rhythm obtained, shockable rhythm, bystander CPR, telephone CPR, time of call to dispatch center, time of EMS CPR, estimated time of bystander CPR, time of first compression for dispatch-assisted CPR, time of first defibrillation.

3. *Measurement of outcome.* Death at scene, death in hospital, discharge alive (ideally with a determination of neurological outcome).

To obtain critical information on the outcome of all patients admitted to the hospital, a good working relationship with area hospitals is essential. A registry is part of ongoing quality improvement and is considered protected information in most states (and consent from the patient to release medical information is not required). The completeness of the registry can of course vary from the bare minimum of information to hundreds of variables. In King County, we have a registry that is comprehensive and serves as the basis for many studies. The 300 variables we collect from CAD reports, incident reports, defibrillation downloads, voice recordings, hospital records, autopsy reports, and death certificates would be considered excessive for routine quality improvement. A good basic registry can be achieved with 14 event and 3 outcome variables. The list of variables in table 10.3 exhibits a minimal data set. For communities not participating in CARES, information about a free-standing registry may be obtained from the Resuscitation Academy (see Addendum).

Table 10.3 Basic variables comprising a cardiac arrest registry

14 event variables:

- Demographic information
- Age
- Sex
- Collapse before EMS arrival
- Witnessed collapse
- Time of call to 911
- Resuscitation stopped because of DNR orders
- Rhythm on arrival (or shockable rhythm on arrival)
- PAD shock
- Dispatcher-assisted CPR
- Bystander CPR without dispatcher-assisted CPR
- Estimated time from call to 911 and bystander CPR (half of interval from 911 call to scene arrival)
- Time from call to 911 to time to dispatcher-assisted CPR (first compression)
- Time from call to 911 to time to EMS CPR
- Time from call to 911 to time to first shock

3 outcome variables:

- Died at scene
- Admitted to hospital
- Discharged alive
- Discharge location (optional)
- CPC score on discharge (optional)

Step 2. Implement Dispatcher-Assisted CPR with Ongoing Training and QI

Most dispatch centers claim to have dispatcher-assisted CPR protocols in place, but in practice they don't offer CPR instructions very often. (Synonymous terms are telephone CPR, dispatcher CPR, and dispatcher-assisted telephone CPR.) Admittedly, it is difficult and stressful for dispatchers to determine the presence of cardiac arrest and provide CPR instructions; it is far easier simply to reassure the caller that help is on the way. But the center whose culture supports its dispatchers to assertively offer callers CPR instructions over the telephone is a center that has the chain of survival firmly in its grasp. This kind of culture can exist only if someone has responsibility for teaching dispatcher-assisted CPR, monitoring the program, and watching it like a hawk. Someone has to listen to recorded information from all cardiac arrest calls and give feedback to individual dispatchers as well as to the entire staff. It is as important to review the calls in which instructions were provided (how could it be done faster, better?) as it is to review the calls in which cardiac arrest was not recognized (how can we do a better job identifying cardiac arrest?)

The adjective "assertive" describes a useful mindset for dispatchers when fielding possible cardiac arrest calls.[6] A take-charge attitude that moves ahead with CPR instructions, when there is reasonable likelihood that cardiac arrest is present, is the attitude needed for this program to succeed. If the dispatcher is overly cautious or holds back in the face of uncertainty, the instructions will seldom be given or there will be considerable delay in their implementation. One element of any successful dispatcher-assisted CPR program is training, which should include continuing education. Dispatchers in King County receive an initial forty hours of training in emergency medical dispatching and are thereafter required to complete eight hours of continuing education every year. Special emphasis is placed on recognizing cardiac arrest and delivering CPR instructions.

Recently, a five-year randomized clinical trial in King County and Thurston County (a county south of King) in Washington State and in London, England, looked at whether dispatcher-assisted CPR achieved better survival with standard CPR (mouth-to-mouth with compressions) instructions than with chest-compression-only instructions. The trial found no difference overall in survival, but there were non-statistical improvements in survival and neurological recovery with chest compression only.[7] As a result, we now provide chest-compression-only instructions for all adult cardiac arrests. The dispatchers provide standard CPR instructions (mouth to mouth combined with chest compressions) for cardiac arrest in children and infants (fortunately, rare events) and when there is an obvious respiratory cause of arrest such as drowning, hanging, or inhaling smoke.

In King County we stress the expectation that every call is a cardiac arrest until proven otherwise. Although only 1 percent of the calls will actually be for a cardiac arrest, nevertheless this expectation primes the dispatcher always to ask the two screening questions (unless the caller is the patient) as quickly as possible: Is the patient conscious (awake)? Is the patient breathing normally?

Dispatchers learn the significance of agonal respirations and how to recognize them. It is particularly important that they offer CPR instructions when there are agonal respirations, since these patients are the ones most likely to be resuscitated and discharged from the hospital. Agonal breathing is present in 56 percent of patients with VF cardiac arrest.[8] Yet the presence of agonal breathing will often confuse the caller and/or dispatcher into thinking the patient is not in cardiac arrest. Despite our considerable training on how to recognize agonal breathing, it remains a challenge. When asked "Is the patient breathing normally?" the caller often responds with "a little" or "sometimes" or "I'm not sure" or "I think so." The dispatcher is seeking a yes or no response to the question and instead receives an ambiguous reply. When the

---

CPR/Adults

1. Is there an AED (Automatic External Defibrillator) on the premise?

2. Does anyone there know **CPR**? *(Trained bystanders may still need instructions. **Ask!**)*

3. Get the phone **NEXT** to the person.

4. Listen carefully. I'll tell you what to do.
   - Get them **FLAT** on their **back** on the **floor**.
   - **BARE** the chest.
   - **KNEEL** by their side.
   - Put the **HEEL** of your **HAND** on the **CENTER** of their **CHEST**, right **BETWEEN** the **NIPPLES**.
   - Put your **OTHER HAND ON TOP** of **THAT** hand.
   - **PUSH DOWN FIRMLY, ONLY** on the **HEELS** of your hands, 2 inches.
   - Do it **50** times, just like you're PUMPING the chest. Count **OUTLOUD 1-2-3...50**. ***(correct rate if needed)
   - **KEEP DOING IT: KEEP PUMPING** the **CHEST UNTIL HELP TAKES OVER**. I'll stay on the line.

   If rescuer becomes too tired to continue instruct them to rest a short time then continue **compressions as soon as possible**.

Ventilation Instructions: (for use when suspected cardiac arrest secondary to respiratory arrest)
   - **PINCH** the **NOSE**: With your other hand, **LIFT** the **CHIN** so the head **BENDS BACK**.
   - Completely **COVER** their **MOUTH** with your **MOUTH**.
   - **GIVE TWO BREATHS OF AIR** (come back to the phone).

   Then back to compression instructions (#4 above) but give **30** compressions between breaths.

Foreign Body Airway Obstruction: (*confirmed* choking now unconscious)
   - After each set of **30** compressions *"Look inside the mouth, remove any obvious obstruction"*. If object is removed give two ventilations between each set of 30 compressions. If object not seen continue with compressions.

NOTE: IF CALLER REPORTS VOMITING, INSTRUCT CALLER TO:
   - Turn their head to one side.
   - Sweep out contents with your fingers before you resume.

10.2 Protocol for dispatcher-assisted CPR instructions used in King County. Prior to delivering these instructions the dispatcher has determined the likely presence of cardiac arrest by asking two critical questions: Is the patient conscious (awake)? Is the patient breathing normally? Note that the instructions call for chest-compression-only CPR. If respiratory arrest is the suspected cause of cardiac arrest then ventilation instructions are provided. There are slightly different protocols for children and infants, as well as protocols for choking patients.

dispatcher asks the caller to describe the breathing, the replies are varied and include gasping, snoring, slow grunting, groaning, and gurgling. Often the agonal breathing can be heard in the background, but if not, the dispatcher may ask the caller to bring the phone to the patient in order to better hear the breathing.

In terms of training and motivation, the director of a dispatch center should do whatever is necessary to ensure that the center achieves a 50 percent rate of offering dispatcher-assisted CPR instructions in cases of cardiac arrest. This is not an unrealistic target. Achieving such a target will require a sponsor—someone who takes charge of the desired change, has the authority to mandate it, and establishes training, professional expectations, and ongoing audits to see that the change is fully implemented (see Addendum on the Resuscitation Academy). Once dispatchers realize how vital they are to the chain of resuscitation, and especially when they see concrete evidence of their success, they will become the staunchest advocates of dispatcher-assisted CPR.

As with high-performance CPR the quality of dispatcher-assisted CPR can be measured. At a minimum, every cardiac arrest call must be reviewed, with the following elements measured:

Was cardiac arrest recognized?

Were the two basic questions asked:

Is the patient conscious (awake)?

Is the patient breathing normally?

Were agonal respirations (if present) recognized?

What was the time from call to recognition of cardiac arrest? (this should be less-than one minute)

Were telephone CPR instructions offered?

What was the time from call to beginning chest compressions (this should be less than two minutes)

Attainable goals should be the provision of dispatcher CPR in 50 percent of all cardiac arrest calls (excluding calls in which bystanders are performing CPR at the time of the call), recognition of cardiac arrest within one minute, and first compression started within two minutes in over 75 percent of dispatcher CPR calls. Feedback must be provided to the dispatcher following every event.

The American Heart Association in 2012 issued a Scientific Statement strongly endorsing dispatcher-assisted CPR, including the importance of asking the two identifying questions, special training in the recognition of agonal respirations, and a vigorous ongoing QI program.[9]

Step 3. Implement High-performance CPR with ongoing training and QI

Recent studies demonstrate the connection between quality CPR and survival from cardiac arrest. Not only is the time interval from collapse to onset of CPR predictive of survival but also the quality of the CPR is just as important. The better the CPR, the better the outcome. Since 2005, when we trained every EMT in our system in high-performance CPR, we have seen a significant increase in survival.[10] Resuscitations that go on for 50 or 60 minutes, with a pharmacy of medications, 10-20 defibrillatory shocks, and a patient who survives—with excellent neurological recovery—used to be the exception but now seem commonplace. It is as though the onset of high-performance CPR suspends death and gives a better opportunity for the defibrillatory shocks and medications to work their magic.

High-performance CPR is as much a construct as a measurable skill.[11] The construct says that letter-perfect CPR is the goal of all resuscitations. This skill can be achieved in training as well as through review of real events. We believe training on manikins with "strip recorders" is the best teaching tool as it provides instant feedback about the quality of CPR. Elements of high-performance CPR include:

- Correct hand position
- Compression rate of 100-120 beats per minute
- Depth of compression of 2 inches
- Full recoil on the upstroke
- 50:50 duty cycles
- Ventilations of one second each
- Minimal interruptions of CPR (no pause to exceed 10 seconds)
- Intubation and IV start without pausing chest compressions

Last, and perhaps most important, is that there is an ongoing QI program that provides feedback with specifics about CPR performance to EMTs following every cardiac arrest. A QI program should among other things measure the percentage of time chest compressions are performed during each two-minute interval between rhythm assessments. Well-trained EMTs should be able to provide chest compressions for at least 90 percent of the available time. Most defibrillators allow digital downloads following the resuscitation, including precise measurements of CPR percentage and quality.

Another aspect to high-performance CPR is the choreography between the EMTs and the paramedics. Other terms used to describe this flawless team performance are the "dance of resuscitation," the "CPR ballet," and the "pit-stop approach to CPR." Observing well-trained rescuers engaged in high-performance CPR is indeed like watching a well-choreographed dance. The term pit-stop refers to the pre-defined role of each rescuer and the very minimal waste of time. Like a professional racecar pit crew, each member of the team knows exactly what to do and does it with minimal wastage of time and effort. This choreography means that members switch or rotate roles with minimal interruptions—current protocols call for rhythm analysis every two minutes. Thus the chest compressor and the ventilator can switch roles every two minutes. With sufficient personnel at the scene, one EMT can start compression, the second attaches the AED pads, the third provides ventilation, while the fourth feels the femoral pulse (in order to define the location of the artery and determine if a shock leads to a perfusing rhythm). A fifth EMT, if present, could be the "captain" of CPR and provide direction to the crew (typically the person providing overall direction is the one who operates the automated external defibrillator). Paramedics should optimally intubate and place the IV with no interruption in chest compressions. Clearly, if there are fewer rescuers the responsibilities must be aggregated. In our system, we think of the EMT crew as owning CPR, meaning that they are responsible for the quality and directing of assignments. The paramedics own advanced life support; in other words, they are responsible for intubating, starting an IV, and administering medications. Upon arrival, paramedics become the overall team captains, but they know to delegate CPR to the EMTs. The EMT team not only keeps track of the quality of CPR but also keeps track of the timing of interventions. Since there is a rhythm analysis every two minutes, an EMT is the official timekeeper, literally using a stopwatch. (In King County, we go slightly beyond two minutes of CPR in order to end with 30 chest compressions prior to every rhythm analysis.)

For the EMTs and paramedics to understand why high-performance CPR is so critical, part of our training includes instruction in the science of CPR. My colleague, Dr. Peter Kudenchuk, has developed a compelling 30-minute video on the science of CPR and why letter-perfect CPR is so important. (This video is freely available at the Resuscitation Academy website). This video is part of every King County EMT's training.

Step 4. Implement Rapid Dispatch

With rapid dispatch, the closest EMT-staffed vehicle is dispatched within seconds when specific medical emergencies are reported to the 911 dispatcher. The dispatch should occur even while additional information is being gathered from the caller. The quick arrival of at least the EMT vehicle allows the EMTs to perform CPR and deliver the first defibrillatory shock. On the other hand, it may be immediately clear that both EMTs and paramedics are required (such as a report of ongoing CPR) and, thus, both vehicles should be rapidly dispatched. If additional information from the caller suggests that paramedics will not be needed after all, the dispatcher can call off the paramedic unit with a "code green" message.

The symptoms or complaints that should trigger a rapid dispatch are: unconscious or suspected cardiac arrest, chest pain, difficulty breathing, stroke symptoms, ongoing seizure, and significant trauma. A community should carefully measure its current time interval from first ring into the alarm center to specific dispatch of the first responding unit (EMT or paramedic unit or EMT/paramedic unit). This time interval is variously labeled but here will be called "dispatch time." The National Fire Protection Association (NFPA) sets a dispatch time standard of 60 seconds for "critical" events. Rapid dispatch can do much better than that. The rapid dispatch target time in King County dispatch centers is 15 seconds or less, especially when the address is auto populated in the dispatcher CAD (computer aided dispatch) system (which applies to most dispatch centers in the United States). The first mention of a critical symptom mandates an immediate dispatch. Dispatch centers that place priority on a rigid, predefined protocol over rapid dispatch are doing their communities a disservice and in the case of cardiac arrest are delaying life-saving therapy.

The concept of rapid dispatch applies to tiered-response EMS systems as well as single-response systems. Many EMS systems' dispatch protocols require full information before even a single rescue vehicle can be sent. That may be an acceptable procedure for the majority of calls, but speed is of the essence in a life-or-death situation, and in those cases usual dispatching protocols must be short-circuited. In Seattle and King County, we train dispatchers to use rapid dispatch when they hear certain key words and phrases from callers—either the short list of symptoms in the preceding paragraph or words such as "collapsed," "unconscious," "can't breathe," and "heart attack." We also urge the dispatcher to use common sense and immediately send EMTs whenever a caller otherwise conveys the likelihood of a critical event. In King County rapid dispatch is used in approximately 30 percent of EMS calls. From personally reviewing hundreds of calls, I am convinced that rapid dispatch saves 30-60 seconds in dispatch time for the most critical medical emergencies. Given the fact that survival falls about 10 percent for every minute of delay in CPR and defibrillation, rapid dispatch can add 5-10 percent to a community's survival rate. All of this can happen with no additional staffing or resources. Not bad. Now you see why I consider this to be one of the low-hanging fruits.

One more point: EMS dispatch centers (whether stand-alone centers or part of larger combined centers, such as fire and police) must have protocols authorized by medical directors. Medical expertise is necessary to provide pre-arrival instructions as well as to determine the urgency of the callers' complaints and how quickly units must be dispatched. The logical person to fill this roll is the EMS medical director. Unfortunately, many dispatch centers still do not involve the EMS medical director in the writing or approval of protocols for medical emergencies, which bizarrely disconnects the patient from the EMS system.

TARGETED COMMUNITY SCORE CARD

Chapter 7 included a Community Score Card to determine the presence or absence of important elements in managing cardiac arrest. Based on the four easy steps discussed above, I propose a targeted community scorecard that emphasizes each of these elements.

Cardiac Arrest Registry
- One point for an ongoing registry of every cardiac arrest that receives EMS care
- One point for determination of outcomes (primarily, discharged alive)
- One point for ability to calculate the Utstein metric (survival from witnessed VF)

High-performance CPR
- One point for specific training and testing with a printout strip
- One point for dedicated person to measure performance from real events
- One point for feedback to EMTs

Assertive dispatcher-assisted CPR
- One point for specific training including recognition of agonal breathing
- One point for a dedicated person who listens to all cardiac arrest tapes and measures performance, such as: Was cardiac arrest recognized (two questions asked)? When was it recognized? What was the time to first compression?
- One point for feedback to dispatchers

Rapid Dispatch
- One point for rapid dispatch program with first-in unit dispatched within 30 seconds of the call for 90 percent of cardiac arrests

There are a total of 10 points. I make no claim that this scorecard is validated or linearly scaled (a score of 8 is not necessarily twice as good as a score of 4). Rather, I am trying to offer a simple metric that anyone can quickly apply to his or her own EMS system. It would be an interesting study to correlate a community's VF survival rate with its number of points. My prediction is that a strong correlation exists.

A PLAN OF ACTION: THE HIGHER-HANGING FRUIT

I am confident that if the above four easy steps are taken, there will be a measurable improvement in survival. Now it is time to go after the higher-hanging fruit (Table 10.4). These more difficult steps will also likely lead to improved survival but their implementation is more challenging and resource intensive.

Step 5. Voice record all attempted resuscitations

Step 6. Begin a program in police defibrillation

Step 7. Establish a public access defibrillation program

Step 8. Establish a local foundation to raise funds for training and QI

Step 9. Institute hypothermia in all receiving hospitals

Step 10. Work toward a culture of excellence

Step 5. Voice Record All Attempted Resuscitations

AEDs and newer manual defibrillators automatically record the patient's heart rhythm and all defibrillatory shocks during a cardiac arrest. In addition, these devices have the option to simultaneously digitally record all voices during the resuscitation.

Though some EMTs and paramedics may think that the recorded information will be used for disciplinary purposes, the goal of recording is simply to reconstruct the actual events of the resuscitation with accuracy. In King County, for example, we have analyzed thousands of voice and ECG recordings and have never used them for any disciplinary action. Listening to a voice recording while viewing the patient's cardiac rhythm makes the event vivid. I have listened to hundreds of recordings and always felt as if I was at the scene. You can tell the moment when the AED was attached and when ventilations were given. You can piece together the sequence and timing of events and deduce the reason for any delays (the dog was growling at the EMT, the patient had to be moved from the bathroom to the hallway, the oxygen tank ran out, and so on). A post-event digital readout of the heart rhythm, with the timing of the shocks, is clearly useful; however, nothing beats a voice recording of the event. Some people believe that the only thing better might be a video recording, like those made by police cams, but I find this suggestion problematic. Such a recording would be logistically challenging and intrusive, not to mention a violation of privacy. It would be only a matter of time before resuscitation videos began appearing on YouTube.[12] Frankly, though, the most important objection to video recording is that they are not needed. A voice recording is enough to allow adequate reconstruction of the event.

Voice and ECG recordings provide the crucial data allowing for the event to be accurately reviewed. When shared with EMTs and paramedics it provides beneficial QI and teaching material. And it makes everyone want to do better the next time. I remember quite vividly listening to a cardiac arrest and hearing the paramedic ask the EMT to stop CPR so he could intubate. Then a long pause ensued that lasted 65 seconds (with no CPR) before the paramedic asked the EMT to resume chest compression. The paramedic, when the tape was reviewed with him, could not believe how long the pause was. You can be sure this paramedic will do better the next time. Many training officers in King County fire departments use the recordings for internal teaching. There is nothing like a real event to grab your attention—to breathe a sigh of relief when things go well and to cringe when they don't.

Step 6. Begin a Program Training Police in Defibrillation

Providing police officers with CPR skills and training in the use of an AED has the potential to increase survival rates from cardiac arrest. Though the promise exists, law enforcement's role in resuscitation and early defibrillation has been modest and inconsistent. Yet some communities that have embraced police defibrillation have seen dramatic improvements in survival. Perhaps the most notable community is Rochester, MN (see chapter 6). Our system in King County has also seen benefit with police response to cardiac arrest.

Embarking on a police defibrillation program is not without challenges, and some communities that have tried have not seen much benefit.[13] There are many issues to address: Support from the police chief and buy-in from the rank and file, support from the fire-department and or EMS agency, initial and ongoing training and its costs, cost of AEDs, supervision, QI, and integration with EMS dispatching. In early 2010 we undertook police AED programs in Bellevue and Kent, two cities in suburban King County, Washington, each with approximately 100,000 residents. The program has contributed to the successful resuscitation of a handful of lives, though not the number we had hoped for. If we set our goals too high, we will try recalibrating aspects of the program.

A few critical lessons we have learned might help other communities as they embark on police defibrillation. First, there must be total support from the police and EMS agencies. I personally taught every police officer in the two Washington departments and I found them to be very willing and supportive. Second, the training message must be simple and involve two checks: "If the person does not respond (check one) and is not breathing normally (check two), attach the AED. Let it analyze and or shock and then follow the CPR prompt." We teach the police to provide chest compression only (most are relived that they do not have to perform mouth-to-mouth ventilation). Third, the dispatch center is key to achieving rapid police response. The police must be dispatched simultaneously with the first-responding EMS agency. This is perhaps the most challenging issue in achieving a successful police defibrillation program. Our goal is for police to be dispatched only for true cardiac arrest events. Many times it is clear that the caller is reporting a cardiac arrest, but other times it can take some seconds (or longer) to confirm an arrest (remember that the EMT unit has already been dispatched under rapid dispatch). When the dispatcher waits to confirm cardiac arrest before dispatching police, the fire department will have had enough of a jump start to arrive before police. How to send police quickly but not oversend is a challenge we continue to work on.

Step 7. Establish a Public Access Defibrillation Program

Public access defibrillation (PAD) refers to placing AEDs in public locations and using them as elements of a community's resuscitation chain. I consider PAD to be a difficult step not necessarily because it is technically challenging but rather because the effects are likely to be modest. Even with widespread dissemination of AEDs in public locations there will be only a modest increase in survival. The Public Access Defibrillation Trial was a multicenter trial demonstrating that sites with AEDs on the premises, and with staff trained in their use, had higher survival rates for VF than comparable sites without AEDs (the non-AED sites relied on the fire department or an EMS agency to bring an AED to the scene).[14] Other studies, reporting the use of AEDs in casinos and on airplanes, also showed benefit.[15]

There is an active PAD program in Seattle and King County, with more than 3,000 AEDs registered with EMS as of 2012. Sites with AEDs include such places as airports, health clubs, jails, community centers, senior centers, shopping malls, office buildings, and ferryboats. The number of AEDs has increased significantly over the past decade. A study from Seattle and King County reporting on eight years' experience with PAD, found that 1.8 percent of VF arrests had an AED applied in 1999 compared to 8.8 percent of VF arrests in 2006. Survival among PAD cases was approximately 60 percent.[16]

The strategy of using public AEDs has merit, but enthusiasm must be tempered with awareness of the relatively small number of cardiac arrests—only 15 percent—that occur in public places (approximately 150 of 1,000 arrests per year in King County). Though the absolute number is small, these are great saves. A cardiac arrest in public usually befalls an active person who is out in the community, and since most collapses in public are witnessed, CPR is often started quickly. The fact that these arrests have everything going for them—they usually involve VF, they are witnessed, CPR and defibrillation are started quickly, and there is probably less comorbidity—explains the excellent survival rate (and the typically good neurological recovery).

Residential facilities offer great potential for PAD programs. As incentives, an EMS agency could provide free training to residents and personnel and could offer to register the facility's AED with the local dispatch center. The agency could also offer advice on where in the facility to place the AED. A residential community or an apartment or condominium building could establish an AED security system. In such a system, the AED would be placed in a locked box (all the residents would know the combination) in a central accessible location. This location would be registered with the dispatch center, and if a cardiac arrest occurred on the premises, someone at the scene would be instructed to get the AED.

Existing computer-aided dispatch programs allow dispatch centers to identify

AEDs at particular locations (assuming that these AEDs are registered with the center), as well as any in close proximity. Wouldn't it be amazing if a caller to 911 were informed that the doorman in the next building had an AED in his building's lobby and was being called to bring it over? This idea is currently being tested in the King County Norcom Communications Center and, though this is not a formal test, I offer this suggestion as one idea for how a community can be creative with AEDs. And what if the dispatcher could automatically alert all staff responsible for AEDs within a certain radius? Thus a security guard in an adjoining building would get a phone text telling him or her that there was a cardiac arrest next door. This technology is commercially available and deployed in a few cities. New smart-phone applications can pinpoint (registered) AED locations. Clearly, AEDs in the community have the potential to save lives. The challenge is to maximize their potential.

There is interest on the part of some national sudden cardiac arrest foundations and prevention advocacy groups to revise building codes to mandate placement of AEDs in multiple-occupancy dwellings and business establishments. The reasoning is that an AED is a lifesaving technology that should be built into the structure of the building, just like a sprinkler system.

Another innovative idea is to use social networking and crowd sourcing (using the public to engage in community data collection) both to identify the locations of AEDs and to volunteer to respond to a cardiac arrest event if notified by the dispatch center. Dr. Raina Merchant, in a recent commentary in *Circulation Cardiovascular Quality and Outcomes*, describes both the challenges and potential benefits of crowd sourcing and the potential ability to retrieve AED location information on smart phone mobile apps. With over one million AEDs sold in the United States wouldn't it be nice to determine the precise location of these AEDs and then have this information readily available for witnesses to a cardiac arrest? Perhaps future AEDs could have embedded geographic transponders.[17]

Step 8. Establish a Local Foundation to Raise Funds for Training and QI

When times are tight financially, usually the first things to be eliminated or reduced are budgets for training and QI. While these decisions may be penny-wise and pound-foolish, they nevertheless reflect the harsh realities and the need to preserve basic operational personnel. Thus, it is important to find additional sources of revenues. Most public agencies are not able to solicit funds directly from the public they serve. But it is possible to establish foundations or engage in other types of fund raising. Charitable gifts can provide needed funds to support activities such as training and QI. These in turn provide the margin of excellence to boost a program to a higher level of performance. The Medic One Foundation (mediconefoundation.org) is an example of how a foundation can supplement a public EMS system. This foundation supports

100 percent of paramedic training and cardiac arrest QI for the Seattle Fire Department. In addition, it funds paramedic training for other agencies and provides equipment and research grants.

EMS agencies may not have the resources or staff necessary to create a separate foundation. One can instead team up with a local public charity that has a similar mission and can act as a fiscal sponsor. For example, an EMS agency could partner with a hospital foundation or auxiliary, fire department auxiliary or benevolent fund, or local community foundation.

Step 9. Institute Hypothermia in All Receiving Hospitals

Hypothermia is the standard of care for resuscitated VF patients when they arrive at the hospital in a coma. Cooling the patient's body for twenty-four hours after resuscitation offers the promise of a modest improvement in the chances of survival, and to date there is no indication of harm from this practice. The American Heart Association and the International Liaison Committee on Resuscitation have both endorsed it. Like any complex hospital procedure, proficiency requires written protocols, practice, and accountability.

As of 2012, most hospitals that receive resuscitated patients have hypothermia protocols in place. Lance Becker, director of the Center for Resuscitation Science at the University of Pennsylvania Perelman School of Medicine (www.med.upenn.edu/resuscitation), is a leading proponent of hypothermia. He and his colleagues, on the basis of laboratory studies, have come to believe that the cells of vital organs do not die from insufficient oxygen; rather, they say, the harm occurs when oxygen is reintroduced. The benefit of cooling is that it inhibits many of the destructive reactions associated with reperfusion of blood and the reintroduction of oxygen. The University of Pennsylvania Hypothermia and Resuscitation Training (HART) Institute offers an annual two-day "boot camp" designed to educate care providers on in-hospital care of cardiac arrest patients (www.med.upenn.edu/resuscitation/hypothermia/hypothermiatraining).

Hypothermia is a relatively recent addition to the armamentarium of resuscitation therapy. In 2002, two studies of hypothermia were published in the *New England Journal of Medicine*. Both studies randomized patients either to receive hypothermia or to have hypothermia withheld (called "normothermia"), for VF patients who had been successfully defibrillated but were comatose when they arrived at the hospital. One of the studies, reporting data obtained from several centers in Europe, demonstrated favorable neurological outcomes six months after cardiac arrest when hypothermia treatment had been delivered: 55 percent of patients in the hypothermia group had favorable outcomes, compared to 39 percent in the control group. Mortality was also significantly lower in the hypothermia group than in the control group—41 percent and 55 percent, respectively.[18] The other study, this one from Australia, did not demonstrate a significant difference in survival (the main outcome of the study) among the hypothermia and normothermia groups, although the authors did report better neurological outcomes in the hypothermia group.[19] This was a smaller study, with only 77 patients as opposed to the 275 patients in the European study. On the basis of these two studies, several national and international organizations, including the International Liaison Committee on Resuscitation and the American Heart Association, now recommend hypothermia for patients who have suffered ventricular fibrillation and are initially resuscitated but are still in a coma when they reach the hospital.

Unresolved issues are whether patients should receive hypothermia in the prehospital setting and whether only VF patients should be eligible for hypothermia therapy. It is for this reason I place hypothermia in the difficult-steps category. Though the therapy is reasonably straightforward, the difficult part comes in determining whether it is beneficial for prehospital use. There are currently no data to clarify whether hypothermia should begin in the field, either after return of spontaneous circulation or in the middle of a resuscitation, in other words prior to return of a pulse and blood pressure. Dr. Francis Kim at the University of Washington is currently studying the potential benefits of prehospital hypothermia for resuscitated VF patients. This is a randomized trial, and the results will not be known until 2013. Also unresolved is whether hospital hypothermia benefits patients who are resuscitated from asystole or pulseless electrical activity. Stay tuned on this issue.

Step 10. Work toward a Culture of Excellence

Creating and nurturing a culture of excellence is perhaps the most difficult step. What is a culture of excellence? It is an implicit awareness perceived by most or all members of the organization that high expectations and high performance define the standard of care. A culture of excellence requires a leader (or leaders) with an uncompromising vision. Ideally, the administrative director and the medical director should share this vision. Practically, they should meet regularly, perhaps weekly, to jointly administer and plan all aspects of the EMS program. The two of them together should establish a long-term plan to create and maintain a culture of excellence. Some people would argue that a high-quality EMS system demands such a culture. An equal number would claim that creating a culture of excellence is extremely challenging. No doubt it is. Nevertheless, a culture of excellence, hard though it may be to define or measure, is probably a key factor separating great systems from those that are satisfactory.

Administrative and medical leadership together must enhance training and continuing education and make medical QI the means of constant improvement. Excellence also requires buy-in from the extended EMS "family" of dispatchers, EMTs, and paramedics. When EMS providers recognize the presence of sincere, mission-driven leadership as opposed to lip service, they respond to the positive culture and contribute to it as well.

THE MEDICAL MODEL

A culture of excellence can be achieved in any organization model. However, I believe such a culture can more easily be accomplished in a system that is based on a medical model. What I mean by a medical model is a system in which a medical director plays a large role in determining and supervising the quality of medical care. Specifically, a medical model of EMS is a system in which the medical director is responsible for the following seven areas: (1) protocols for dispatchers, EMTs, and paramedics; (2) medical supervision online and offline; (3) evidence-based practice; (4) ongoing medical QI; (5) training and continuing education; (6) controlled substance policies, and (7) medical discipline. I'd like to suggest an eighth optional area of responsibility, namely, ongoing research studies. Continuing studies (to push the envelope of knowledge) create a sense of being part of a larger enterprise and help foster a desire to contribute new evidence-based knowledge to the world of EMS. These studies do not have to be randomized clinical trials. One can embark on small-scale projects and still make a contribution. The studies need not necessarily be published in peer-reviewed journals—merely sharing the findings with the personnel can be rewarding and help to achieve a sense of pride.

A medical model does not require that the physician director "run" the entire system—in fact, the less administrative involvement by the medical director, the better. The medical director should be responsible for the quality of medical care and establish high expectations and see that they are being met. The EMTs and paramedics must be accountable to the medical director for the quality of their care. The ideal system would have the administrative director responsible for budget, operations, and personnel matters and the medical director responsible for patient care. And in the best of all words the two would work closely in partnership since their responsibilities complement each other. I don't expect medical directors to deal with hiring, though I expect them to have a say in who is hired. And I don't expect doctors to directly "fire" anyone, though I expect them to work with the administrative director to limit, suspend, or terminate an EMT or paramedic whose medical care is substandard. In Seattle and King County there is a phrase that encapsulates the critical role of the medical director: "The EMT or paramedic practices under the medical license of the medical director." In essence, the clinical buck stops with the medical director.

How does one create a medical model? Certainly there is no guidebook to follow and probably many if not most EMS programs think they already have a medical model. But I think the test is whether the medical director has responsibility for all the seven areas above. Why stress the concept of the medical model? Because the medical director is so importantly involved in every link in the chain of survival and every piece of the frame of survival.

Medical directors are appointed in various ways. Whatever the process, the medical director must have the authority to supervise a system that uses a medical model of EMS care. The medical director must clearly state and constantly promote high expectations, and the EMTs and paramedics must be accountable to the medical director for their patient care.

It is desirable (though I know not always possible) that the medical director be jointly appointed by the EMS administrative director and the academic dean or department chair. An academic appointment ensures accountability. Moreover, an academic physician is generally one who is committed to furthering learning and one who probably has knowledge about epidemiological principles and research methodologies. This is not to say that every medical director must conduct research—far from it—but only that the director must understand the benefits and limitations of data and know how to interpret (and not overinterpret) them. An academic medical director has access to all the expertise of an academic medical center. Many a time I have turned to colleagues in cardiology, anesthesiology, pediatrics, obstetrics, trauma surgery, endocrinology, biostatistics, epidemiology, preventive medicine, health services, and toxicology to get answers about clinical issues and to seek help in guiding policy.

What can a community do if it is geographically distant from an academic medical center? Many centers offer clinical appointments to individuals who are in service roles in the community or who help with the teaching mission of the university. I think that many deans and department chairs in emergency medicine would welcome a conversation with a community's elected officials or its EMS administrative director and would be pleased to help establish a clinical appointment for the community's medical director. It is also advantageous for a community to partner with an academic medical center, which probably already staffs the region's trauma center. A partnership between a local community and an academic medical center can be a win-win proposition. The EMS program can provide training opportunities for emergency medical residents and help partner with the medical school on EMS fellowships. The medical center can provide clinical and communications expertise, database management, and managerial experience and can cooperate with local medical directors to establish regional consortia of EMS medical directors and programs. An academic medical center, after all, has a mission to serve the larger community, and the good will and reciprocity generated by this kind of effort can reap big dividends.

CONTINUOUS QUALITY IMPROVEMENT

A culture of excellence also demands ongoing quality improvement. The medical director, with the support of the administrative director, is responsible for conducting QI audits of the EMS system. The cultural norm says we (all of us who provide care) are measuring how we perform in order to perform even better.

Medical QI can involve any aspect of EMS care. As it relates to cardiac arrest, however, the substrate for continuous QI is the cardiac arrest registry. Without QI, the cardiac arrest registry is just a collection of facts. With QI, the registry becomes the basis for improvement. QI can occur at the macro (system) level or micro (components of the system) level and even at the level of an individual resuscitation. At the system level, one should be able to determine the survival rate for witnessed VF. For the micro level, QI bores down to the components of the system. For example: What is the average time to CPR? Defibrillation? What percentage of arrests have bystander CPR? Telephone CPR? What is the average time to deliver CPR instructions?

The time intervals from the 911 call to CPR and defibrillation are critical to measure. As discussed in chapter 4, measuring these time intervals can be challenging, but without this information it will be like trying to solve a puzzle with several key pieces missing. Most EMS systems report response time (time from call to arrival at scene). In many centers, the actual call occurs seconds (sometimes a minute or more) before being keyed as an EMS call. Thus the call occurred before the response time clock started ticking. And arrival at scene occurs a minute or several minutes before someone touches the patient. Measuring time intervals in EMS is a maze. The point, however, is that there are unmeasured time intervals prior to the so-called response time and unmeasured time intervals after the response time. What really matters is the interval from the first ring in the primary PSAP to contact with the patient, including who starts CPR, when it starts, and the exact time of the first defibrillatory shock.

At the level of individual cases QI should routinely try to piece together the key interventions. This is particularly important for VF cases when the patient did not survive. If one starts with a mindset that every case of VF should survive, then when the patient does not survive, the question becomes, "Why not?" The following may help address this question:

Who started CPR?
What was the time to CPR?
What was the time to first defibrillation? (total number of defibrillatory shocks)
Were telephone CPR instructions offered?
Did the dispatcher recognize agonal respirations?
How long did it take for the dispatcher to recognize the need for CPR and begin telephone instructions?
Was there rapid dispatch? (What was the time to dispatch the first-in unit?)
What was the interval between EMTs' arrival at the patient's side and delivery of the first shock?
What was the density of CPR between two shocks?

After the first defibrillatory shock, how long did it take to resume chest compressions?

Did CPR occur for two minutes between shocks?

Was the patient intubated? (How many attempts were required for intubation?)

Was an alternate airway used? (Such as laryngeal mask airway)

Was an intravenous line started? (Was it peripheral, central, or interosseous?)

When was hypothermia started?

Every link and every sublink in the chain of survival can be studied; the number of possible QI projects is limited only by resources and by the accuracy of the registry's data. An EMS system should never become complacent. There are always opportunities for improvement, and continuous QI is the way to bring it about.

IMPROVE SKILLS AMONG PARAMEDICS, EMTS, AND DISPATCHERS

Improvement in skills is another part of a culture of excellence—training for excellence. The cultural norm says that we (again, all of us who provide care) train in order to improve our skills. Paramedics' skills improve with a combination of training, continuing education, and actual performance. In Seattle and King County, paramedics are required to perform 12 intubations and 36 IVs every year to maintain certification. Paramedic staffing correlates directly with opportunities to perform critical skills. There are strong advocates for various types of paramedic staffing in EMS programs. In Seattle and King County a tiered response system is utilized and paramedics are sent only to the most serious calls. Thus, they are able to maintain critical skill such as endotracheal intubation and central-vein IV placement. In other systems, a paramedic is sent to all EMS calls. These programs assume that service is thereby improved, since every call, regardless of the seriousness of the emergency, will have a paramedic in attendance. But the unintended consequence is less opportunity for any single paramedic to practice critical skills. As discussed in chapter 5, it is unclear whether a high or low ratio of paramedics to total population served is associated with community cardiac arrest survival.

As for EMTs, the care provided by these personnel is the foundation for all subsequent care delivered during an attempted resuscitation. If that foundation is of poor quality, the entire care structure is jeopardized. EMTs can do a great deal to treat ventricular fibrillation definitively, or to prime the patient's body with high-performance CPR for further intervention by paramedics. The details of CPR and defibrillation often determine the outcome, and the key to positive outcomes is training.

Emergency dispatchers are also members of the EMS team. They have the critical role of mobilizing the EMTs and paramedics and seeing that telephone CPR begins before EMS personnel show up. Dispatchers' training, practice, and skill review are as important to positive outcomes as are high-performance CPR and defibrillation. A highly trained dispatcher can, with rapid dispatch, easily save 30 to 60 seconds in the initial dispatch and, by offering telephone CPR instructions, can significantly increase the likelihood of the patient's survival.

A NATIONAL ACTION PLAN

The last steps transcend local initiative and involve programmatic initiatives at the national level (see Table 10.5). The five national steps will not lead to immediate increases in cardiac arrest survival but are nevertheless important infrastructure changes that will indirectly improve programs. These steps may be the most difficult to implement as they require national political consensus—always a challenging task to secure—not to mention the matter of funding. Several organizations, such as the Sudden Cardiac Arrest Foundation, the Sudden Cardiac Arrest Coalition, and the Sudden Cardiac Arrest Association, are working to bring these issues before Congress.

Table 10.5 National Initiatives to Improve Survival

Step 11. Create a national lead agency for prehospital emergency care

Step 12. Mandate national reporting of cardiac arrest

Step 13. Establish national performance standards for cardiac arrest care

Step 14. Create an Institute of Resuscitation Research within the National Institutes of Health

Step 15. Establish guidelines for compassionate withholding of resuscitation

Step 11. Create a National Lead Agency for Prehospital Emergency Care

Some agency at the federal level has to champion emergency medical services, thereby helping to create standards of care and gathering the necessary resources. The idea for a lead federal agency gained momentum with a 2006 report from the Institute of Medicine, Emergency Medical Services at the Crossroads.[20] This report's massive size was matched by its political impact. Covering the entire spectrum of prehospital care, the report convincingly documented major challenges, including fragmentation of services, incompatible communication equipment, lack of coordination between EMS systems and hospitals, lack of uniform training and supervision, lack of accurate data, irrational funding mechanisms, lack of readiness for disasters, and a limited evidence base (in other words, there is a dearth of good information about what works and what does not). In short, the report said, it's a mess out there.

Clearly, cardiac arrest is a major component of prehospital emergency care, and it received a fair amount of attention in the report. Although the report was not written exclusively to improve resuscitation rates but rather to improve prehospital care in general, many of its twenty specific recommendations are relevant to cardiac arrest and resuscitation. One of these is that a lead federal agency should be established for prehospital emergency care, ideally within the U.S. Department of Health and Human Services. I would like to believe that this recommendation will eventually be adopted. The Institute of Medicine is a respected institution. Its reports have high credibility, and Congress often follows its advice (though not always immediately, since it can take time for ideas to incubate and percolate up through the political process).

EMS has long been an orphan in the federal system, relegated to a rung far down the administrative ladder of the U.S. Department of Transportation (DOT), within the National Highway Traffic and Safety Administration (NHTSA).[21] Although it would undoubtedly be helpful to have a lead federal agency for emergency medical services, that will not address the fundamentally ambiguous nature of EMS. The Institute of Medicine report clearly nails the issue, in stating that EMS operates at the intersection of health care (the hospital system), public health, and public safety. It has responsibilities in all three spheres and yet has not been well integrated into any of them. As the report states, "EMS has a foot in many doors but no clear home." This ambiguity diffuses any focus on solving the problem—if there are too many agencies, there will be too many opportunities to ignore the problem as well as to pass the buck.

A lead agency, if it ever comes into being, should require communities to publicly disclose how they measure up against performance standards for cardiac arrest, in the same way that state and federal regulations require hospitals to report their rates of hospital-acquired infections and complications following major surgery. The lead agency might even promote a bit of friendly competition. How about an award for any community that achieves a 50 percent rate of survival (meaning discharge from the hospital) for witnessed VF?[22]

Step 12. Mandate National Reporting of Cardiac Arrest

As we saw in chapter 6, Graham Nichol thinks that the way to mobilize public action around what he calls the "dirty little secret" of cardiac arrest—the fact that survival rates vary tremendously, even outrageously, from one community to another—is to make cardiac arrest a reportable disease. Only mandatory reporting, he says, can focus public awareness on the situation.

In theory, making cardiac arrest a reportable disease is a good idea. In practice, however, it would be problematic, for many reasons. Which cardiac arrests would be defined as reportable—all out-of-hospital cardiac arrests that end in the patient's death, or only those in which EMS personnel attempt resuscitation? Would reportable cardiac arrests be only those with cardiac etiology, or would any etiology be reportable? And what data elements should be reported? Any attempt to define cardiac arrest as a reportable disease would have to address these questions. A national database on cardiac arrest could help in this effort.

Earlier in this chapter, CARES was described; though it has the potential to serve as a national registry of cardiac arrest it is unlikely to happen without mandatory reporting. Another potential resource is the National EMS Information System (NEMSIS), which is a national effort to create a uniform data system for reporting responses to EMS calls, including cardiac arrest. NEMSIS has achieved consensus on the need for a national data set and is making progress toward adoption by states and EMS programs. NEMSIS is not without its detractors. Chief among the criticisms is the lack of funding to support data system upgrades and training. But the biggest challenge to NEMSIS becoming a vehicle for cardiac arrest reporting is the lack of outcome information. Information on discharge and neurological status is not collected by NEMSIS. Any national data system that included cardiac arrest would have many problems to solve before universal adoption.[23] Nevertheless, momentum for cardiac arrest as a reportable disease appears to be growing. The American Heart Association issued a scientific statement in 2008 describing the essential features of making cardiac arrest a reportable disease.[24]

Step 13. Establish National Performance Standards for Cardiac Arrest Care

There are regrettably few, if any, national performance standards for resuscitation. Standard 1710 of the National Fire Protection Association (NFPA) does posit response times, but such standards are voluntary in most of the United States. A 2011 consensus paper from the American Heart Association calls for specific benchmarks and quality improvement goals for out-of-hospital cardiac arrest.[25] These goals span the spectrum from medical leadership to dispatch to EMS and hospital care. Whether one agrees with the specific goals is in some ways less important than the fact that performance standards are becoming part of the national dialogue on how to improve survival rates. The following are possible standards for an urban EMS system and are meant to complement the 10 specific local implementation steps at the beginning of this chapter. Note how the standards are weighted heavily toward bystander CPR (whether by a trained person or as a result of dispatcher assistance) and the rapid delivery of CPR and defibrillation—standards that will surely lead to improved survival:

Bystander CPR in more than 60 percent of witnessed cardiac arrests
Dispatcher-assisted CPR in more than 50 percent of all cardiac arrests (excluding arrests when bystander CPR is in progress at the time of call)

Less than five minutes between pickup of the call to 911 and the arrival of EMTs at
the patient's side more than 90 percent of the time

Less than six minutes between pickup of the call to 911 and the first defibrillatory
shock more than 90 percent of the time

Less than ten minutes between pickup of the call to 911 and the arrival of paramedics at the patient's side 90 percent of the time

Use of voice and heart rhythm recordings in all resuscitations

Medical director's review and critique of all resuscitations

A community survival rate (discharge from hospital) of 25 percent for patients
with witnessed VF

Just as the NFPA holds career and voluntary fire departments to different standards
for response times, different standards could apply to urban and rural EMS systems.
But whatever the standards are, adherence to them should be mandatory, and every
EMS organization, every year, should be required to report its performance to the relevant agency (perhaps the national lead agency discussed in the previous section).

I realize that any set of federal performance standards is likely to engender a storm
of resistance. There is the issue of unfunded mandates, and also of centralized versus
local control. And will there be consequences if a community falls short of the standards? Should the standards be linked to receipt of federal dollars, such as national
highway funding or Medicare reimbursement? (Most EMS services bill Medicare when
possible for transportation to local hospitals.) The data reported should also be available to public scrutiny. Citizen groups and the news media should celebrate when EMS
agencies meet the standards, and they should demand explanations when agencies
fall short. And, again, a little friendly competition might not be a bad thing. Perhaps
a national magazine could publish an annual guide to America's top ten cardiac-safe
cities. We have such rankings for most-livable cities, best colleges, and best hospitals.
Why not for surviving cardiac arrest?

Step 14. Create an Institute of Resuscitation Research within the NIH

It would be wonderful if the National Institutes of Health included an institute called,
say, the National Institute of Resuscitation Research (NIRR). But the likelihood of establishing a new research entity within the National Institutes of Health is approximately equal to the likelihood of seeing pigs fly. Nevertheless, concerted efforts by
resuscitation researchers have placed this idea on the national agenda and did convince the National Heart, Lung, and Blood Institute to contribute to funding for the
Resuscitation Outcomes Consortium, or ROC (https://roc.uwctc.org).[26] Despite some
initial frustrations, the ROC is a good initiative; it does not, however, have the permanence of an Institute. Creation of a National Institute of Resuscitation Research would

allow the research agenda to cross traditional lines, since research on resuscitation and emergency medical services necessarily involves basic science, clinical science, health services, epidemiology, economics, and ethics.[27]

One of the first tasks of a newly created NIRR would be to establish a clearing-house for research on resuscitation. It would be useful if the leading research issues could summate and disseminate the latest clinical and health services findings. So many issues remain unresolved that it may be time to establish a national research agenda. It would not take much to begin reaping big dividends from an institute like an NIRR. If national survival rates for cardiac arrest could be improved by a mere two percentage points that would mean 3,000 fewer Americans dying of cardiac arrest every year.

A second task would be to designate national centers of EMS research. Not every EMS agency should do research, but a few centers in the United States have excellent reputations for resuscitation research and should be supported. There is a National Institutes of Health model for providing grants to research centers, usually for a renewable term of five years, as well as awards to midcareer investigators for the same term (these awards provide support for established clinicians to further their research programs and give them opportunities to mentor junior investigators). Is this a self-serving recommendation? To an extent, yes, of course. But I'm not alone in thinking that good research centers deserve to be supported. The National Highway Traffic Safety Administration's National EMS Research Agenda has as its second recommendation the establishment of at least five "centers of excellence" to facilitate EMS research. Good idea.

Step 15. Establish Guidelines for Compassionate Withholding of Resuscitation

Chapter 8 discussed the problems that arise when EMS personnel do not have access to a patient's advance directive. Establishing guidelines for compassionate withholding of resuscitation, modeled on those used in King County, would be humane and simply the right thing to do. Discussions about end-of-life issues can be contentious. Perhaps the best way to move this agenda forward would be for national EMS organizations, such as the National Association of EMS Physicians, to take the lead in drafting model policies for compassionate nonresuscitation. This step will not per se increase survival from cardiac arrest but it can lead to "improved survival" in the broadest sense. This is an issue that transcends survival rate. Rather, it touches the core of who we are as emergency responders and how we should behave ethically and with humaneness and compassion. Ah, but isn't it inhumane to withhold resuscitation when 911 is called? I understand the complexity and perceived liability in withholding resuscitation. But respecting a person's wishes in the setting of a life-ending illness is the humane act. Performing resuscitation when it violates patient autonomy—and is futile to boot—should be avoided whenever possible.

It would be easy to sweep this matter under the rug, to assume that everyone who calls 911 wants a full-bore resuscitation. The reality is that many times 911 is called because at the time of an expected death, family members often do not know what to do. I have seen it happen all too often. A patient is enrolled in hospice and the family receives clear directions to call hospice instead of 911 but at the moment of death the family forgets and instead calls 911. Their call to 911 may be a request for information or a request to have death confirmed rather than a plea to bring their loved one back from an expected and hopefully humane death. But there is little nuance when calling 911. It is a system that once activated is full on. It is also not the role of dispatchers to determine if the patient has a valid "do not resuscitate" order before deciding whether to send EMS. Too often, because EMS is programmed to act first and ask questions later, the important issues of patient autonomy and medical futility are ignored. Patients' end-of-life wishes (or family members who convey these wishes in the case of cardiac arrest) must be respected in the setting of the end stages of a terminal illness. How can EMS come to accept a program that recognizes the autonomy of the patient and acknowledges the medical futility of attempting to resuscitate someone who has died from a terminal disease? This issue is too infrequently discussed. Admittedly, when EMS arrives at the scene the situation can be confusing. We always ask our EMTs to start the resuscitation and then try to sort out the situation. Is there a do-not-resuscitation document? Does the family know the patient's wishes? Was 911 called for information instead of wanting a resuscitation? Once the situation is clarified then stop the resuscitation or continue full on. That is the right thing to do.

PUTTING PLANS INTO ACTION

This chapter lists ten local steps and five national steps that will lead to improved survival. At the local level, there are four easy steps (the low-hanging fruit) and six more difficult steps (the higher-hanging fruit). But one community's "easy" may be another community's "difficult." An EMS director or manager, partnering with the medical director, must decide what can be achieved in his or her own community. Success with the low-hanging fruit will create momentum for tackling the higher-hanging fruit. The steps listed above provide the overview and general approach to implementation. Missing are detailed game plans as well as the specific tools to implement the programs. Reading a short description of high-performance CPR, or dispatcher-assisted CPR, or rapid dispatch may convince you of the importance and need of such programs but how do you bring them about?

At the beginning of this chapter, I urged Captain Daniel to attend a Resuscitation Academy session. This is not some fictional teaching program. The Resuscitation Academy really exists and it is offered tuition-free. Academy training is offered twice a year in Seattle, and the goal is to provide the knowledge and tools for EMS leaders to improve survival in their own communities (see the Addendum on the Resuscitation Academy). It was apparent from the first Academy class in 2009 that lectures and breakout sessions and workshops could only go so far. We, the faculty, needed to spell out the details of how to implement the various programs we were talking about. The Resuscitation Academy Tool Kits were developed to do just this. They provide a how-to guide for setting up various programs within local communities. But even tool kits have limitations, and we realize more and more how hard it can be for local communities to implement the various programs. We think more attention must be focused on the challenges of implementation and the need to mobilize local community resources. Thus the last portion of this chapter tries to shine a beacon (perhaps a little flashlight) on the difficult topic of implementation.

IMPLEMENTATION

Hendrika Meischke, PhD, is a professor of Health Services at the University of Washington. We have been colleagues in the world of resuscitation research for over twenty years. We both wonder what it takes for communities to implement some of the recommendations in this chapter as well as the lessons and programs of the Resuscitation Academy. The question is also gaining attention at the national level—the American Heart Association recently published a consensus statement in 2011 appropriately called "Implementation strategies for improving survival after out-of-hospital cardiac arrest in the United States." Why does community A embrace these recommendations and transform their system and why does community B, given the same information, do very little to improve resuscitation? What is the secret sauce? I wish there were definitive answers, though there is no end to possible explanations. Is it individual charisma? Is it leadership? Is it complementary personalities (the chemistry and synergism we saw between Dr. Copass and Dr. Cobb in chapter 6)? Is it legislative mandates (funded or not)? Is it adequate resources? Certainly some or all of these may provide part of the explanation. Common sense says that an effective leader can be a catalyst for change (I have seen very strong county medical directors almost single- handedly make substantive and dramatic changes in their EMS system), but such individuals are relatively rare and often the changes evaporate when that individual leaves or retires.

Dr. Meischke offers a framework to understand successful implementation. For a community to improve its survival rate, she believes there must be three complementary features. First, the core components (cardiac arrest registry, assertive dispatcher-assisted CPR, high-performance CPR, rapid dispatch) must be in place. Second, there must be fidelity to the core components. The best way to achieve fidelity is to define performance standards and use QI to measure the actual performance. This makes sense since, as is all too common, there is a large gap between perceived performance and actual performance. Third, the EMS program must adapt to the local situation. Again, this makes sense since only through mobilization of local resources can there be any chance of undertaking new initiatives. Change, always difficult, is best smoothed with local buy-in and support.

I like Dr. Meischke's framework since it provides structure to the miasma of ideas on this topic. Since this chapter provides a total of 15 steps to improve cardiac arrest survival, let me conclude the chapter with 5 suggested actions on how to implement changes in your local community.

ACTION 1: Form an advisory board. We believe the most important ingredient in the sauce of implementation is a team effort with a shared vision. The vision can be as simple as "Improving survival from out-of-hospital cardiac arrest." The advisory board or steering committee (or whatever term you use) should ideally be led or co-led by the EMS director (or fire chief or chief of EMS operations) and the medical director, with a core group consisting of the dispatch director, the head of EMT and paramedic training, the QI officer (if one exists), a representative of the local hospital (or local hospital association), and ideally a political leader (mayor or council member) and a "citizen." The latter could be the head of a local philanthropic organization, such as the Kiwanis or Rotary club. This core group may be ad hoc or formal (in other words commissioned by the mayor or council with formal appointments), and all it takes is one "fired-up" individual to catalyze the initiative. Large communities should have a full or at least a part-time staff person who is accountable to the advisory board and can keep everyone on task and maintaining forward momentum. I think of the staff person as the site coordinator who works on behalf of the advisory board.

ACTION 2: Determine how to make it happen in your community. Every step in this chapter must be customized to the local system and its strengths. There is no one pattern. Rochester, MN, has a completely different EMS system from Seattle and King County. And yet both achieve high survival rates, proving that there is no ONE system. Each EMS leader must mobilize and strategize based on what is possible locally.

ACTION 3: Set specific goals. This group must be realistic—they will not transform their system overnight and they should set attainable goals achieved by plucking the low-hanging fruits. Progress will likely be slow and iterative (step by step). But once on the path to improvement there is no stopping that community.

ACTION 4: Establish performance standards. For example, earlier in this chapter I listed possible performance standards for dispatcher-assisted CPR and high-performance CPR. Let everyone know what the standards are and why they matter. Then provide the training and support to meet these standards. Constant (and timely) feedback is also part of the equation.

ACTION 5: Measure and improve. Ongoing measurement of survival and ongoing QI are vital. A cardiac arrest registry need not be onerous. It can take as little as 10-15 minutes to register the data. Similarly, analysis of cardiac arrest CPR performance or dispatch performance need not be exhaustive; 10-15 minutes should provide the vital elements of QI and will certainly provide the information needed to monitor the system and allow for feedback to the individual EMS personnel and individual dispatchers. Praise is given for good performance, and, for the "less than good" performance, we always stress the challenges of the task and ask how it can be done better the next time. We have never used QI information in a punitive or disciplinary manner.

These five implementation actions help define the frame of resuscitation. The metaphor of a chain of survival and a frame of survival fit nicely with the concepts of resuscitation. The chain of survival is all about the specific therapy, particularly providing CPR and defibrillation as rapidly as possible and with as much fidelity as possible. The frame of survival is all about the qualitative factors—leadership, culture, ongoing training, and QI. These are the stuff of implementation: establish an advisory board (leadership), set specific goals (vision), establish performance standards (culture), determine how to make it happen (training), measure and improve. Clearly, the links in the chain and the qualities in the frame are integrally linked. Put them together and lives can be saved.

Email from Chief David Daniel

Dr. Eisenberg: Thanks so much for the opportunity to visit. I'm sorry we were unable to meet but I want to share with you a most remarkable resuscitation I viewed during my ride along with Medic 4. What was so remarkable to me was the seamless integration of EMT and paramedic care. It was like watching a finely choreographed ballet. The EMTs did letter perfect CPR and one of them even timed every stoppage of chest compression. The paramedics intubated the patient and started a central line without CPR stopping. Amazing! I have never seen this before. When the paramedics and I arrived the patient had been shocked twice by the EMTs. I was told that the wife had started CPR with assistance of the dispatcher. There was a faint pulse on our arrival but the patient refibrillated and the paramedics gave 7 more shocks. After 45 minutes the patient achieved a sustained return of spontaneous circulation, albeit supported by pressor agents.

My jaw drops in amazement and admiration of such a remarkable resuscitation. I sure hope the patient survives. After we left the hospital the lead paramedic recapped in six words what I had just witnessed. He said, "We never give up on VF."

He did not seem to be bragging; it was offered as a simple fact. The other paramedic mentioned to me that the full resuscitation including rhythm, voice and calculation of CPR fraction would be posted on line within 7 days for all the crewmembers to see. I was told that each crewmember will also receive an email when the outcome is known. I am blown away. So again, I thank you for the opportunity to view first hand your EMTs and paramedics in action. I just signed up for the next Resuscitation Academy – and convinced my medical director to join me.

Best wishes,
Captain David Daniel

ELEVEN

A Vision of the Future

Wouldn't it be amazing if the following news story appeared in the *New World Times* of 2050?

> October 2050, Stockholm
>
> Dr. William Oslerberg accepted the Nobel Prize in Medicine for the discovery of a new class of viruses, named "fibriviruses," that cause ventricular fibrillation. The virus is acquired in childhood. It lies dormant for several decades until fatty deposits in the lining of the coronary artery activate the virus and cause it to invade endothelial cells, reprogramming them to release cardioexcitatory gingykines.
>
> Oslerberg noted in his acceptance speech that the gingykines were named for his dog, Gingy, who became excited every time she saw him. He is confident that a vaccine can be developed against the new virus and that it will eliminate ventricular fibrillation as a cause of death.

Beware the seer who claims to predict the future. Even so, I can't resist the temptation. First, I'll make a short-term prediction and then gaze into the distant horizon for a long-term prediction.

IN THE SHORT-TERM

I believe that survival from VF in many communities could reach 60 percent. Some communities are already near 50 percent.[1] In King County we will approach 60 percent in the near future with meticulous application of high-performance CPR and intensive training in dispatcher recognition of cardiac arrest and delivery of telephone CPR. For communities currently at the 10, 20, 30, or 40 percent survival rates, I cannot guarantee a sudden surge to 60 percent, but I do think dramatic increases in survival are possible.

What is the likelihood that the four easy steps (the low-hanging fruit of cardiac arrest registry, dispatcher-assisted CPR, high-performance CPR, and rapid dispatch) of chapter 10 can be widely implemented and that they would come to define a new standard of care? (Remember I am not talking about communities that perfunctorily establish these programs but rather communities that train to high fidelity and with ongoing QI to ensure that standards are being met.) I am reasonably confident that dispatcher-assisted CPR and high-performance CPR will be embraced as communities learn of their potential and, most important, realize how relatively easy they are to implement. Dispatcher-assisted CPR and high-performance CPR work in synergy to keep the heart and brain "alive" for a precious few minutes and maximize the likelihood of successful defibrillation. These two programs by themselves do not defibrillate the heart but they improve the chances that a defibrillatory shock whenever it comes along will result in a perfusing rhythm. They also help provide nutrients and oxygen to the brain and thus improve neurological outcome.

The other two low-hanging fruits—cardiac arrest registry and rapid dispatch—also are likely to improve survival. Participation in a registry leads to several positive developments. There is the obvious ability to identify areas that need improvement and to respond to deficiencies, but another benefit is the opportunity for peer comparison. Let's assume communities A and B have similar demographics and similar EMS systems. Community A has a witnessed VF survival rate of 30 percent and community B has a survival rate of 10 percent. What is likely to happen? After the congratulations and champagne in A (and laments and eating of crow pie in B), I suspect community B will engage in self-analysis and see what it can do to lessen the gap. A bit of competitiveness can be a good thing. A registry can also lead to improved performance through the motivational power of the Hawthorne effect. Knowing that the EMS medical director is scrutinizing every cardiac arrest and determining outcomes will likely lead to better performance.

The last of the low-hanging fruit is rapid dispatch. In many communities this may be easy to accomplish but in others impediments of culture and proprietary requirements of the computer-aided dispatch (CAD) system may make rapid dispatch more challenging to implement. For one reason, many EMS medical directors do not have authority or influence over dispatch protocols, and for another, most dispatch centers are driven by the needs of police (police calls account for a majority of dispatches) and are cautious in instituting change for fear of adversely affecting police response time. Rapid dispatch by its very nature quickly determines that a serious medical problem is present and that it will become better defined while EMS personnel are en route. Despite these impediments I am optimistic that EMS directors and medical directors will come to realize that rapid dispatch is an easy way to shave time off the response interval. Jonathan Larsen, captain in the Seattle Fire Department (and a leader in the Resuscitation Academy), puts it this way, "It all comes down to time. You can't get into the truck and roll out the door any quicker or drive to the scene any faster. Rapid dispatch is an instant solution to improve response times. It is a no brainer." I agree.

IN THE LONG-TERM

My long-term prediction is that VF will become less of a public health problem than it is today. The lessening of the scourge of VF will likely come about in several ways— through prevention, identification of high-risk patients, reducing the incidence of heart disease, widespread defibrillation, better defibrillation, and better post-resuscitation care.

Can VF Be Prevented?

Although ventricular fibrillation is the final pathway of sudden death, no one really understands why it occurs. Why does a heart that beats normally for millions of beats suddenly go into a chaotic and lethal rhythm? Determining the answer to this question is the greatest challenge facing cardiology today. But the lack of a definitive answer does not preclude speculation. Many possible causes of VF, from irritation in the heart muscle to the influence of emotions and stress, have been suggested. Ventricular fibrillation does not appear out of nowhere. Almost always it is triggered in the context of underlying heart disease and atherosclerosis.

The most widely accepted explanation for VF is that it is triggered by ischemia (insufficient blood supply to the heart). This explanation makes physiological sense, since one assumes that ischemic heart cells will be more susceptible to cellular damage, which in turn can leak enzymes that may irritate the conducting system of the heart and lead to VF. The leaking of these enzymes has an effect comparable to that of a match thrown into a room filled with gasoline fumes.

Another possible VF trigger is a change in the autonomic nervous system's regulation of the heart. The autonomic nervous system comprises the sympathetic system (generally stimulatory) and the parasympathetic system (generally quieting). All the organs of the body have both sympathetic and parasympathetic nerves, which allow the organs to remain in proper balance. It is speculated that VF occurs when there is a sudden increase in sympathetic stimulation of the heart. This stimulation may be the result of stress or of overstimulation (for example, cocaine-induced VF may be caused by this mechanism). A variation on the sympathetic-tone argument comes from re-searchers who speculate that the trigger for VF is regional differences in the tone of the heart muscle, caused by zones of ischemia or infarction.

Sometimes medications can induce VF. In the 1980s, for example, there was a trial for a new drug that was intended to reduce disturbances in heart rhythm but instead had the paradoxical effect of increasing such disturbances, including VF. Some medications lead to potassium depletion in the body, and this in turn can trigger VF. Other medications block the sodium, potassium, or calcium channels within cell membranes, and these blockages in turn may lead to increased disturbances in heart rhythm. There are undoubtedly many drug interactions that are poorly under-stood. Given the polypharmacy which most elderly Americans rely upon daily, not to mention the plethora of vitamins and supplements, it should not be surprising that too much or too little of a particular medication can have adverse effects or produce unexpected interactions.

Genetic predispositions may also play a role in triggering VF. There are known genetic conditions, such as long Q-T syndrome and others, which make an individual more prone to VF (see chapter 3). No doubt there are other genetic factors yet to be identified that make the heart more vulnerable to VF. Many diseases probably result from interactions between environmental factors and the patient's genetic disposi-tion. Consider smoking and lung cancer. Not everyone who smokes gets lung cancer—only 10 to 15 percent. Do the 85 to 90 percent have lucky genes? Does a patient who fibrillates have unlucky genes?

Can VF Be Predicted?

Even if one did not understand the specific triggers of VF, it still might be possible to identify people at risk of having VF and to take preventive steps. One can, with some precision, stratify risks for cardiac arrest and VF. For example, the general population has an incidence of cardiac arrest of 1 arrest per 3,000 people per year. For people with ischemic heart disease, the incidence is 5 arrests per 100 people per year, or 5 percent. For mild congestive heart failure, the figure is 8 percent; for severe congestive heart failure, it is 12 percent. Rates for VF are probably half those given for the preced-ing conditions. For someone who has had one episode of VF, the chance of a repeat episode in any given year is 20 percent. According to national guidelines, someone who has moderate or severe congestive heart failure,[2] or who has had an episode of VF that was not associated with an acute myocardial infarction, should receive an implantable cardioverter defibrillator (ICD), because the risk of VF is so high. Why not put an ICD in everyone at risk? These devices are expensive—$75,000, including the implantation costs—and they are not without serious complications, among them the risk of infection and of the device's misfiring (in other words, it may deliver a shock when a shock is not needed).[3] ICD technology is not perfect, and this is clearly not a strategy for everyone.

While it would be useful to identify who in the general population (or even among those with ischemic heart disease) might be likely to have VF, it would be even more of a challenge to predict when the event would happen. It is one thing to state that someone has a 5 percent chance of VF in any given year, but it is another to know that this person is likely to have VF in the next month or week or day. There is currently no diagnostic procedure or test that can make such a prediction. Until such a day comes, we have no choice when VF occurs but to start CPR and rush a defibrillator to the patient.

Reducing the Incidence of Heart Disease

Despite the lack of understanding about what triggers VF, and the difficulty in knowing when VF will occur, there are still strategies for reducing its incidence and that of sudden cardiac death in general. Perhaps the best strategy is to reduce the risk factors for heart disease in individuals. The usual cast of characters is implicated here, and the approach to them is defined by avoidance (smoking) or control (high cholesterol, high blood pressure, diabetes), but there are also preemptive actions that can be taken—engaging in vigorous exercise, taking a daily aspirin, drinking a daily glass of wine, and consuming omega-3 fatty acids (such as those found in fish) twice weekly. Optimism about modification of risk factors must be tempered by the difficulty of making changes in lifestyle. Nevertheless, modification of risk factors may be our best option until such time as we have a clear understanding of VF. It is, after all, possible to manage a disease without understanding its cause. Cholera was managed by removal of contaminated water sources long before the cholera organism was identified. Scurvy was managed with citrus fruits added to the diet long before the effects of vitamin C deficiency were elucidated. And countless other diseases have been and can be controlled even in the absence of precise knowledge about their causes. Similarly, we can reduce the incidence of VF if we can reduce the incidence of heart disease. The best confirmation of this strategy is the observation that the incidence of VF is indeed falling, and that it parallels the decline in the number of deaths from heart disease. In Seattle, Cobb and his colleagues looked at the incidence of VF over a period of thirty years and noted a dramatic reduction.[4] Other authors have made similar observations.[5]

A strong argument for preemptive modification of risk factors is the fact that cardiac arrest is in many instances the first manifestation of heart disease. In other words, someone has heart disease but it remains totally silent until he or she collapses in cardiac arrest. A detailed review of all cardiac arrest incident reports in King County for the years 2000 and 2001 demonstrated that approximately 60 percent of the patients had known heart disease.[6] This figure may even be slightly low, since there were some events (such as cardiac arrests that occurred in public places) in which paramedics were unable to determine the patient's medical history. Nevertheless, the figure is still remarkable for what it reveals about the large number of people who collapsed suddenly without any known heart disease. The fact that they didn't know about it doesn't mean that they didn't have heart disease—many of the hearts, if autopsies had been performed, would have shown evidence of heart disease—but it does mean that up to 40 percent of the victims of sudden death were unaware that they had heart disease. According to other studies, that figure is approximately 30 percent.[7] Any strategy designed to target high-risk patients would have to take these findings into account.

Widespread Defibrillation

There is a simple causal chain in resuscitation. The more defibrillators there are in a community, the more likely they will be used. The sooner a shock can be delivered, the more likely the patient will survive. The bottom line will be a higher overall survival rate in the community. Making AEDs widely available in public locations is an option with only modest potential, primarily because of the small percentage of cardiac arrests that occur in public places and the challenge of placing AEDs throughout a community. A better strategy might be to place AEDs in high-risk public locations such as exercise facilities, shopping malls, and other locations where large numbers of people congregate.[8] As noted in chapter 10, AEDs are slowly disseminating into the community and beginning to play a small but measurable role in the initial management of VF.[9]

Another strategy might be to encourage AEDs in the homes of high-risk individuals. As noted above, the biggest challenge to the high-risk home strategy is identifying high-risk patients. A small percentage of patients with known high risk (such as moderate to severe congestive heart failure as defined by a low ejection fraction) are eligible to receive implantable defibrillators. The one trial that randomized home AEDS to 7,000 patients with prior anterior wall myocardial infarction (not a particularly high risk event especially since the patients were enrolled months or even years after the myocardial infarction) had far fewer events than anticipated. The study was unable to show a survival difference between the two groups.[10]

Because so many VF events do not have a structural coronary event (acute infarction), symptoms are often not present, and sometimes there is absence of underlying coronary artery disease, a traditional solution seems evasive. The current medical approach categorizes an automated external defibrillator as a medical device. Most are costly, requiring a prescription (one device that is FDA approved for over the counter sale is available for sale on the Web at $1,200), and few insurance companies will cover the expense. Current AEDs are engineered and ruggedized primarily for EMS or first responder situations. They are able to deliver 30 shocks and monitor for an hour.

They also have sophisticated data recording capability. The power demands of current AEDs require sophisticated and expensive batteries. A cardiologist friend of mine has an AED in the trunk of his car but it has had a dead battery for months and he can't seem to get around to ordering a new one for $300 dollars. The hassle factor of online ordering a specialized, expensive battery is sizable.

The above AED requirements result in large and costly devices. Rather than pursue a medical approach of solving unexpected VF, try a consumer model. The consumer model accepts that VF is an unpredictable and infrequent event and that, while there may be hierarchies of risk, any adult is at some risk of dying from sudden and unexpected VF. A consumer model says a defibrillator must be reengineered for consumers. It must be widely available, small, run on disposable batteries, and be engineered for two or three shocks. And, most important, it must be inexpensive. I would love to see a $100 consumer automated external defibrillator that is powered by a 9-volt battery and is no bigger than an iPhone. This would be a game changer. And why not shoot for the moon—how about an AED attachment that could run off a smart phone's operating system and battery. When activated, it would automatically alert the dispatch center and send GPS coordinates.

A consumer AED would be a real breakthrough but it would not solve the entire problem of providing quick defibrillation. The reality remains that half of all cardiac arrests that occur at home are unwitnessed, and so the potential benefit of an AED is considerably lessened. Certainly a simple and reliable alerting device would be very useful, since it would potentially turn many unwitnessed cardiac arrests into incidents in which someone is alerted. For example, a life-sign transmitter worn on the body could be used to indicate, or trigger alarms for, high-risk cardiac arrhythmias or loss of vital signs. As one engineer said, "It should be easy to tell when a pump inside 200 pounds of warm salt water stops moving." It should be easy, but I suspect that we are years away from manufacturing such a device.

Better Defibrillation

Improving defibrillation is another way of improving the science of resuscitation. Regrettably, not every defibrillatory shock is successful. In fact, most shocks are unsuccessful and often multiple shocks are required until the patient is either converted to a sustaining rhythm or eventually reaches asystole (flat line) and the effort is called off. How can the ability of a shock to defibrillate be improved? As discussed in chapter 5, the timing and sequencing of CPR and defibrillation are important. It is also possible for information from the fibrillatory signal to provide useful data to guide the resuscitation. Most people looking at an ECG rhythm strip of ventricular fibrillation see squiggly lines, but a great deal of information is buried within that chaotic pattern.

Electrical aspects of the VF signal can be used to calculate the probability that return of spontaneous circulation (P-ROSC) will be restored by the next shock (survival can be calculated as well).[10] This probability is determined from calculations of spectral densities, frequency, dominant frequency, amplitude, scaling exponents, transformations, and other electrical terms I don't pretend to understand. And since the P-ROSC can be calculated in real time, it will be possible to determine whether it is rising or falling. This calculation in turn can guide the resuscitation. For example, if the P-ROSC is calculated to be 20 percent immediately after pads attachment, the "smart" defibrillator might indicate that CPR should be performed and medications administered instead of an immediate shock delivered. Once the P-ROSC reaches 50 or 60 percent, a shock would be indicated. Shocking for a low P-ROSC is not indicated, since the low likelihood of success will only deprive the heart of CPR during the pause for the defibrillatory shock, and the shock itself is not without potential harm to the heart muscle. To give a concrete example, a defibrillator that can guide therapy will electronically "see" a patient whose VF has a frequency of 400 per minute and an amplitude of 4 millimeters and will then advise the operator to provide (high-performance) CPR instead of defibrillation. The machine will prompt the rescuer to "prime" the heart until the VF signal is ripe for a successful shock. When the threshold for success has been reached and surpassed, the machine will prompt the rescuer to deliver the shock. Or, again, a defibrillator that "sees" a patient whose VF has a frequency of 600 per minute and an amplitude of 6 millimeters will tell the operator to shock immediately. There is much interest in such a technology,[11] and I hope there will be some breakthroughs in the coming decade.

Defibrillators could be improved to "read" the ECG rhythm while CPR is ongoing. Current defibrillators require CPR to cease periodically so that the AED (or the rescuer) can see and interpret the ECG signal without interference. If the defibrillator could sense VF while CPR was in progress, the patient could receive continuous CPR right up to the moment of defibrillation. This in turn would keep the left ventricle filled with blood and allow a defibrillatory shock to be more successful. Ample animal studies have demonstrated that stopping CPR for even fifteen seconds allows blood to drain from the ventricle and makes a shock less likely to defibrillate the heart. Ideally, there would be no pause in delivery of CPR. Several defibrillator manufacturers and scientists at the University of Washington and other universities are working on such an enhanced defibrillator. Scientific articles demonstrating its feasibility are beginning to appear.[12]

Changing the defibrillatory waveform itself may improve the efficiency of defibrillation. Current defibrillators use monophasic or biphasic wave forms, and there are several variations of each. There is no reason to think that better waveforms cannot be found. What about triphasic or quadraphasic waveforms? What about dual-pathway defibrillators using more than two pads? What about defibrillatory pads that abrade the skin to lower impedance and thus require lower energy to defibrillate the heart. Ongoing research will likely shed light on these options. It is clearly in AED manufacturers' interest to find the most efficient method of defibrillation that uses the least amount of energy.

Recent evidence suggests that the current practice of lifting the hands off the chest while defibrillation occurs may not be necessary. It has been conventional wisdom that the rescuers should not be touching the patient (therefore stopping CPR) during defibrillation in order not to receive a shock themselves. A 2008 study in *Circulation* demonstrated that rescuers performing chest compression during the defibrillatory shock are exposed to low levels of current.[13] In other words, even if the rescuer is touching the patient's chest during the exact moment of defibrillation, there is not enough current entering the rescuer to be of any consequence. It should be pointed out that the rescuers in the study were wearing polyethylene medical gloves (the current practice for EMS personnel), which serve as insulators. The study is significant because it suggests that CPR need not stop for defibrillation, which in turn may keep the ventricles more filled with blood, making the defibrillatory shock more likely to succeed.

It is even conceivable that a future device may obtain information other than the heart's ECG signal. It may be able to look at heart wall motion or pick up internal sounds that can be used to guide the rescuer. And let's not stop with heart function. Why not combine a defibrillator with a device for measuring specific blood chemistries? Imagine a defibrillator with a port to accept and analyze a micro drop of a patient's blood (it would be similar to the equipment used for glucose measurement and other point-of-care devices that are increasingly used in and out of hospitals). After the device determined the patient's lactate, potassium, pH, bicarbonate, cardiac enzymes, and a host of other parameters (all in a few seconds), recommended drugs and their dosages would be flashed on a screen along with the sequence and recommended energy level of defibrillation.

Finally, to complete this discussion about improving the science of resuscitation, let us also consider the wearable defibrillator. There is probably a small niche for such a device. It can be used, for example, by the unstable ICU patient waiting for a heart transplant or an ICD, or by the patient who already has an ICD but has developed a problem with it and is awaiting a replacement. Nevertheless, the high cost and inconvenience of a wearable defibrillator make this option an impractical out-of-hospital solution to the problem of sudden cardiac death.

Better Post-Resuscitation Care

Yet another way to improve overall survival rates for sudden cardiac arrest is to improve the survival of individuals who have been successfully defibrillated. Currently, about 30-50 percent of all patients who are initially resuscitated and admitted to a hospital go on to die there. Just imagine if techniques could be devised to improve this survival rate. Extensive research is under way to salvage more defibrillated patients. Most of the time, the term "salvage" is used in connection with the brain and other vital organs. Its use in this context is relevant because most deaths that occur after hospitalization for cardiac arrest are due to brain damage from lack of oxygen and to pump failure of the heart.

New therapies offer some promise of improving survival once the patient has been resuscitated. Hypothermia was the first, and to date only, therapy to improve survival and neurological recovery among resuscitated VF patients (see chapter 10). While this is encouraging, there are still many unresolved issues with hypothermia therapy.

Another possible therapeutic intervention is hemofiltration (filtration of the blood). Hemofiltration attempts to filter out endotoxins and inflammatory molecules that were created when the body was in cardiac arrest. In a French study, investigators assigned sixty-one patients to one of three groups—a control group that received no intervention, a group that received hemofiltration, and a group that received both hemofiltration and hypothermia. Survival was better in the two hemofiltration groups than in the control group, and hypothermia was found to confer no additive benefit.[14] Lest everyone rush to perform hemofiltration, however, there are some downsides—it is expensive and cumbersome, and it may lead to abnormal lowering of potassium and other electrolytes in the blood.

I'm sure other post-resuscitative measures will be proposed and studied in the future. Let's hope some are beneficial.

THE PARADOX OF TECHNOLOGY

There are remarkable technologies to recognize and treat ventricular fibrillation but the fundamental understanding of what causes VF eludes us. AEDs and ICDs and other high-tech devices can stave off death and improve the quality of life. Internal and external automated defibrillators—truly a marvel of design and engineering— have saved thousands of lives. But within the "gee whiz" aspects of the technology there is a paradox not appreciated by most people: ICDs and AEDs actually represent our failure to understand and prevent heart disease. We treat the final expression of the disease—in this case, sudden death—long after the disease first appears. Similar paradoxes exist with respect to the sophisticated medical technologies used in renal dialysis, cancer therapy, and a host of other treatments.

AEDs and ICDs share a trajectory characteristic of many other emerging medical technologies: initial skepticism, successful human application, exaggerated expectations, extended indications, clinical trials demonstrating limitations, and, finally, redefined applications. Meanwhile, the device in question becomes increasingly sophisticated as each new generation incorporates additional features, all of them housed in a smaller package. All too often, however, this reduction in size is not accompanied by a parallel reduction in cost.

By contrast with the situation in what is perceived to be high-technology medicine, a more fundamental understanding of disease often characterizes the interventions of what most people would consider to be low-technology medicine. For example, vaccinations, medications for high blood pressure, and insulin for diabetes are simple, inexpensive therapies based on deep understanding of the underlying disease.[15] Defibrillation is both awesome and impressive. The technology is truly remarkable, as are the advances made in recent decades. But our inability to understand the triggers and causes of ventricular fibrillation is humbling.

Someday we will achieve a fundamental understanding of VF and its causes, and such understanding will lead to effective therapies to prevent its onset. In the meantime, there is a bottom line of sorts. We can take action, as individuals and communities, to reduce the likelihood of VF and to treat it should it occur. Individuals can reduce their risks.[16] Communities can improve their EMS responses. For now, that is all we can do. But it may be enough to ensure the continued beating of many hearts too good to die.

NEW YORK CITY, REVISITED—DECEMBER 31,

FIVE YEARS IN THE FUTURE

The onset of Clarence's symptoms was almost imperceptible at first. He just had a little more difficulty breathing. Initially he attributed the trouble to a mild stomach upset. But it got worse and worse, and he found himself leaning forward to try to take in more air. Soon beads of perspiration covered his forehead.

Clarence rang his neighbor and asked for help. By the time his neighbor got down the corridor to Clarence's apartment, there was no answer, and the neighbor had to run back to his own apartment to get the key Clarence had given him. When he finally entered, Clarence was on the floor.

The neighbor dialed 911. The dispatcher confirmed the address and asked if the patient was conscious? "No" was the reply. Was the patient breathing normally? Again "no." The dispatcher informed the neighbor that there was an AED in the lobby of the apartment building and that someone else at the dispatcher center was calling the doorman and would tell the doorman to rush the device up to Clarence's apartment. Meanwhile, the dispatcher gave Clarence's neighbor instructions for performing chest compression CPR. "Push hard and fast in the center of the chest, right between the nipples. Count just like me. One, two, three, four, five. Keep going."

Within two minutes, the doorman, breathless, arrived with the AED (little bigger than an iPhone) and applied it to Clarence's chest, following the machine's electronic voice instructions (and taking a little prompting from the dispatcher). The first shock was successful, and shortly after it was delivered, Clarence began to moan. The EMTs arrived within seven minutes from the time the neighbor had called 911. Soon after they arrived, Clarence refibrillated. The EMTs performed two minutes of high-performance CPR and delivered a second shock, which resulted in an organized rhythm and faint pulse. The paramedics placed an LMA (laryngeal mask airway) to insure an open airway and started an IV line. Just as they were administering an anti-arrhythmic medication, Clarence went into ventricular fibrillation yet again, and a third shock was successfully applied.

Clarence was transported to Bellevue hospital. In the emergency department he was started on the hospital's hypothermia protocol. Eight days later, Clarence was discharged home with excellent neurological recovery.

Two weeks after Clarence's cardiac arrest, the EMS medical director reviewed Clarence's case and sent "attaboys" to the crew and dispatcher. Since the case was the last for the calendar year, she pulled up her spreadsheet, quickly did a few calculations, and proudly announced that the survival rate for witnessed VF in New York was 46 percent for the year.

Addendum: Resuscitation Academy

Measure, improve, measure, improve . . .

If you've seen one EMS system, you've seen one EMS system

It's not complicated, but it's not easy

Change occurs step by step

Performance, not protocol

Everyone in VF survives

It takes a system to save a victim

—"Mantras" at the Resuscitation Academy

The tag line for the Resuscitation Academy is "improving cardiac arrest survival, one community at a time." Since the first Academy class in 2009, we have been trying to do just that. The Resuscitation Academy, held twice a year in Seattle, is a joint effort of King County EMS (Public Health—Seattle and King County), Seattle Medic One (Seattle Fire Department), and the Medic One Foundation. Additional support comes from Harborview Medical Center, University of Washington, Medtronic Foundation HeartRescue Program, Asmund S. Laerdal Foundation for Acute Medicine, and Life Sciences Discovery Fund. Many of the faculty you have met in chapter 6—Drs. Cobb, Copass, Rea, Kudenchuk, Nichol, and Sayre. The executive director is Ann Doll, head of the Medical QI Section in King County EMS, who provides direction, leadership, and tremendous organizational skills. The strong partnership between Seattle Medic One and King County EMS is personified by the contributions of Captain Jonathan

Larsen and Senior Paramedic Norm Nedell, both from the Seattle Fire Department; Linda Culley, Randi Phelps, Steve Perry, Jennifer Blackwood, Megan Bloomingdale, and Susan Damon from King County EMS; Michele Olsufka from Seattle Medic One; Dr. Hendrika Meischke from the University of Washington, and Jan Sprake, executive director of the Medic One Foundation. The faculty members are veterans in directing EMS programs and distinguished researchers in resuscitation science. My back of the envelope calculation says that the faculty members collectively represent 300 years of EMS experience.

The Resuscitation Academy is offered tuition-free and attendees come from throughout the country and the world. The small class size allows for a two-way exchange of information—the faculty provides evidence-based information and tools to improve cardiac arrest survival and the attendees share the real-life challenges they face. Every community has a different constellation of culture, leadership, resources, and opportunity. Above all we (the faculty) have learned that change is very challenging and one should never assume that a good idea will always be embraced and implemented. Impediments to change, whether they stem from habit, inertia, malaise, or lack of resources, can overwhelm the best of intentions. We have also learned that no system will transform itself overnight. Change is not only difficult, it occurs slowly—tiny step by tiny step. (I use "we" throughout this description of the Resuscitation Academy to acknowledge the fantastic team effort.)

RESUSCITATIONACADEMY.ORG

Information about the Academy may be found at resuscitationacademy.org. The most recent curriculum is posted on the site, as well as upcoming Academy classes and registration information. Though we have experimented with different lengths for the Academy, ranging from five days to one day, we have settled into a two-day length that allows a nice mixture of lectures, small group discussions, workshops, and breakout sessions. We expect every student to select a project to implement in his or her home community upon return from the Academy. We limit each Academy to 35-40 students in order to maintain a small-group seminar feel to the class. Plus the small class allows the faculty to get to know the individuals and vice versa.

THE ACADEMY'S MANTRAS

The Academy's mantras, although bordering on the simplistic, attempt to encapsulate a kernel of wisdom. The first, "Measure, improve, measure, improve . . . ," defines the essence of ongoing quality improvement. If you don't measure something you can't improve it. And once you measure it you will reveal things that need improving. And once you improve the system, measure it again to see if it has improved. And so on and so on. Measurement and improvement can apply to many elements of an EMS system. First and at the most basic level, they refer to measuring cardiac arrest events and outcomes (death, survival, neurological recovery). But they also apply to components of the EMS system, such as time metrics (time for dispatch, time for response, time for scene arrival, time for patient arrival), high-performance CPR metrics (CPR density, depth of compression, full recoil, duration of pauses), and dispatcher assisted CPR metrics (recognition of agonal breathing, time to recognition of cardiac arrest, time to delivery of chest compression instructions).

The next mantra, "If you've seen one EMS system, you've seen one EMS system," reminds both the faculty and the students that there exists incredible variety among EMS systems. No two systems are the same; what may be easy to accomplish in one may be difficult if not downright impossible in another. One example: in some Washington State counties, the EMS medical director has no authority in setting dispatch standards or guidelines for dispatching of EMS. Thus, even if the medical director wishes to establish a dispatcher-assisted CPR program, it would be impossible without the full cooperation of the dispatch director. If the dispatch center does not welcome physician involvement (unfortunately too commonly true), an impasse exists unlikely to be brokered. But that same community may have a mandatory CPR training program for high school students—something other EMS systems wish they had. The differing strengths and limitations of every EMS community are legion.

"It's not complicated, but it's not easy" is a favorite mantra of my colleague Dr. Tom Rea. The science behind the programs is not difficult to grasp and the program requirements are fairly straightforward. An understanding of quantum mechanics is not required. But there may be logistical, cultural, political, resource, union, and a variety of other obstacles that block easy implementation. We believe strongly that change must start at the local level. It is the local medical, administrative, training, operations, and other personnel who are most accountable and can best decide how to bring about change. The Academy faculty can provide the tools and describe roadblocks other communities have encountered, but ultimately each attendee must determine what is doable and how much effort it will take.

The message "change occurs step by step" is pretty clear. EMS systems are complex organizations and not likely to be transformed overnight, no matter what the leadership may wish. Dr. Rea offers the analogy of not trying for a home run on your first at bat in the Majors. A single would do just fine. Even a walk will move the effort forward. With each change (improvement) one should remember the first mantra and continue to measure to see if the change really improved matters.

"Performance, not protocol" is a favorite mantra of Captain Jonathan Larsen, supervisor of the Seattle Medic One program. What counts during a resuscitation is the actual performance of the dispatchers, EMTs, and paramedics. A perfect example is dispatcher-assisted CPR. Most dispatch centers claim to have protocols for telephone

CPR but, in fact, when you measure their performance they come up lacking. There is either infrequent or delayed recognition of cardiac arrest,or both. The bottom line is that these centers may have the protocols but are lacking in performance. Another example might be EMS systems that have protocols defining a standard of high-performance CPR. But unless the system trains and requires its EMTs to achieve letter-perfect performance, the protocol will be so many empty words. Of course, the best way to identify and correct poor performance is through ongoing QI, which circles back to the first mantra— "measure, improve."

The next mantra is "Everyone in VF survives." This pithy expression makes the point that expectations become reality. Of course, not everyone in VF will survive out of hospital cardiac arrest but if there is a mindset that they will, behavior will subtly be altered to make it happen. The crew will work a little harder and not give up. They will assume the patient will make it to the hospital alive. In our EMS system, losing a patient in VF is simply unacceptable. I have seen patients receive over 20 defibrillatory shocks with the resuscitation lasting over an hour before achieving a sustaining pulse and blood pressure. Amazing! Remember the cardiologist in chapter 9 who depicted VF as a benign rhythm? His tongue was in his cheek, since VF means a patient is clinically dead, but he was also making the important point that all that is needed to treat this rhythm is quickly applied electricity. Therein lies the challenge. Quickly applied defibrillation is easy for a cardiologist in a cath laboratory but a bit more difficult out in the community. Nevertheless, if one keeps the mantra in mind—everyone in VF survives—a kind of self-fulfilling prophecy is created. Another aspect to this slogan is that medical directors and EMS directors will begin to scrutinize cases more closely, particularly those in which survival did not occur. The relevant question to ask is "Why did this patient in VF not survive?" Asked this way, it forces one to look at the system factors that may have contributed to the patient's death. Was there a delay in responding? Was there a delay in dispatcher recognition of cardiac arrest? Were telephone CPR instructions provided? Was there bystander CPR? Were there excessive pauses in chest compression? Were there delays in defibrillation?

"It takes a system to save a victim." Given the unpredictable and catastrophic nature of sudden cardiac arrest, not to mention the brief therapeutic window of opportunity, it is remarkable that anyone can be resuscitated. It is amazingly complicated and difficult to save a victim of sudden cardiac arrest. Though it may be individuals who perform CPR, attach the defibrillator, secure the airway, and administer medications it is a system that makes it all possible. The system is made up of a complex web of interacting agencies—dispatch centers, fire departments, paramedic programs, EMS agencies, and hospitals—and literally hundreds of dispatchers, EMTs, paramedics, fire chiefs, medical services officers, medical services administrators, training officers, QI staff, medical director, hospital nurses, doctors, and staff. Implied in this mantra is the modifier "excellent." Every part of the Academy, directly or indirectly, is about building an excellent system.

THE ACADEMY'S MAIN MESSAGE

The Academy encapsulates the collective experience of decades of running the Seattle Medic One and King County EMS programs. Chapter 9, "Putting It All Together," offered the message that quantitative and qualitative factors explain a system's success or failure in managing cardiac arrest. The combination of measurable and "soft" factors was conveyed in the figure of the chain of survival (measurable quantitative factors) surrounded by a frame of survival ("softer" qualitative factors). The operant message is that the chain of survival and the frame of survival provide a complete package for success. The Academy offers concrete instruction on how to build that package.

Quantitative Programs: Improving the Chain of Survival

The Academy starts with the need to measure cardiac arrest survival. We encourage all attendees to enroll their community in a national cardiac arrest database such as CARES (Cardiac Arrest Registry to Enhance Survival—mycares.net). The CARES website is packed with useful information including the data dictionary and examples of auto generated reports. CARES staff will help—with training and guided instruction—any EMS system wishing to join the CARES network.With training complete, it requires about 15 minutes for the registrar to enter a case and about 5 minutes for designated hospital staff to provide outcome data. An upgrade in 2011 added optional data elements. Participation in the registry provides an excellent snapshot of a system's performance as well as comparison data with national averages. The registry comes with templates so communities can review their statistics in any manner they choose. The Utstein template provides the survival rate for witnessed cases of VF, generally considered to be the best summary metric of cardiac arrest survival in a community.

If a community is unable to enroll in CARES the Academy can supply attendees with a stand-alone database called CATS—Cardiac Arrest Tracking System. This registry uses an Access program to capture the key variables for cardiac arrest events, including hospital outcomes. The system is almost identical to CARES in terms of data elements, and it comes with a complete data dictionary. Users of CATS are able to retrieve Utstein and customized reports. Since it is a freestanding registry, there is no opportunity to automatically compare performance with other communities or with a national average.

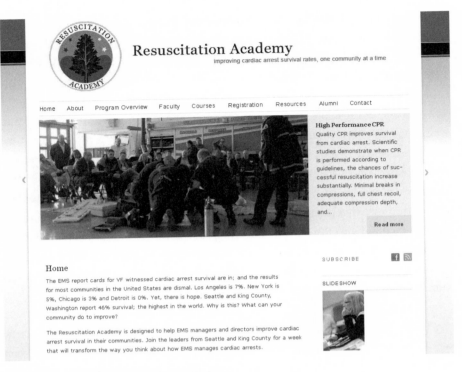

Screen shot of Resuscitation Academy web site

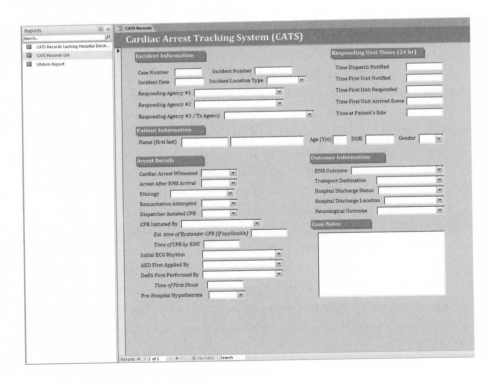

Cardiac Arrest Tracking System (CATS)

Because of the importance of CPR and defibrillation much attention is given to these two topics. Lectures and tool kits are provided on how to begin or improve dispatcher-assisted CPR (synonymous terms are telephone CPR, dispatcher CPR, and dispatcher-assisted telephone CPR), high-performance CPR, bystander CPR, public access defibrillation, and police AED. We know that not every part of each tool kit will apply to every community. We encourage the attendees to pick and choose that which is most relevant to their situation. As described in chapter 10, the two programs with the best payoff for the least investment of resources are assertive programs in dispatch-assisted CPR and training in high-performance CPR. As a result, the Academy devotes extra time to describe the importance of these programs and provides separate workshops to supplement lecture material. In order to explain why high-performance CPR is so critical, the first morning of the Academy includes a lecture on the science behind CPR. This lecture is a convincing portrayal of why fidelity to letter-perfect CPR maximizes blood flow to the brain and heart, which in turn provides the substrate for a successful defibrillatory shock.

QUALITATIVE PROGRAMS: IMPROVING THE FRAME OF SURVIVAL

Since QI is such a vital part of the Frame of Survival we place particular emphasis on QI for dispatcher-assisted CPR and high-performance CPR. Attendees see the QI system for each of these programs and learn in workshops the details of how they operate.

Tool Kits

The Resuscitation Academy provides toolkits on the following topics:

Cardiac Arrest Registry
High Performance CPR: Training, Implementation, and QI
Dispatcher Assisted CPR: Training, Implementation, and QI
Community Public Access Defibrillation
Police Defibrillation
End of Life Issues
Foundation and Fundraising

The tool kits are not recipe books with specific steps for each program. Rather, they provide the information, background, training materials, sample letters, sample forms, references, and resources, as well as a general approach to achieving buy-in from directors, managers, dispatchers, EMTs, paramedics, and police. While they provide important tools, the contents of each kit must be applied and/or modified based upon resources and leadership within the attendee's community.

While most of the kits are directed toward the chain and frame of survival, there are two kits that provide supplemental information. One is on End of Life Issues (See chapters 8 and 10) and the other tackles the challenging matter of raising funds. Most EMS programs face increasing demand for services and programs, while grappling with decreasing resources. When EMS personnel are being laid off, it seems hardly the right time to take on new programs requiring new staff or additional resources. But we think there are ways to create additional resources. Call it the margin of excellence to make the system better even in the face of difficult economic conditions. One of the tool kits specifically addresses how to establish a local foundation and engage in fundraising. Several communities have used the information in this kit to find resources for new equipment and to fund additional staff time for QI activities.

The tool kits are publicly available on the Resuscitation Academy website: resuscitationacademy.org. PDFs of each tool kit may be downloaded at no charge. All the information on the website is free.

The faculty considers the Resuscitation Academy to be a work in progress. We strive to make each Academy better than the one before. In addition to the two-day full Academy, we offer one-day mini Academies focused on dispatcher-assisted CPR and high-performance CPR. Such mini Academies can better reach the folks directly responsible for training and QI. We continually learn from attendees what works best and what needs to be dropped or modified. We have welcomed the opportunity to partner with EMS leaders in other states to assist with regional Resuscitation Academies.

Notes

ONE **How We Die Suddenly**

1 The ratio of ventilations to chest compressions was two to fifteen when this event occurred. Now the ratio is two to thirty. In addition, EMTs and paramedics now follow every shock with two minutes of CPR before assessing the patient's rhythm.

2 C. S. Fox, J. C. Evans, M. J. Larson, W. B. Kannel, and D. Levy, "Temporal Trends in Coronary Heart Disease Mortality and Sudden Cardiac Death From 1950 to 1999: The Framingham Heart Study," *Circulation* 110 (2004), 522–27.

3 R. Davis, "Doctors in Charge Rarely Call the Shots: Most Medical Directors in Big Cities Lack the Power to Improve the System," *USA Today*, July 29, 2003.

4 T. D. Rea, M. S. Eisenberg, G. Sinibaldi, and R. D. White, "Incidence of EMS-Treated Out-of-Hospital Cardiac Arrest in the United States," *Resuscitation* 63 (2004), 17–24.

5 R. D. White, T. J. Bunch, and D. G. Hankins, "Evolution of a Community-Wide Early Defibrillation Programme: Experience over 13 Years Using Police/Fire Personnel and Paramedics as Responders," *Resuscitation* 65 (2005), 279–83; T. D. Rea, M. Helbock, S. Perry, et al., "Increasing Use of Cardiopulmonary Resuscitation During Out-of-Hospital Ventricular Fibrillation Arrest: Survival Implications of Guideline Changes," *Circulation* 114 (2006), 2760–65.

6 R. B. Dunne, S. Compton, R. J. Zalenski, R. Swor, R. Welch, and B. F. Bock, "Outcomes from Out-of-Hospital Cardiac Arrest in Detroit," *Resuscitation* 72 (2007), 59–65. There was only one cardiac arrest survivor in the Detroit report and this patient had a rhythm other than VF. There were actually no survivors from VF. It is not technically accurate to speak of a 46–fold difference in survival when one of the numbers is zero. Thus, I have taken the liberty to state the survivor rate was <1 percent. As if it weren't bad enough that Detroit has the lowest survival rate for VF, a recent FBI report listed Detroit as the most dangerous city in the

country in terms of crime; see D. N. Goodman, "Detroit Is the Most Dangerous City in Nation, Report Finds," *Seattle Post-Intelligencer*, Nov. 18, 2007. I don't wish to pick on Detroit, especially since I have a soft spot for the city where I was born and spent the first eighteen years of my life. Rather, I admire Dunne and colleagues for their courage in conducting their study and publicizing its findings.

7 G. Nichol, E. Thomas, C.W. Callaway, et al., "Regional Variation in Out-of-Hospital Cardiac Arrest Incidence and Outcome," *JAMA* 300 (2008), 1423–31.

8 The Leapfrog Group (www.leapfroggroup.org) provides national comparison information on issues of hospital safety and quality. In September 2007, the group reported that 87 percent of 1,256 U.S. hospitals that were surveyed did not have recommended policies in place to prevent hospital-acquired infections.

9 A variety of other rhythms can cause cardiac arrest, but these are much less common than the big three–VF, asystole, and pulseless electrical activity. Pulseless ventricular tachycardia (VT) is one of these other rhythms. Most researchers lump VT with VF because VT usually degenerates to VF in a matter of minutes. Two more rhythms that uncommonly lead to cardiac arrest are fast atrial tachycardia and atrial fibrillation.

10 C. M. Pratt, M. J. Francis, J. Luck, C. R. Wyndham, R. R. Miller, and M. A. Quinones, "Analysis of Ambulatory Electrocardiograms in 15 Patients During Spontaneous Ventricular Fibrillation with Special Reference to Preceding Arrhythmic Events," *Journal of the American College of Cardiology* 2 (1983), 789–97.

11 Potentially correctable causes of PEA include severe volume loss, severe acidosis, hypothermia, severe high or low potassium, severe low blood sugar, toxins and drug overdoses, cardiac tamponade (fluid in the sac surrounding the heart), a collapsed lung, large myocardial infarction, and pulmonary embolus. It may be possible to correct some of these causes with field therapy.

12 Clinicians often speak of coarse, medium, and fine ventricular fibrillation. These are on a continuum, since VF is likely to begin as coarse and then progress to fine and finally to flatlining. Coarse VF has an amplitude of approximately 7–10 mm. and occurs early in cardiac arrest. Medium VF has an amplitude of 3–7 mm. and is likely to occur five to ten minutes into the arrest. Fine VF has an amplitude of 1–2 mm. and is likely to occur after ten to fifteen minutes of cardiac arrest. Coarse VF is most responsive to a defibrillatory shock, and fine VF is least responsive.

13 See M. Holmberg, S. Holmberg, and J. Herlitz, "Incidence, Duration, and Survival of Ventricular Fibrillation in Out-of-Hospital Cardiac Arrest Patients in Sweden," *Resuscitation* 44 (2000), 7–17. This study found that very fine VF can last as long as forty minutes. There is a problem, however, in estimating the duration of VF in humans. Many instances of long-duration VF may not actually have started as VF. For example, the initial rhythm that led to the collapse may have been ventricular tachycardia (VT), and there may have been a weak pulse and low blood pressure, but after ten or twenty minutes the VT may have converted to VF (as it usually does). Therefore, the patient in this situation may have been in VF for only a few minutes, though the time from collapse to rhythm determination may have been twenty minutes. For part of this time, the patient may actually have had a perfusing rhythm.

14 See T. D. Valenzuela, D. J. Roe, S. Cretin, D. W. Spaite, and M. P. Larsen, "Estimating Effectiveness of Cardiac Arrest Interventions: A Logistic Regression Survival Model,"

Circulation 96 (1997), 3308–13; Holmberg, Holmberg, and Herlitz, "Incidence, Duration, and Survival of Ventricular Fibrillation in Out-of-Hospital Cardiac Arrest Patients in Sweden." The rate of this fall with delays in defibrillation is not clear, however. Data from King County suggest that the fall in the survival rate is approximately 4 percent per minute when the delay lasts between four and thirteen minutes. The differences between the King County rate and other reported rates may be due to the statistical tests that were used to compute this figure for King County.

15 It is not completely clear whether small amounts of oxygen prevent cell death or whether a small amount of circulation removes acids and other toxic by-products of cell metabolism. Perhaps both mechanisms play a role, or they may play different roles at various stages in the process of cell death.

16 S. J. Diem, J. D. Lantos, and J. A. Tulsky, "Cardiopulmonary Resuscitation on Television: Miracles and Misinformation," *New England Journal of Medicine* 334 (1996), 1578–82.

17 See T. D. Rea, M. S. Eisenberg, G. Sinibaldi, and R. D. White, "Incidence of EMS-Treated Out-of-Hospital Cardiac Arrest in the United States."

18 Furthermore, when CPR is shown in movies or on television, it is usually portrayed incorrectly, with the wrong hand position, the wrong depth of compression, the wrong rate, or all three of these errors. The media may be in the business of entertaining, not educating, but it seems that both ends could be accomplished with relatively little effort.

TWO A History of Resuscitation

1 P. V. Karpovich, *Adventures in Artificial Respiration* (New York: Association Press, 1953).

2 London's Royal Humane Society has no connection with the U.S. animal welfare organization known as the Humane Society.

3 A. Johnson, *An Account of Some Societies at Amsterdam and Hamburg for the Recovery of Drowned Persons*, London, 1773, 119.

4 The society's description of mouth-to-mouth or mouth-to-nostril respiration included the advice that "a cloth or handkerchief [could] be used to render the operation less indelicate."

5 M. Eisenberg, *Life in the Balance: Emergency Medicine and the Quest to Reverse Sudden Death* (New York: Oxford University Press, 1997), 251.

6 Sudden death by drowning is manifestly different from sudden death caused by heart disease. In drowning, the initial problem is that the victim has stopped breathing; for the first five to ten minutes, however, the heart is still beating, so if the victim can be extracted from the water and induced to breathe, the outcome will be good. But in a sudden cardiac arrest, both the heart and respiration have stopped. In this case, it is futile to induce respiration without restarting the heart.

7 The natural history of a disease need not inevitably lead to death. It can lead to any intermediate outcome, such as remission or disability, or even cure. A more accurate term might be natural progression.

8 Interview with James Elam, Aug. 6, 1990, cited in Eisenberg, *Life in the Balance*.

9 Interviews with Peter Safar, Dec. 23, 1988, and Aug. 19, 1990, cited in ibid.

10 D. D. Dill, "Symposium on Mouth-to-Mouth Resuscitation (Expired Air Inflation), Council on Medical Physics," *Journal of the American Medical Association* 167 (1958), 317–19.

11 Interview with James Jude, Nov. 1, 1990, cited in Eisenberg, *Life in the Balance*.

12 W. B. Kouwenhoven, J. R. Jude, and G. G. Knickerbocker, "Closed-Chest Cardiac Massage," *Journal of the American Medical Association* 173 (1960), 94–97.

13 Cited in Donald W. Benson, "Recent Advances in Emergency Resuscitation," *Maryland State Medical Journal* 34 (1961), 398–411.

14 P. Safar, T. C. Brown, and W. J. Hotley, "Failure of Closed-Chest Cardiac Massage to Produce Pulmonary Ventilation," *Diseases of the Chest* 41 (1962), 1–8.

15 Committee on CPR of the Division of Medical Sciences, National Academy of Science–National Research Council, "Cardiopulmonary Resuscitation," *Journal of the American Medical Association* 198 (1966), 372–79. See also the Web site of the American Heart Association (http://www.americanheart.org), which contains links to CPR training resources in local communities.

16 In 1967, Western Reserve University created a federation with Case Institute of Technology to become Case Western Reserve University.

17 This early research had been funded by the electric industry, which was concerned about fatal accidents involving linemen.

18 Ironically, twenty years after Beck's accomplishment, the management of cardiac arrest was returned to fire departments.

19 C. S. Beck et al., "Ventricular Fibrillation of Long Duration Abolished by Electric Shock," *Journal of the American Medical Association* 135 (1947), 985.

20 P. M. Zoll, A. J. Linenthal, W. Gibson, M. H. Paul, and L. R. Norman, "Termination of Ventricular Fibrillation in Man by Externally Applied Electric Countershock," *New England Journal of Medicine* 254 (1956), 727–32.

21 B. Lown, R. Amarasingham, and J. Neuman, "New Method for Terminating Cardiac Arrhythmias: Use of Synchronized Capacitor Discharge," *Journal of the American Medical Association* 182 (1962), 548–55.

22 Based on written reply from Frank Pantridge to questions, September 25, 1991. Cited in Eisenberg, *Life in the Balance*.

23 Ibid.

24 Interview with John Geddes, June 10, 1990, cited in Eisenberg, *Life in the Balance*.

25 J. Pantridge and J. S. Geddes, "A Mobile Intensive-Care Unit in the Management of Myocardial Infarction," *The Lancet* 2 (1967), 271–73. This article has historical importance because it served to stimulate prehospital emergency cardiac care programs throughout the world. In Belfast on May 19, 1967, Pantridge had presented these results in person at a meeting of the Association of Physicians of Great Britain and Ireland. "We were disbelieved and, indeed, to some extent ridiculed," he said as he described having met with a "cannot do" attitude. But that skepticism probably fueled his determination—Pantridge loved to tilt at conventional wisdom. As a historical footnote, August 1967 was exactly 200 years after the founding of the Society for Recovery of Drowned Persons. That rescue effort, begun in Amsterdam to resuscitate victims of the typical eighteenth-century sudden death, culminated two centuries later in the Belfast achievement—a system for resuscitating victims of cardiac arrest, the typical twentieth-century sudden death.

26 W. J. Grace, "Out-of-Hospital Care for Cardiac Emergencies: Prevention of Sudden Death in the Community," *Heart & Lung: The Journal of Acute and Critical Care* 3 (1974), 733–35.

27 W. J. Grace and J. A. Chadbourn, "The Mobile Coronary Care Unit," *Diseases of the Chest* 55 (1969), 452–55.

28 E. Nagel, J. C. Hirschman, P. W. Meyer, and F. Dennis, "Telemetry of Physiologic Data: An Aid to Fire Rescue Personnel in a Metropolitan Area," *Southern Medical Journal* 61 (1968), 598–601; E. Nagel, J. C. Hirschman, S. R. Nussenfeld, D. Rankin, and E. Lundblad, "Telemetry-Medical Command in Coronary and Other Mobile Emergency Care Systems," *Journal of the American Medical Association* 214 (1970), 332–38.

29 Interviews with Eugene Nagel, July 2, 1989, and July 6, 1992, cited in Eisenberg, *Life in the Balance.*

30 Ibid.

31 Ibid.

32 L. A. Cobb and A. P. Hallstrom, "Community-Based Cardiopulmonary Resuscitation: What Have We Learned?," *Annals of the New York Academy of Science* 382 (1982), 330–42.

33 Interviews with Leonard Cobb, March 27, 1989, cited in Eisenberg, *Life in the Balance.*

34 Ibid.

35 Ibid.

36 M. Eisenberg, M. Copass, A. Hallstrom, et al., "Treatment of Out-of-Hospital Cardiac Arrests with Rapid Defibrillation by Emergency Medical Technicians," *New England Journal of Medicine* 302 (1980), 1379–83.

37 R. O. Cummins, M. Eisenberg, P. Litwin, et al., "Automatic External Defibrillators Used by Emergency Medical Technicians: A Controlled Clinical Trial." *Journal of the Americal Medical Association* 257 (1987), 1605–10.

38 The idea for an automated defibrillator was first conceived by Arch Diack, a surgeon in Portland, Oregon. His prototype, literally assembled in a basement, utilized a unique defibrillatory pathway—tongue to chest. A breath detector embedded in the defibrillator's tongue electrode was intended to prevent the operator from accidentally shocking a person who was breathing. Diack's device was essentially a rate counter, far cruder than today's sophisticated VF detectors. The production model weighed thirty-five pounds and was programmed to give verbal instructions. It was an idea ahead of its time, and most people who were aware of it viewed it as a curiosity. By the late 1980s, however, other manufacturers had entered the field, and this development led to the creation of the automated external defibrillators that we have today. Current AEDs, like regular defibrillators, use electrode pads attached to the chest. AEDs are programmed to guide the operator, with a series of voice prompts, through the defibrillation procedure. The pads, once attached, automatically detect the type of heart rhythm, and if VF is present, the AED instructs the operator to press a button (usually flashing red or orange) to shock the patient. From the use of automated external defibrillators by EMTs, there was a natural and logical progression to first their use by first responders (police or security personnel), by laypersons in public locations (such as airports, schools, and exercise facilities, in an approach known as "public access defibrillation"), and by people in their own homes, using AEDs purchased over the counter without a prescription.

39 W. B. Carter, M. Eisenberg, and A. Hallstrom, "Development and Implementation of Emergency CPR Instruction via Telephone," *Annals of Emergency Medicine* 13 (1984), 695–700.

40 T. D. Rea, M. S. Eisenberg, L. L. Culley, and L. Becker, "Dispatcher-Assisted Cardiopulmonary Resuscitation and Survival in Cardiac Arrest," *Circulation* 104 (2001), 2513–16.

THREE   Causes of Sudden Cardiac Death

1   These data reflect only cases of community cardiac arrest in which resuscitation efforts were made by EMS personnel. The data do not accurately portray all deaths in King County. Cancer deaths, for example, account for only a small minority of all resuscitation efforts, but they represent a much higher proportion of all deaths in the county.

2   Though the victim of cardiac arrest usually has a known diagnosis of heart disease, his or her sudden collapse is totally unexpected. In some instances, however (estimates range from 10 to 30 percent), cardiac arrest is the first manifestation of underlying heart disease. In other words, the person had coronary artery disease but didn't know it. How is this possible? The blockage may not have been large enough to cause symptoms, or the person may have learned to avoid painful symptoms of angina—say, by walking up stairs more slowly, or by never running to catch a bus. In the context of underlying heart disease, while the person's death is of course unexpected, at least it is comprehensible. But in the context of no known disease, his or her death may appear at first to have no explanation.

3   Heart ischemia (a reduction in blood flow with a concomitant reduction in oxygen to the heart muscle caused by a partial or complete blockage in a coronary artery) leads to the symptoms of angina (a muscle cramplike sensation). Ischemia is a descriptive term of what is happening inside the heart muscle. Angina is one of the manifestations of ischemia. Other manifestations may be fatigue or difficulty breathing.

4   Fluid in the lung is called "congestion," hence the term "congestive heart failure." Fluid in the feet and ankles is referred to as "edema."

5   American Heart Association Statistics Committee and Stroke Statistics Subcommittee, "Heart Disease and Stroke Statistics: 2006 Update," *Circulation* 113 (2006), e85–e151.

6   The flow of electric current in the heart is affected by the concentration and flux, in and out of heart cells, of substances called "electrolytes," including sodium, potassium, magnesium, and calcium. Tiny channels on the surfaces of heart cells permit the flow of such electrolytes. When the function of these channels is altered by a genetic abnormality, by an abnormal concentration of electrolytes, or by certain drugs, rhythm problems can result.

FOUR   A Profile of Sudden Cardiac Arrest

1   King County's paramedic program was implemented sequentially, region by region, between 1973 and 1979.

2   EMTs, paramedics, and emergency dispatchers in Seattle and King County participate in many studies. Among studies currently in progress are the Resuscitations Outcome Consortium Trial (Seattle–King County is one of eleven sites in North America selected for this federally funded consortium); the DART Trial, a study of dispatcher-assisted telephone CPR involving regular CPR as compared to instructions for chest compression only; and the SPHERE project, for identification of patients with high blood pressure and high blood sugar by EMTs. Other studies in progress deal with hypothermia for patients after resuscitation,

the use of troponins in the identification of patients with acute coronary syndrome, the benefits of changes in CPR and defibrillation protocols, and genetic study of patients who have suffered cardiac arrest. Past studies in which dispatchers, EMTs, and paramedics have participated include studies on the following topics: defibrillation performed by EMTs; widespread training of citizens in CPR; innovative ways to teach CPR; dispatcher-assisted telephone CPR; public access defibrillation; benefits of prehospital thrombolysis; use of 12-lead electrocardiograms; use of bretylium versus lidocaine; use of high-dose epinephrine; benefits of distributing information to older adults to alert them to signs and symptoms of a heart attack; use of devices for chest compression; glucometry and pulse oximetry performed by EMTs; computer-based training and online continuing education for EMTs; alternate transport destinations for patients; compelling reasons for terminating CPR; use of nurse-staffed advice lines for callers to 911; use of AEDs in the homes of high-risk patients; delivery of CPR before defibrillation; and use of brain protectants after cardiac resuscitation.

3. The King County cardiac arrest registry is the heart of every regional and local effort to improve the EMS system in the King County area. One person works full time, more or less, to collect, code, and report cardiac arrest data for the county's population of 1.4 million (a separate registry is maintained by the Seattle Medic One program for the 600,000 residents of Seattle). Other individuals assist part time with collecting the dispatching digital recordings and the digitized AED tapes.

4 A 2003 report from Seattle and King County, which studied all out-of-hospital deaths due to heart disease, reveals the magnitude of these events; see T. D. Rea, M. S. Eisenberg, L. J. Becker, et al., "Emergency Medical Services and Mortality from Heart Disease: A Community Study," *Annals of Emergency Medicine* 41 (2003), 494–99. The study reports on a total of 3,705 cardiac deaths that occurred in out-of-hospital community settings, and in 1,428 of these cases there was a call to EMS. (In 2,277 of these cardiac deaths, there was no call to EMS; these deaths occurred in hospitals or were expected deaths that occurred at the victims' homes.) Of the 1,428 deaths in which there was EMS involvement, EMS personnel attempted to resuscitate 808 victims (57 percent), whereas EMS personnel made no attempt to resuscitate 620 victims (43 percent) who were considered dead on arrival. Thus, to summarize, EMS personnel responded to many cases of cardiac fatal arrest, but in only about 60 percent of these cases did they attempt to resuscitate the victim.

5 I use the term *dispatchers* to refer to both call receivers and dispatchers. Technically, in large communications centers, the call receiver takes the call and speaks with the caller while another individual, the dispatcher, sends the proper units. The call receiver would normally provide the telephone CPR instructions. In small centers, the role of call receiver and dispatcher is wrapped up in one person. Dispatchers and call receivers are also known as "telecommunicators."

6 L. A. Cobb, C. E. Fahrenbruch, M. Olsufka, and M. K. Copass, "Changing Incidence of Out-of-Hospital Ventricular Fibrillation, 1980–2000," *Journal of the American Medical Association* 288 (2002), 3008–13; J. Herlitz, J. Engdahl, L. Svensson, M. Young, K. A. Angquist, and S. Holmberg, "Decrease in the Occurrence of Ventricular Fibrillation as the Initially Observed Arrhythmia after Out-of-Hospital Cardiac Arrest During 11 Years in Sweden," *Resuscitation* 60 (2004), 283–90.

7 L. A. Cobb and A. P. Hallstrom, "Community-Based Cardiopulmonary Resuscitation: What Have We Learned?," *Annals of the New York Academy of Science* 382 (1982), 330–42.

8 T. D. Rea, M. S. Eisenberg, L. L. Culley, and L. Becker, "Dispatcher-Assisted Cardiopulmonary Resuscitation and Survival in Cardiac Arrest," *Circulation* 104 (2001), 2513–16; L. L. Culley, J. J. Clark, M. S. Eisenberg, and M. P. Larsen, "Dispatcher-Assisted Telephone CPR: Common Delays and Time Standards for Delivery," *Annals of Emergency Medicine* 20 (1991), 362–66; J. J. Clark, L. Culley, M. Eisenberg, and D. K. Henwood, "Accuracy of Determining Cardiac Arrest by Emergency Medical Dispatchers," *Annals of Emergency Medicine* 23 (1994), 1022–26.

9 J. Herlitz, M. Eek, M. Holmberg, and S. Holmberg, "Diurnal, Weekly, and Seasonal Rhythm of Out-of-Hospital Cardiac Arrest in Sweden," *Resuscitation* 54 (2002), 133–38.

10 It is known that stress can exacerbate certain diseases. For example, during the Iraqi missile attacks on Israel that accompanied the 1991 Persian Gulf War, there was an increase in acute myocardial infarction and sudden cardiac arrest among Israelis. Similar increases have been observed elsewhere after earthquakes.

11 Herlitz, Eek, Holmberg, and Holmberg, "Diurnal, Weekly, and Seasonal Rhythm of Out-of-Hospital Cardiac Arrest in Sweden."

12 Rea, Eisenberg, Culley, and Becker, "Dispatcher-Assisted Cardiopulmonary Resuscitation and Survival in Cardiac Arrest."

13 Herlitz, Eek, Holmberg, and Holmberg, "Diurnal, Weekly, and Seasonal Rhythm of Out-of-Hospital Cardiac Arrest in Sweden."

14 P. E. Litwin, M. S. Eisenberg, and A. P. Hallstrom, "The Location of Collapse and Its Effect on Survival from Cardiac Arrest," *Annals of Emergency Medicine* 16 (1987), 787–91.

15 One study has demonstrated that even though doctors' offices and clinics are a setting for only 1 percent of all cardiac arrests, not all offices are equal—the offices of cardiologists and internists are associated with the highest risk. See L. Becker, M. Eisenberg, and C. Fahrenbruch, "Cardiac Arrest in Medical and Dental Practices: Implications for AEDs," *Archives of Internal Medicine* 16 (2001), 1509–12.

16 L. Becker, M. Eisenberg, C. Fahrenbruch, and L. Cobb, "Public Locations of Cardiac Arrest: Implications for Public Access Defibrillation," *Circulation* 97 (1998), 2106–09.

17 Seattle and King County are on Puget Sound, and ferries are a common means of transportation around the area.

18 This means that it would take 500 restaurants to produce a rate of one cardiac arrest per year in a restaurant. Another way of saying the same thing would be to say that only once in 500 years is a cardiac arrest likely to occur in any given restaurant.

19 C. M. Albert, M. A. Mittleman, C. U. Chae, I. M. Lee, C. H. Hennekens, and J. E. Manson, "Triggering of Sudden Death from Cardiac Causes by Vigorous Exertion," *New England Journal of Medicine* 343 (2000), 1355–61.

20 W. Whang, J. E. Manson, F. B. Hu, et al., "Physical Exertion, Exercise, and Sudden Cardiac Death in Women," *Journal of the American Medical Association* 295 (2006), 1399–1403.

21 If EMTs regularly synchronized their AEDs' clocks with dispatchers' clocks, that practice would allow precise measurement of the interval between the victim's collapse (or the call to a PSAP) and the first defibrillatory shock. It is not a particularly high-tech approach, but without periodic synchronization (perhaps weekly) it will never be possible to ensure that the automatic time stamp for the shock is accurate. Some current AEDs can automatically resynchronize their internal clocks every time digital recordings are downloaded. In the future I suspect automatic synchronization will be a feature of every AED sold. Knowing the

time interval from calling 911 to the precise moment of defibrillation is simply too important a piece of information not to be routinely collected.

22 My biostatistician colleagues tell me that new techniques of imputing data—that is, substituting plausible values for missing information—can be used to combine estimated intervals with objectively recorded ones.

23 Information about NG911 can be found at http://www.its.dot.gov/ng911/index.htm.

FIVE Who Will Live and Who Will Die?

1 T. D. Rea, M. S. Eisenberg, G. Sinibaldi, and R. D. White, "Incidence of EMS-Treated Out-of-Hospital Cardiac Arrest in the United States," *Resuscitation* 63 (2004), 17–24. If the national survival rate for ventricular fibrillation were double what it is now, or 36 percent, an additional 13,000 individuals would survive every year.

2 These laws—known as HIPAA laws, since they came into being with passage of the Health Insurance Portability and Accountability Act of 1996—do in fact provide ample opportunity for hospitals to release patients' information when it is requested in connection with programs for quality assurance, and when safeguards on patients' confidentiality are in place.

3 I have great respect for the researchers in New York, Chicago, Los Angeles, and Detroit who had the courage to document and publish their communities' underwhelming performance. The Chicago research led that city to take several concrete steps to remedy the situation, including the addition of four new paramedic units and renewed training. But it has been more than a decade and half since that research was published, and no follow-up study was ever performed to determine whether conditions had improved.

4 M. Eisenberg, R. Cummins, and M. Larsen, "Numerators, Denominators, and Survival Rates: Reporting Survival from Out-of-Hospital Cardiac Arrest," *American Journal of Emergency Medicine* 9 (1991), 544–46.

5 R. O. Cummins, D. A. Chamberlain, N. S. Abramson, et al., "Recommended Guidelines for Uniform Reporting of Data from Out-of-Hospital Cardiac Arrest: The Utstein Style: A Statement for Health Professionals from a Task Force of the American Heart Association, the European Resuscitation Council, the Heart and Stroke Foundation of Canada, and the Australian Resuscitation Council," *Circulation* 84 (1991), 960–75.

6 I. Jacobs, V. Nadkarni, J. Bahr, et al., "Cardiac Arrest and Cardiopulmonary Resuscitation Outcome Reports: Update and Simplification of the Utstein Templates for Resuscitation Registries: A Statement for Healthcare Professionals from a Task Force of the International Liaison Committee on Resuscitation (American Heart Association, European Resuscitation Council, Australian Resuscitation Council, New Zealand Resuscitation Council, Heart and Stroke Foundation of Canada, Interamerican Heart Foundation, Resuscitation Council of Southern Africa)," *Resuscitation* 63 (2004), 233–49.

7 In this chapter, I do not pretend to provide an exhaustive review of all the scientific literature on the factors associated with survival of cardiac arrest. Instead, I have tried to select one or two representative articles for each of the various factors.

8 R. A. Swor, R. E. Jackson, J. E. Tintinalli, and R. G. Pirrallo, "Does Advanced Age Matter in Outcomes after Out-of-Hospital Cardiac Arrest in Community-Dwelling Adults?," *Academy of*

Emergency Medicine 7 (2000), 762–68.

9 C. Kim, L. Becker, and M. S. Eisenberg, "Out-of-Hospital Cardiac Arrest in Octogenarians and Nonagenarians," *Archives of Internal Medicine* 160 (2000), 3439–43.

10 L. B. Becker, B. H. Han, P. M. Meyer, et al., "Racial Differences in the Incidence of Cardiac Arrest and Subsequent Survival: The CPR Chicago Project," *New England Journal of Medicine* 329 (1993), 600–606.

11 K. Chu, R. Swor, R. Jackson, et al., "Race and Survival after Out-of-Hospital Cardiac Arrest in a Suburban Community," *Annals of Emergency Medicine* 31 (1998), 478–82.

12 M. R. Cowie, C. E. Fahrenbruch, L. A. Cobb, and A. P. Hallstrom, "Out-of-Hospital Cardiac Arrest: Racial Differences in Outcome in Seattle," *American Journal of Public Health* 83 (1993), 955–59.

13 The term "inversely correlated" means that the two factors are associated but move in opposite directions. Therefore, the more comorbidity, the lower the likelihood of survival.

14 A. P. Hallstrom, L. A. Cobb, and B. H. Yu, "Influence of Comorbidity on the Outcome of Patients Treated for Out-of-Hospital Ventricular Fibrillation," *Circulation* 93 (1996), 2019–22.

15 There are undoubtedly subpopulations within a community (for example, people who suffer cardiac arrest in public locations) for whom the maximum survival rate is higher than 50 percent.

16 D. S. Siscovick, T. E. Raghunathan, I. King, et al., "Dietary Intake and Cell Membrane Levels of Long-Chain N-3 Polyunsaturated Fatty Acids and the Risk of Primary Cardiac Arrest," *Journal of the American Medical Association* 274 (1995), 1363–67.

17 D. Edelson, B. S. Abella, S. Kim, T. L. Vanden Hoek, and L. Becker, "The Effects Of Obesity on CPR Quality and Survival after Cardiac Arrest," presented at the Resuscitation Science Symposium, annual meeting of the American Heart Association, Chicago, 2006.

18 R. D. White, T. H. Blackwell, J. K. Russell, and D. B. Jorgenson, "Body Weight Does Not Affect Defibrillation, Resuscitation, or Survival in Patients with Out-of-Hospital Cardiac Arrest Treated with a Nonescalating Biphasic Waveform Defibrillator," *Critical Care Medicine* 32 (2004), S387–92.

19 R. Bresalier, R. Sandler, H. Quan, et al., "Cardiovascular Events Associated with Rofecoxib in a Colorectal Adenoma Chemoprevention Trial," *New England Journal of Medicine* 352 (2005), 1092–1102.

20 Cardiac Arrhythmia Suppression Trial (CAST) Investigators, "Preliminary Report: Effect of Encainide and Flecainide on Mortality in a Randomized Trial of Arrhythmia Suppression after Myocardial Infarction," *New England Journal of Medicine* 321 (1989), 406–12.

21 S. Feero, J. R. Hedges, and P. Stevens, "Demographics of Cardiac Arrest: Association with Residence in a Low-Income Area," *Academy of Emergency Medicine* 2 (1995), 11–16.

22 K. Reiner, E. D. Stecker, C. Vickers, K. Gunson, J. Jui, and S. S. Chugh, "Incidence of Sudden Cardiac Arrest Is Higher in Areas of Low Socioeconomic Status: A Prospective Two-Year Study in a Large United States Community," *Resuscitation* 70 (2006), 186–92.

23 A. Hallstrom, P. Boutin, L. Cobb, and E. Johnson, "Socioeconomic Status and Prediction of Ventricular Fibrillation Survival," *American Journal of Public Health* 83 (1993), 245–48.

24 S. O. Clarke, G. D. Schellenbaum, and T. D. Rea, "Socioeconomic Status and Survival from Out-of-Hospital Cardiac Arrest," *Academy of Emergency Medicine* 12 (2005), 941–47.

25 A. J. Sayegh, R. Swor, K. H. Chu, et al., "Does Race or Socioeconomic Status Predict Adverse

Outcome after Out-of-Hospital Cardiac Arrest? A Multi-Center Study," *Resuscitation* 40 (1999), 41–46.

26 N. Wade, "Gene Identified as Risk Factor for Heart Ills," *New York Times*, May 4, 2007.

27 The survival rate for pulseless electrical activity is slightly higher than for asystole; for both, however, the rate is usually in the low single digits. I also suspect that surviving PEA or asystole carries a higher risk of neurological complications than does surviving ventricular fibrillation.

28 These patients form the denominator for all this book's cross-community comparisons, as recommended in the Utstein guidelines. Ventricular fibrillation may be the initiating rhythm after cardiac arrest, but it will degenerate to asystole after twenty minutes or so. Therefore, in calculating the likelihood of survival, it would have been problematic to use in the denominator the rhythms of patients who collapsed without witnesses. When there was no witness, the fact that the patient was found in asystole reveals nothing about the rhythm that caused the cardiac arrest.

29 R. O. Cummins, M. S. Eisenberg, A. P. Hallstrom, and P. E. Litwin, "Survival of Out-of-Hospital Cardiac Arrest with Early Initiation of Cardiopulmonary Resuscitation," *American Journal of Emergency Medicine* 3 (1985), 114–19.

30 A. P. Hallstrom, J. P. Ornato, M. Weisfeldt, et al., "Public-Access Defibrillation and Survival after Out-of-Hospital Cardiac Arrest," *New England Journal of Medicine* 351 (2004), 637–46.

31 R. W. Simons, T. D. Rea, L. J. Becker, and M. S. Eisenberg, "The Incidence and Significance of Emesis Associated with Out-of-Hospital Cardiac Arrest," *Resuscitation* 74 (2007), 427–31. This study reported emesis in 32 percent of 1,000 cardiac arrests in King County. Two-thirds of the vomiting episodes occurred before the arrival of EMS personnel. Patients who vomited had a survival rate of 13 percent, as compared to 18 percent for those who did not vomit. The difference was statistically significant.

32 J. J. Clark, M. P. Larsen, L. L. Culley, J. R. Graves, and M. S. Eisenberg, "Incidence of Agonal Respirations in Sudden Cardiac Arrest," *Annals of Emergency Medicine* 21 (1992), 1464–67.

33 A variant of the occurrence of agonal breathing is seizure activity associated with cardiac arrest. With cardiac arrest, the brain is deprived of oxygen, and this situation can lead to a seizure. The exact incidence of this phenomenon is not known. If I had to guess, I would say that it occurs in 5 to 10 percent of cardiac arrests. The occurrence of a seizure may lead a bystander to conclude that the victim has epilepsy, and this mistaken conclusion may in turn cause a delay in calling 911, or a delay in dispatchers' recognizing the true nature of the problem. It is not known whether seizure activity at the time of cardiac arrest is associated with a better or a worse outcome.

34 C. M. Albert, M. A. Mittleman, C. U. Chae, I. M. Lee, C. H. Hennekens, and J. E. Manson, "Triggering of Sudden Death from Cardiac Causes by Vigorous Exertion," *New England Journal of Medicine* 343 (2000), 1355–61.

35 K. A. Miller, D. S. Siscovick, L. Sheppard, et al., "Long-Term Exposure to Air Pollution and Incidence of Cardiovascular Events in Women," *New England Journal of Medicine* 356 (2007), 447–58. This is not specifically a study of cardiac arrest; presumably, however, cardiovascular events are correlated with cardiac arrests.

36 R. B. Low, S. Lamba, W. Gluckman, T. Cocuzza, and L. Bielory, "The Effect of Weather and Air Pollution on EMS Calls for Complaints of Chest Pain in an Urban City," *Annals of*

Emergency Medicine 48 (2006), S69 (abstract).

37 For example, a two-year study of 404 cardiac arrests in King County examined the reasons why dispatcher-assisted telephone CPR was not delivered. Altogether, 166 victims did not receive bystander CPR, either from a trained bystander or through the intervention of a dispatcher giving CPR instructions over the telephone, and in this group of 166 cardiac arrests there were eight situations (5 percent) in which CPR could not be started because the victim could not be moved into the proper position. The study also reported that 25 percent of the 404 patients did receive CPR from a bystander, and 34 percent received CPR through instructions communicated over the telephone by a dispatcher, whereas the remaining 41 percent did not receive CPR before the fire department arrived. See S. R. Hauff, T. D Rea, L. L. Culley, F. Kerry, L. Becker, and M. S. Eisenberg, "Factors Impeding Dispatcher-Assisted Telephone Cardiopulmonary Resuscitation," *Annals of Emergency Medicine* 42 (2003), 731–37.

38 The medical director of a midwestern EMS program told me that his paramedics took virtually everyone they found in cardiac arrest to the hospital, invariably with ongoing CPR. As a result of this policy, his community had a very low survival rate. Enhancing or diminishing the denominator by means of policies concerning whom to resuscitate does affect the community's survival rate, though of course it does little to save more patients in cardiac arrest. But it does make cross-community comparisons very challenging, since the criteria governing the decision about when to initiate resuscitation are so different. This is yet another reason why survival rates for a community should be calculated on the basis of witnessed cardiac arrests in which ventricular fibrillation is present, since resuscitation is always attempted for a patient in VF unless the patient has a valid DNR (do not resuscitate) order. Another, more subtle possibility for variance in the criteria governing the decision to resuscitate — in this case, the decision to defibrillate — concerns the specific brand of automated external defibrillator used by a particular EMS system. Four companies manufacture the AEDs that are commonly used in the United States, and each AED has its own proprietary system for detecting ventricular fibrillation. (One might think that all VF-detection algorithms would meet a national or industry standard, but that is not the case.) Therefore, the specific criteria for detecting VF may differ from one community to another, and this difference may have no other basis than the brand of AED being used in a particular community. This possibility is mostly speculative, and it would be a real challenge to conduct a study directly comparing different AEDs. Nevertheless, the possibility exists that subtle differences in VF-detection algorithms may be influencing decisions about the types of VF that are considered shockable, and these decisions in turn may be influencing some patients' likelihood of survival.

39 See M. L. Weisfeldt and B. Becker, "Resuscitation after Cardiac Arrest: A 3–Phase Time-Sensitive Model," *Journal of the American Medical Association* 288 (2002), 3035–38. Support for this model has come from Gilmore and her colleagues, who demonstrated that although CPR offers no benefit during the first four minutes when cardiac arrest includes ventricular fibrillation, it is nevertheless of considerable benefit between four minutes and approximately twelve minutes into the arrest. See C. M. Gilmore, T. D. Rea, L. J. Becker, and M. S. Eisenberg, "Three-Phase Model of Cardiac Arrest: Time-Dependent Benefit of Bystander Cardiopulmonary Resuscitation," *American Journal of Cardiology* 98 (2006), 497–99.

40 E. J. Gallagher, G. Lombardi, and P. Gennis, "Effectiveness of Bystander Cardiopulmonary Resuscitation and Survival Following Out-of-Hospital Cardiac Arrest," *Journal of the American Medical Association* 274 (1995), 1922–25; R. J. Van Hoeyweghen, L. L. Bossaert, A. Mullie, P. Calle, P. Martens, W. A. Buylaert, and H. Delooz, "Quality and Efficiency of Bystander CPR: Belgian Cerebral Resuscitation Study Group," *Resuscitation* 26 (1993), 47–52; L. Wik, P. A. Steen, and N. G. Birche, "Quality of Bystander Cardiopulmonary Resuscitation Influences Outcome after Prehospital Cardiac Arrest," *Resuscitation* 28 (1994), 195–203.

41 T. P. Aufderheide, G. Sigurdsson, R. G. Pirrallo, et al., "Hyperventilation-Induced Hypotension During Cardiopulmonary Resuscitation," *Circulation* 109 (2004), 1960–65.

42 M. Zuercher, R. W. Hilwig, J. Nysaether, et al., "Incomplete Chest Recoil During Piglet CPR Worsens Hemodynamics," presentation at the Resuscitation Science Symposium, annual meeting of the American Heart Association, Orlando, Florida, 2007.

43 P. T. Morley, "Monitoring the Quality of Cardiopulmonary Resuscitation," *Current Opinion in Critical Care* 13 (2007), 261–67.

44 M. Eisenberg, A. Hallstrom, M. Copass, L. Bergner, F. Short, and J. Pierce, "Treatment of Ventricular Fibrillation: Emergency Medical Technician Defibrillation and Paramedic Services," *Journal of the American Medical Association* 251 (1984), 1723–26; M. Eisenberg, M. Copass, A. Hallstrom, et al., "Management of Out-of-Hospital Cardiac Arrest: Failure of Basic Emergency Medical Technician Services," *Journal of the American Medical Association* 243 (1980), 1049–51; M. Eisenberg, L. Bergner, and A. Hallstrom, "Cardiac Resuscitation in the Community: Importance of Rapid Provision and Implications for Program Planning," *Journal of the American Medical Association* 241 (1979), 1905–7.

45 J. H. Indik, C. M. Peters, R. L. Donnerstein, et al., "Direction of Signal Recording Affects Amplitude-Based Measures of VF in Humans Undergoing Defibrillation Testing During ICD Implantation," presented at Resuscitation Science Symposium, annual meeting of the American Heart Association, Orlando, Florida, 2007.

46 The lack of blood deprives the heart of oxygen, and any blood that is present may be very acidotic. Therefore, the shock may work for a second or two, but the heart will not stay defibrillated, because there is no oxygenated blood in the heart muscle—the coronary artery is empty because the left ventricle is empty, on account of CPR's having been delayed or stopped.

47 T. D. Rea, M. Helbock, S. Perry, et al., "Increasing Use of Cardiopulmonary Resuscitation During Out-of-Hospital Ventricular Fibrillation Arrest: Survival Implications of Guideline Changes," Circulation 114 (2006), 2760–65. Since the Rea article numerous articles have reinforced the importance of quality CPR as a determinant of survival. We have come to use the term high-performance CPR to designate high-quality CPR. All the EMTs in Seattle and King County are trained in high-performance CPR.

48 L. A. Cobb, C. E. Fahrenbruch, T. R. Walsh, et al., "Influence of Cardiopulmonary Resuscitation Prior to Defibrillation in Patients with Out-of-Hospital Ventricular Fibrillation," *Journal of the American Medical Association* 281 (1999), 1182–88; L. Wik, T. B. Hansen, F. Fylling, et al., "Delaying Defibrillation to Give Basic Cardiopulmonary Resuscitation to Patients with Out-of-Hospital Ventricular Fibrillation: A Randomized Trial," *Journal of the American Medical Association* 289 (2003), 1389–95.

49 I. Jacobs, J. C. Finn, H. F. Oxer, and G. A. Jelinek, "CPR Before Defibrillation in Out-of-Hospital Cardiac Arrest: A Randomized Trial," *Emergency Medicine Australasia* 17 (2005), 39–45.

50 M. S. Eisenberg, B. T. Horwood, R. O. Cummins, R. Reynolds-Haertle, and T. R. Hearne, "Cardiac Arrest and Resuscitation: A Tale of 29 Cities," *Annals of Emergency Medicine* 19 (1990), 179–86.

51 I. G. Stiell, G. A. Wells, B. J. Field, et al., "Improved Out-of-Hospital Cardiac Arrest Survival through the Inexpensive Optimization of an Existing Defibrillation Program: OPALS Study Phase II: Ontario Prehospital Advanced Life Support," *Journal of the American Medical Association* 281 (1999), 1175–81.

52 Several studies from King County have demonstrated the highest rates of survival for cardiac arrests involving VF when paramedics respond; see M. Eisenberg, L. Bergner, and A. Hallstrom, "Out-of-Hospital Cardiac Arrest: Improved Survival with Paramedic Services," *The Lancet* 1 (1980), 812–15. See also Wik, Steen, and Bircher, "Quality of Bystander Cardiopulmonary Resuscitation Influences Outcome after Prehospital Cardiac Arrest"; Aufderheide, Sigurdsson, Pirrallo, et al., "Hyperventilation-Induced Hypotension During Cardiopulmonary Resuscitation"; Zuercher, Hilwig, Nysaether, et al., "Incomplete Chest Recoil During Piglet CPR Worsens Hemodynamics."

53 Eisenberg, Bergner, and Hallstrom, "Out-of-Hospital Cardiac Arrest: Improved Survival with Paramedic Services." Fortunately, EMT services lacking defibrillation capability no longer exist.

54 R. Davis, "Many Lives Are Lost across USA Because Emergency Services Fail," *USA Today*, July 28, 2003.

55 T. D. Rea, M. S. Eisenberg, L. L. Culley, and L. Becker, "Dispatcher-Assisted Cardiopulmonary Resuscitation and Survival in Cardiac Arrest," *Circulation* 104 (2001), 2513–16.

56 L. H. Soo, D. Gray, T. Young, A. Skene, and J. R. Hampton, "Influence of Ambulance Crew's Length of Experience on the Outcome of Out-of-Hospital Cardiac Arrest," *European Heart Journal* 20 (1999), 535–40.

57 D. M. Williams, "JEMS Salary and Workplace Survey," JEMS 31 (2006), 38–49. JEMS conducts and publishes annual surveys of salary and workplace conditions. The survey from 2010 showed only modest changes in salaries from 2006.

58 Ibid.

59 Ibid.

60 Rea, Eisenberg, Culley, and Becker, "Dispatcher-Assisted Cardiopulmonary Resuscitation and Survival in Cardiac Arrest."

61 Hallstrom, Ornato, Weisfeldt, et al., "Public-Access Defibrillation and Survival after Out-of-Hospital Cardiac Arrest."

62 L. L. Culley, T. D. Rea, J. A. Murray, et al., "Public Access Defibrillation in Out-of-Hospital Cardiac Arrest: A Community-Based Study," Circulation 109 (2004), 1859–63. Culley and her colleagues studied the initial experience of communities with public access AEDs, examining fifty episodes in which an AED was used before the fire department arrived, and finding a 50 percent survival rate in this cohort. See also T. D. Rea, M. Olsufka, B. Bemis, L. White, L. Yin, and et al: "A Population-Based Investigation of Public Access Defibrillation: Role of Emergency Medical Services Care," *Resuscitation* 81 (2010), 163-67

63 CPR and defibrillation, since they are also therapies, could have been discussed in this

section. Given their intimate association with the system of care, however, and with the criticality of time in a cardiac arrest, they are discussed in the section on system factors. As for therapy itself, it begins in the field, but it continues in the emergency room and on the cardiac floor of the hospital. One could argue that the evaluation clock of an EMS system should stop upon the patient's admission to the hospital, since hospital care surely must be a separate determinant of the outcome, but the counterargument is that hospital admission without discharge is an empty victory. The only meaningful statistic is the one that reflects discharge from the hospital, and virtually all researchers in the field accept this as the only important outcome. Therefore, it is important to add hospital therapy to the mix of factors predicting the outcome for the patient.

64 M. E. C. Ong, E. H. Tan, F. S. Peng, et al., "Survival Outcomes with the Introduction of Intravenous Epinephrine in the Management of Out-of-Hospital Cardiac Arrest," *Annals of Emergency Medicine* 50 (2007), 635–42.

65 In animals, an ITD raises blood pressure during CPR. ITDs have been approved by the FDA for use in shock. The question of whether ITDs help in CPR was studied by the Resuscitation Outcomes Consortium (ROC) and no benefit was seen (see note 66).

66 T. Aufderheide, G. Nichol, T. D. Rea, S. P. Brown, B. G. Leroux, P. E. Pepe, P. J. Kudenchuk, J. Christenson, M. R. Daya, P. Dorian, C W. Callaway, et al., "A Trial of an Impedance Threshold Device in Out-of-Hospital Cardiac Arrest," *New England Journal of Medicine* 365 (2011), 798-806.

67 A. Hallstrom, T. D. Rea, M. R. Sayre, et al., "Manual Chest Compression vs. Use of an Automated Chest Compression Device During Resuscitation Following Out-of-Hospital Cardiac Arrest: A Randomized Trial," *Journal of the American Medical Association* 295 (2006), 2620–28.

68 Twelve cities—Atlanta, Austin, Chicago, Cleveland, El Paso, Fort Worth, Los Angeles, Nashville, New Orleans, New York, San Antonio, and San Francisco—have decided to adopt chest compression only for their dispatch centers' telephone instructions. These cities have followed the lead of seven others, including Seattle and Richmond, that had already changed to chest-compression-only instructions. Thus nineteen cities are providing this type of telephone instruction. See R. Davis, "Simpler Method for CPR Coming," *USA Today*, Feb. 23, 2004.

69 M. Sayer, R. A. Berg, D. M. Cave, R. L. Page, J. Potts, and R. D. White, "Hands-Only (Compression-Only) Cardiopulmonary Resuscitation: A Call to Action for Bystander Response to Adults Who Experience Out-of-Hospital Sudden Cardiac Arrest," *Circulation* 117 (2008), 2162–67. The American Heart Association's endorsement of hands-only CPR is not without controversy. The European Resuscitation Council (www.erc.edu) issued a statement in response to the AHA Science Advisory. The Council stated that there is insufficient evidence to make any changes at this time and confirmed its recommendation that CPR should consist of mouth-to-mouth ventilation and chest compression. The ERC concluded its statement, "For those rescuers who are unwilling or unable to give mouth-to-mouth ventilation, chest compression-only is more acceptable than performing no CPR at all." (www.erc.edu/index.php /docLibrary/en/viewDoc/775/3/)

70 P. Safar, T. C. Brown, and W. J. Hotley, "Failure of Closed-Chest Cardiac Massage to Produce Pulmonary Ventilation," *Diseases of the Chest* 41 (1962), 1–8.

71 A. Hallstrom, L. Cobb, E. Johnson, and M. Copass, "Cardiopulmonary Resuscitation by Chest Compression Only or with Mouth-to-Mouth Ventilation," *New England Journal of Medicine* 289 (2000), 1389–95.

72 K. Nagao et al., "Cardiopulmonary Resuscitation by Bystanders with Chest Compression Only (SOS–KANTO): An Observational Study," *The Lancet* 369 (2007), 920–26.

73 One trial is the Dispatcher Assisted Resuscitation Trial (DART) involving King County, Thurston County (in Washington State), and the London Ambulance Service. The other trial, the TANGO study, is taking place in Sweden and parts of Finland. Results may be available as early as 2009.

74 P. A. Steen, "Does Active Rescuer Ventilation Have a Place During Basic Cardiopulmonary Resuscitation?," *Circulation* 116 (2007), 2514–16.

75 B. D. Shy, T. D. Rea, C. Edwards, L. J. Becker, and M. S. Eisenberg, "Time to Intubation and Survival in Prehospital Cardiac Arrest," *Prehospital Emergency Care* 8 (2004), 394–99.

76 The EMS world is conflicted about the type of airway management that paramedics should be allowed to perform. The Cadillac of airway management, and the type performed in emergency rooms and operating rooms, is endotracheal intubation with paralytic medications, and yet probably fewer than 10 percent of EMS systems authorize paramedics to use paralytics. Other systems allow intubation without paralytics, and still others allow airway-adjunctive airways, such as laryngeal mask airways or combitube airways, which are considered less effective than endotracheal intubation.

77 Hypothermia after Cardiac Arrest Study Group, "Mild Therapeutic Hypothermia to Improve the Neurologic Outcome after Cardiac Arrest," *New England Journal of Medicine* 346 (2002), 549–56; S. A. Bernard, T. W. Gray, M. D. Buist, et al., "Treatment of Comatose Survivors of Out-of-Hospital Cardiac Arrest with Induced Hypothermia," *New England Journal of Medicine* 346 (2002), 557–63.

78 F. Kim, M. Olsufka, D. Carlbom, et al., "Pilot Study of Rapid Infusion of 2 L of 4 Degrees C Normal Saline for Induction of Mild Hypothermia in Hospitalized, Comatose Survivors of Out-of-Hospital Cardiac Arrest," *Circulation* 112 (2005), 715–19.

79 M. Skrifvars, M. Castrén, S. Aune, A. Thoren, J. Nurmi, and J. Herlitz, "Variability in Survival after In-Hospital Cardiac Arrest Depending on the Hospital Level of Care," *Resuscitation* 73 (2007), 73–81.

80 K. Sunde, M. Mytte, D. Jacobson, et al., "Implementation of a Standardised Treatment Protocol for Post-Resuscitation Care after Out-of-Hospital Cardiac Arrest," *Resuscitation* 73 (2007), 29–39.

81 The interaction of CPR and defibrillation involves the timing and sequence of defibrillation as well as the quality of CPR and defibrillation. New types of recording monitors are now able to monitor the quality of CPR with accuracy.

82 As of 2007, hypothermia was only beginning to become standard care in King County.

83 As already noted, the formula somewhat arbitrarily sets the maximum potential for prehospital resuscitation at 50 percent, though the exact ceiling may be higher; for the purposes of illustration, however, the particular ceiling is less important than the influence of various therapies.

84 What do I mean by the word "timely"? I mean that paramedics, at least 50 percent of the time, should arrive within five minutes after the EMTs arrive. In setting five minutes as the

target time, I assume that the EMTs are providing high-quality CPR and are delivering one or more shocks to the patient.

85 All the determinant factors are influenced and nurtured by quality improvement, which is a common denominator of the contributory factors. In essence, quality improvement is simply a tool for measuring whether or not performance is meeting expectations, and whether or not attempted improvements are having the intended effects. Are things getting better? Worse? Are they staying the same? An EMS system without an active and vigorous program of quality improvement is like a mountaineer without a compass.

SIX Location, Location, Location: Best Places to Have a Cardiac Arrest

For this chapter, I conducted the following interviews, listed here in chronological order: Leonard Cobb, Dec. 21, 2006, Seattle; Mike Helbock, Jan. 5, 2007, Seattle; Michael Copass, Jan. 12, 2007, Seattle; Tom Rea, Jan. 25, 2007, Seattle; Graham Nichol, Feb. 6, 2007, Seattle; Al Hallstrom, Feb. 27, 2007, Seattle; Tom Hearne, Feb. 28, 2007, Seattle; Mario Trevino, March 9, 2007, Bellevue, Washington; Roger White, March 12, 2007, Rochester, Minnesota (telephone); Michael Sayre, March 14, 2007, Columbus, Ohio (telephone); Tod Levesh, March 20, 2007, Seattle (telephone); Peter Kudenchuk, March 22, 2007, Seattle; A. D. Vickery, Apr. 3, 2007, Seattle; Terry Sinclair, Nov. 13, 2007, Seattle; Mark Morgan, Nov. 18, 2007, Seattle (telephone); and Cleo Subido, Nov. 20, 2007, Seattle.

1 During 2010 and 2011, survival rates in Seattle, King County, and Rochester, MN, have reached 50 percent. T. D. Rea, M. Helbock, S. Perry, et al., "Increasing Use of Cardiopulmonary Resuscitation During Out-of-Hospital Ventricular Fibrillation Arrest: Survival Implications of Guideline Changes," Circulation 114 (2006), 2760–65. See also R. D. White, T. J. Bunch, and D. G. Hankins, "Evolution of a Community-Wide Early Defibrillation Programme: Experience over 13 Years Using Police/Fire Personnel and Paramedics as Responders," Resuscitation 65 (2005), 279–83.

2 Over the decades, Leonard Cobb has been my teacher, my mentor, my co-investigator, and my colleague. Several years ago he stepped down as a full-time professor—his current title is professor emeritus—and as director of the Medic One program. He recently celebrated his eighty-second birthday and is still very much involved in the Medic One research program, to which he devotes 50 percent of his time.

3 In my opinion, shared by Cobb and Copass, no system without strong medical control can possibly excel. It is difficult, of course, to define what strong medical control is; you know it when you see it, but it is something of a challenge to put it into words. For me, it is defined by the qualities of presence (being actively involved in the program), command (letting everyone know who is the medical boss), leadership (always being out in front), loyalty (defending and standing by the paramedics), integrity (never compromising on the quality of care for patients), experience (being streetwise), and professionalism (conveying respect and dignity for every patient).

4 The medical director is not the chief administrative authority, however. That role falls to the fire chief, who in turn delegates administrative authority to battalion chiefs and lieutenants, and to duty officers.

5 In Seattle and King County, six medical directors are in charge of six separate paramedic

programs (one in Seattle, five in King County), supervising a combined total of 255 paramedics for an average director-to-paramedic ratio of about 1 to 42. One of the six programs serves a rural island and has only a few paramedics; the remaining five programs have an average of 50 paramedics each. My own bias is that the optimal director-to-paramedic ratio is between 1 to 50 and 1 to 100. I'm sure that there are medical directors in large programs who would strongly disagree, but my own view is that when the medical director and the line paramedics stop knowing each other well, things start to fray at the edges. By way of analogy, consider a first-year survey course at the college level—when class size grows to more than 100, it is the rare professor who is able to recognize his students by name and by sight, let alone know much about their strengths and weaknesses.

6 According to Cobb, only twice has it been necessary to remove anyone from the role of paramedic, and both times it was because of an attitudinal problem rather than dereliction of duty or a grievous medical error. When the Medic One program began, paramedics were recertified every two years, and if the fire chief was unable to deal with a troublesome paramedic, Cobb was given the power to decertify that individual or decline to renew his or her certification. But Cobb never had to exercise that option. Perhaps just the knowledge that he could was enough to deter substandard paramedic care.

7 Each of the six paramedic programs (one in Seattle, five in King County) has one or more base-station hospitals, and in each of these hospitals an attending physician in the emergency department provides line medical control. In other cities and states, however, specially trained nurses in base-station hospitals may provide medical authorization.

8 In Seattle, the average response time for EMTs is three and a half minutes; in King County, it is five minutes. The average response times for paramedics in Seattle and King County are seven minutes and ten minutes, respectively. Some idea of the scale of the Seattle and King County EMS systems is captured by the following figures. The area's combined population is approximately 2 million—600,000 in Seattle, and 1.4 million in suburban and rural King County. Thirty fire departments in urban, suburban, and rural King County provide the first-tier EMT response; thus firefighters respond to every 911 call. In Seattle and King County, in 2006, firefighter EMTs responded to 167,000 calls, and paramedics were involved in 52,000 calls. Therefore, approximately 30 percent of all calls in 2006 were considered serious enough to involve paramedics.

9 As described in chapter 4, the effort to maintain a cardiac arrest registry is labor-intensive. It would be pleasant to think that all this effort could be automated on the basis of downloading computer-based records. In reality, however, few databases are linked; considerable effort is needed to obtain hospital records, and dispatch records are not automatically linked to EMS reports, at least not in many communities. My best estimate is that maintaining a cardiac arrest registry for a community of approximately 1 million people will require one full-time-equivalent employee. This person must clarify ambiguous information, resolve discrepancies among pieces of information, and, most important, prepare reports and summarize data. Clearly, the administrative agency must provide support for this kind of activity.

10 In Seattle and King County, the annual revenue generated by a countywide EMS property tax is approximately $60 million. This comes to a cost of $30 annually per person. Six different individuals, who together comprise two FTEs, provide medical supervision for the county's six paramedic programs. The communities served by the programs vary in size,

and so the time for medical supervision varies; on average, however, a half-time doctor is needed for medical supervision of the paramedics serving a population of 500,000. In addition, there is a half-time-equivalent medical director for EMT-level care. Approximately six FTE positions staff the QI programs in Seattle and King County. The total cost for medical supervision and quality improvement is less than $1.2 million. Thus the combined cost of medical supervision and quality improvement, including the ongoing surveillance of cardiac arrests, is 2 percent of the total annual EMS operating cost, equivalent to $0.60 annually per person for these vital functions. For the history of the EMS property tax, see note 16.

11 The 2006 *JEMS* survey was actually based on responses from 104 cities. *JEMS* also publishes an annual survey of salaries; D. M. Williams, "*JEMS* Salary and Workplace Survey," *JEMS* 31 (2006), 38–49, gives an average starting salary for EMTs as $28,000, whereas he reports that the average starting salary for paramedics is $35,000. EMS personnel in fire departments earn higher salaries than workers in private ambulance companies. For example, paramedics in fire departments earn $42,000, as compared to $32,000 for paramedics in private ambulance companies.

12 D. M. Williams, "2006 *JEMS* 200–City Survey," *JEMS* 32 (2007), 38–54.

13 The King County EMS system, for example, which covers 1.4 million people, is one of those that were not included. The system comprises thirty-two communities that, taken individually, are not among the 200 largest in the United States.

14 Williams, "2006 *JEMS* 200–City Survey."

15 The 2006 *JEMS* 200–City Survey reported that EMS agencies collected an average of 56 percent of billed charges for transport; that the average charge for BLS (basic life support) emergency transport was $473, with $700 for ALS (advanced life support) emergency transport; and that the payment sources were Medicare (32 percent), Medicaid (14 percent), private insurance (27 percent), patients themselves (17 percent), and other funding (17 percent). See ibid.

16 The Seattle and King County systems are tax supported. Because funding for paramedic services and for a portion of EMT services comes from a countywide property tax levy, there is generally no charge to the patient for either care or transport. (One exception is made when fire department EMTs call a private ambulance to provide transportation to the hospital for a stable patient who is not critically ill; the patient is then billed by the ambulance company.) As for the levy, it has averaged $0.25 per $1,000 of assessed valuation annually since 1979, when it was first approved. It is now put up for reapproval every six years, and voters have continued to support it by overwhelming margins. The most recent vote on this levy, which called for a slightly increased annual rate of $0.30 per $1,000 of assessed valuation, took place in November 2007. The levy passed with the support of 83 percent of the voters. The next levy vote will occur in 2013.

17 The U.S. Department of Transportation curriculum is used to train police as first responders, and firefighters are trained as EMTs.

18 By comparison, Seattle and King County do not use police in any uniform way, though in a few of the area's cities police do act as first responders in the case of a cardiac arrest. In Redmond, for example, police have been involved in several dramatic saves.

19 The Gold Cross Ambulance Service is affiliated with the Mayo Foundation, which encompasses the Mayo Clinic.

20 In 1998, Rochester's firefighters also began to be trained in AED operation.

21 On negative attitudes, see W. J. Groh, M. R. Lowe, A. D. Overgaard, J. M. Neal, W. C. Fishburn, and D. P. Zipes, "Attitudes of Law Enforcement Officers Regarding Automated External Defibrillators," *Academy of Emergency Medicine* 9 (2002), 751–53. On the experience in Miami, see R. J. Myerburg, J. Fenster, M. Velez, et al., "Impact of Community-Wide Police Car Deployment of Automated External Defibrillators on Survival from Out-of-Hospital Cardiac Arrest," *Circulation* 106 (2002), 1058–64.

22 A perfect example of resistance comes from six rural counties in Indiana with a total population 465,000, where a new police AED program did not improve survival rates, largely because police vehicles responded to only 26 of 388 cardiac arrests, or 6.7 percent; one can only assume that police in these rural counties did not view their job description as including defibrillation. See W. J. Groh, M. M. Newman, P. E. Beal, N. S. Fineberg, and D. P. Zipes, "Limited Response to Cardiac Arrest by Police Equipped with Automated External Defibrillators: Lack of Survival Benefit in Suburban and Rural Indiana: The Police as Responder Automated Defibrillation Evaluation (PARADE)," *Academic Emergency Medicine* 8 (2001), 324–30.

23 R. Davis, "Many Lives Are Lost Across USA Because Emergency Services Fail," *USA Today*, July 28, 2003, makes the same point. Davis reports that in Seattle the paramedic-to-population ratio is 13.5 to 100,000, and that in Milwaukee it is 17.9 to 100,000; both communities have high survival rates—45 percent and 27 percent, respectively. By contrast, in Nashville the ratio is 33.3 to 100,000 and in Omaha it is 44.6 to 100,000; Nashville and Omaha have survival rates of 5 percent and 3 percent, respectively.

24 The sevenfold difference cited by Nichol is specific to the ten communities participating in the ROC trial, which are, for the most part, not the same ones mentioned in chapter 1 in connection with the statement that an individual is forty-six times more likely to survive a cardiac arrest in some communities than in others.

25 A. Hallstrom, T. D. Rea, M. R. Sayre, et al., "Manual Chest Compression vs. Use of an Automated Chest Compression Device During Resuscitation Following Out-of-Hospital Cardiac Arrest: A Randomized Trial," *Journal of the American Medical Association* 295 (2006), 2620–28.

26 Sayre is also collaborating with physician colleagues in St. Cloud, Minnesota, and Austin, Texas, in a multisite effort to improve survival rates for cardiac arrest. "Take Heart America" is the name of a program that aims to increase CPR training, place more AEDs in public locations, and increase the use of hypothermia for resuscitated patients. The fact that three communities are engaged and working together for these ends is encouraging. See R. Davis, "A Plan: 'Take Heart America': Program Aims to Improve Cardiac-Arrest Survival Rates," *USA Today*, Feb. 20, 2007.

27 Intravenous succinylcholine is a potent medicine that immediately paralyzes the patient. This is what emergency physicians often use before emergency intubation. Once the patient is paralyzed, a paramedic can more easily visualize his or her vocal cords and correctly place the tube. In the rare event that intubation is not achieved after several attempts, the paramedic must ventilate with a bag-valve mask until the paralysis wears off (usually within several minutes), all the while assessing other options.

28 E. M. Bulger, M. K. Copass, R. V. Maier, J. Larsen, J. Knowles, and G. J. Jurkovich, "An Analysis

of Advanced Prehospital Airway Management," *Journal of Emergency Medicine* 23 (2002), 183–89.

29 Mario Trevino retired from the Bellevue Fire Department in 2010.

30 The National Fire Protection Association (NFPA), a member-funded nonprofit organization, is not a federal agency but enjoys wide national recognition. With 7,000 members all volunteering their time and expertise, NFPA has 300 committees that issue impressively detailed consensus statements and standards for building safety codes, life safety codes, and EMS matters. NFPA standard 1710, for example, issued in 2001, recommends response times for fire department – based EMS systems, and standard 1720 recommends response times for volunteer fire departments.

31 Mark Morgan retired from Valley Communications Center in 2011.

32 W. B. Carter, M. S. Eisenberg, A. Hallstrom, and S. Schaeffer, "Development and Implementation of Emergency CPR Instructions via Telephone," Annals of Emergency Medicine 13 (1984), 695–700; M. Eisenberg, A. Hallstrom, W. Carter, et al., "Emergency CPR Instructions via Telephone," American Journal of Public Health 75 (1985), 47–50; M. S. Eisenberg, W. Carter, A. Hallstrom, R. O. Cumming, P. Litwin, and T. Hearne, "Identification of Cardiac Arrest by Emergency Dispatchers," American Journal of Emergency Medicine 4 (1986), 299–301.

33 Tom Hearne died in November 2010 at the age of 67. He helped build one of the best EMS systems in the World. In 1979 I hired Tom to be a program coordinator on a research project in the EMS Division. Over the next 15 years he rose in responsibilities to become the EMS Division Director and in 2003 he returned the favor to hire me as medical director. Tom was one of the most decent and kindhearted individuals I have ever known. We were the best of friends. I miss him.

34 The glue that holds the system together is the countywide EMS strategic plan, a long-range policy document created every six years to coincide with the six-year term of the EMS countywide tax levy (see n. 16). All the constituent agencies participate in creating the plan, which is circulated in draft form until it is finalized. The plan gives detailed goals for EMT and paramedic services as well as for dispatching, oversight, and projected new programs, and it includes a six-year financial plan. Hearne believes that the strategic plan also keeps the system transparent and accountable.

35 An EMS advisory board, whose function is like that of a board of directors, approves or disapproves Hearne's proposals. Hearne himself is accountable to the director of the health department and to the county executive.

36 For more about the chain of survival, see chapter 7 and figure 7.1.

SEVEN **What Can Your Community Do?**

1 T. D. Valenzuela, D. J. Roe, G. Nichol, L. L. Clark, D. W. Spaite, and R. G. Hardman, "Outcomes of Rapid Defibrillation by Security Officers after Cardiac Arrest in Casinos," *New England Journal of Medicine* 343 (2000), 1206–9. Terry Valenzuela, medical director of the Tucson Fire Department and lead author of this study, has presented these findings at several scientific meetings. He says that the two questions he hears most often after his presentation are "Were they winning or losing at the time of collapse?" and "What were they playing?"

2 For defibrillation on airplanes, see R. L. Page, J. A. Joglar, R. C. Kowal, et al., "Use of Automated External Defibrillators by a U.S. Airline," *New England Journal of Medicine* 343 (2000), 1210–16.

3 Advanced care can continue in the emergency room and in the hospital's cardiac ICU or cardiac floor. For example, hypothermia can be used to lower the patient's body temperature after he or she regains a spontaneous pulse and blood pressure (see chapters 9 and 10). Hypothermia typically begins in the emergency room and continues in the ICU, but some communities are studying the feasibility of beginning hypothermia in the field, which can be accomplished if paramedics administer two liters (about two quarts) of chilled IV fluids. Thus a good case can be made for a fifth link in the chain of survival—"early post-recuscitation care"—and in fact this fifth link is added in chapter 9

4 The only practical way to achieve a rapid time to CPR is for bystanders to begin CPR in a large proportion of cardiac arrests. And the quickest way to achieve more bystander CPR in a community is to institute an assertive dispatcher-assisted CPR program. .

5 There are regional and state efforts under way to report survival information for cardiac arrest. For example, the State of California now has a public Web site listing numbers of patients with witnessed VF and numbers of discharges from hospitals (http://www.emsa .ca.gov/Data_inf/defib05.asp). The figures for 2005 were pretty grim: there were 918 patients who received a defibrillatory shock, and there were 660 who suffered a witnessed cardiac arrest; the overall survival rate was 2 percent. Most communities in California simply did not report data related to cardiac arrest survival rates.

6 The report card contains thirty-five elements, each worth 3 points, and a perfect score is 105 (clearly, not all elements have equal weight). While hardly a precise grading system, the report card does list the key components of a high-quality EMS system. Many of these are not all-or-nothing elements, so partial scores may be appropriate. At any rate, grading is on the honor system. It may prove enlightening to grade your community's EMS system, but the real purpose of the report card is to point the way toward improvement.

7 The paramedics in the Seattle Medic One program always lived in dread of receiving a copy of an incident report with "See me" scribbled across the top in the handwriting of Michael Copass, the medical director. Few paramedics ever received a "See me" notice more than once, and the second notice was certainly not for the same problem.

EIGHT **A Completed Life**

1 C. S. Beck and D. S. Leighninger, "Death after a Clean Bill of Health," *Journal of the American Medical Association* 1960 (174), 133.

2 P. Safar, "Concluding Statement by the Editor," in P. Safar, ed., *Advances in Cardiopulmonary Resuscitation*, 1st ed. (New York: Springer-Verlag: 1977), 296–97.

3 M. Eisenberg, *Life in the Balance: Emergency Medicine and the Quest to Reverse Sudden Death* (New York: Oxford University Press, 1997), 251.

4 L. Bergner, M. Bergner, A. P. Hallstrom, M. Eisenberg, and L. A. Cobb, "Health Status of Survivors of Out-of-Hospital Cardiac Arrest Six Months Later," *American Journal of Public Health* 74 (1984), 508–10; M. Eisenberg, L. Bergner, and A. Hallstrom, "Survivors of Out-of-Hospital Cardiac Arrest: Morbidity and Long-Term Survival," *American Journal of Emergency Medicine* 2 (1984), 189–92.

5　T. J. Bunch, R. D. White, G. E. Smith, et al., "Long-Term Subjective Memory Function in Ventricular Fibrillation Out-of-Hospital Cardiac Arrest Survivors Resuscitated by Early Defibrillation," *Resuscitation* 60 (2004), 189–95.

6　A "show" resuscitation is carried out primarily for the benefit of bystanders—EMS personnel may demonstrate an effort and go through the motions even though they know that there is no chance of a successful outcome. Some have argued that resuscitations like these should not be performed, and that EMS personnel should either go full bore or declare the patient dead instead of wasting resources, placing themselves at risk for exposure to infectious disease, and creating false hope among bystanders. Though I agree that "show" resuscitations should be discouraged, I can see circumstances in which they may be appropriate. Some sudden deaths in infants and children, for example, or certain trauma deaths may warrant a resuscitation effort even when circumstances offer no chance of success.

7　Nevertheless, EMS personnel can withhold resuscitation efforts when certain physical findings are present, including rigor mortis, lividity, coolness of the body, and trauma incompatible with life (see chapters 4 and 5). The regulations regarding who can declare a patient dead vary from program to program. Some programs require that the patient be brought to a hospital before death can be officially declared, but most allow death to be declared at the scene. Usually a physician, communicating with EMS personnel by telephone or radio, is involved in the decision.

8　Exceptions could be made if there was a valid DNR order or official advance directive, or if the EMTs found conditions that were not compatible with life.

9　S. Feder, R. L. Matheny, R. S. Loveless Jr., and T. D. Rea, "Withholding Resuscitation: A New Approach to Prehospital End-of-Life Decisions," *Annals of Internal Medicine* 144 (2006), 634–40.

10　*POLST* was developed over a four-year period by a multidisciplinary task force of the Center for Ethics in Health Care at Oregon Health & Science University. A number of other localities, encouraged by the success of the Oregon *POLST* program, have also formed coalitions and adopted *POLST*-like paradigms. Efforts like these have now been adopted statewide in four states and are in development in another seventeen states or portions of states.

11　P. Safar, "Concluding Statement by the Editor," 297.

NINE　Putting It All Together

1　See chapter 5, note 77. The American Heart Association in its 2010 Guidelines for CPR and ECC also recognizes the fifth link in the Chain of Survival. The Association calls it "integrated post-cardiac arrest care."

2　The metaphor of a chain (consisting of quantifiable factors) embedded in a frame (consisting of qualitative factors) like all metaphors can never be 100 percent on target. The two key concepts are that measurable and unmeasurable factors contribute to understanding an EMS system's performance and that both groups of factors are intertwined. Perhaps a gumbo soup might be a better metaphor, with all the quantifiable and qualitative factors swimming together in the broth of the community. But the gumbo metaphor misses the concept of the chain, which is definitely temporally connected. So I keep coming back to the chain and the frame. Plus the frame is both a noun and verb. The frame frames the chain. Oh well, I welcome your ideas. One last thing, allow me a little poetic license to use the term "unmeasurable"—it just sounds more appropriate than "not measurable" or "immeasurable."

3   S. J. Diem, J. D. Lantos, and J. A. Tulsky, "Cardiopulmonary Resuscitation on Television: Miracles and Misinformation," *New England Journal of Medicine* 334 (1996), 1578–82.

4   This chapter ends on an optimistic note, and, indeed, I fervently believe that changes in a system, large changes as well as small ones, can dramatically improve a community's survival rate for VF cardiac arrest. Short of an EMS system's success in improving itself, there are other possible scenarios that may ultimately improve survival rates for VF and these are discussed in the final chapter, "A Vision of the Future."

TEN   A Plan of Action

1   B. McNally, R. Robb, M. Mehta, et at. Out-of-Hospital Cardiac Arrest Surveillance – Cardiac Arrest Registry to Enhance Survival (CARES), United States, October 1, 2005-December 31, 2010. Centers for Disease Control and Prevention. *Morbidity and Mortality Weekly Report* 60 (2011) (No. SS#8), 1–19. See also B. McNally, A. Stokes, A. Crouch, A. L. Kellerman, "CARES: Cardiac Arrest Registry to Enhance Survival," *Annals of Emergency Medicine* 54 (2009), 674–83.

2   A registry that lacks access to hospital information is all but useless. Hospital information is vital in determining whether a patient was discharged and the nature of his or her neurological status, as well as in determine the cause of the cardiac arrest. In the HIPAA era, hospitals are concerned about releasing patients' medical information to EMS agencies, yet many states allow this information to be provided in connection with EMS quality improvement. In Washington, for example, state law establishes the right of a "health care provider [to] disclose health care information about a patient without the patient's authorization to the extent a recipient needs to know the information, if the disclosure is . . . to any other person who requires health care information for health care education, or to provide planning, quality assurance, peer review, or administrative, legal, financial, or actuarial services to the health care provider." The CARES staff can help an EMS program navigate its way to obtaining hospital information.

3   The forms can be completed electronically or on paper. If the paper version is used, one copy is left with the receiving hospital. Electronic versions can be freestanding or Web-based. Some communities use a mix of paper-based and electronic reporting. The wave of the future appears to be tablet-based electronic entry of data directly in the field. The reports can be forwarded to hospitals and supervisors and QI managers, as well as stored in the record-management system.

4   Defibrillation downloads are usually sent electronically and dispatch center CAD reports and recordings of cardiac arrest calls can usually be obtained electronically. Clearly, the dispatch center would have to authorize the EMS QI person accessing the information.

5   See chapter 4, note 21.

6   The first edition of *Resuscitate!* used the term "aggressive." I think the term "assertive" better defines the proper attitude.

7   L. White, J. Rogers, M. Bloomingdale, C. Fahrenbruch, L. Culley, C. Subido, et al.: "Dispatcher-Assisted Cardiopulmonary Resuscitation—Risks for Patients Not in Cardiac Arrest," Circulation 121 (2010), 91–97.

8   See chapter 5, note 32.

9   E. B Lerner, T. D. Rea, B. J. Bobrow, J. E. Acker III, R. A. Berg, S. C. Brooks, D. C. Cone, et al., "Emergency Medical Service Dispatch Cardiopulmonary Resuscitation Prearrival Instructions to Improve Survival from Out-of-Hospital Cardiac Arrest: A Scientific Statement From the American Heart Association Circulation." Published online January 9, 2012.

10 See chapter 5, note 47. The change in King County's EMS CPR protocol occurred in January 2005. Later in 2005, the AHA published new CPR and ECC guidelines based in part on the Rea et al. King County study. The 2005 guidelines stressed the importance of increased CPR and rhythm assessments every two minutes. In the 2010 guidelines, the importance of high-quality CPR was further stressed. The guidelines also remarked on the wide variation in cardiac arrest survival rates across EMS systems and noted the lack of bystander CPR for most cardiac arrests.

11 High-performance CPR is similar in concept to what the AHA calls high-quality CPR. We think the concept of "high-performance" better defines each parameter of CPR (for example, we offer a specific range of 100–120 instead of greater than 100 and strive for minimal interruptions in CPR—none to exceed 10 seconds). We also make the EMT responsible for the quality of CPR (the EMT owns CPR).

12 Our tapes are part of our formal registry and QI program and are therefore protected from public disclosure.

13 See chapter 6, notes 21 and 22.

14 A. P. Hallstrom, J. P. Ornato, M. Weisfeldt, et al., "Public-Access Defibrillation and Survival after Out-of-Hospital Cardiac Arrest," New England Journal of Medicine 351 (2004), 637–46.

15 On the use of AEDs in casinos and airplanes, see these two articles from the New England Journal of Medicine 343 (2000): T. D. Valenzuela, D. J. Roe, G. Nichol, L. L. Clark, D. W. Spaite, and R. G. Hardman, "Outcomes of Rapid Defibrillation by Security Officers after Cardiac Arrest in Casinos," 1206–9; and R. L. Page, J. A. Joglar, R. C. Kowal, et al., "Use of Automated External Defibrillators by a U.S. Airline," 1210–16.

16 T. D. Rea, M. Olsufka, B. Bemis, L. White, L. Yin, et al., "A Population-Based Investigation of Public Access Defibrillation: Role of Emergency Medical Services Care," Resuscitation 81 (2010), 163–67. See also L. L. Culley, T. D. Rea, J. A. Murray, et al., "Public-Access Defibrillation in Out-of-Hospital Cardiac Arrest: A Community-Based Study," Circulation 109 (2004), 1859–63.

17 R. M. Merchant and D. A. Asch, "Can You Find an AED If a Life Depends on It?" Circulation Cardiovascular Quality and Outcomes 5 (2012), 1-3.

18 See chapter 5, note 77.

19 See chapter 5, note 77.

20 The Institute of Medicine advises the federal government and other national agencies on medical matters. Institute of Medicine reports may be commissioned by specific agencies or by the organization itself. "Emergency Medical Services at the Crossroads" is one of a trio of reports commissioned by the Josiah Macy Jr. Foundation and four federal agencies. (The other two reports are: "Hospital-Based Emergency Care: At the Breaking Point," about the

crisis in emergency departments; and "Emergency Care for Children: Growing Pains," about deficiencies in emergency care for children.) The report discussed here is available online at http://www.iom.edu/CMS/3809/16107/35010.aspx.

21 It is an historical anomaly that DOT is the agency currently in charge of defining the EMT curriculum. This arrangement stems from a 1968 National Academy of Sciences report on the tragedy of trauma and the development of an EMT curriculum.

22 That figure is not entirely arbitrary; it is the rate reported for the very first prehospital cardiac care program in 1966; see J. Pantridge and J. S. Geddes, "A Mobile Intensive-Care Unit in the Management of Myocardial Infarction," *The Lancet* 2 (1967), 271–73. Moreover, several communities are already pushing that figure. The rules for the competition should be simple—one calendar year, with all consecutive cases (witnessed VF, minimum of fifty cases), and with clinical data confirmed by an outside reviewer. However, as I will argue in chapter 11, I think a survival rate of 60 percent is attainable.

23 The National EMS Information System (NEMSIS), an effort to define the elements that all EMS systems should collect, was conceived in 2001 by the National Highway Traffic Safety Association, the National Association of EMS Physicians, and the Maternal and Child Health Bureau of the Health Resources and Services Administration (since then, the Centers for Disease Control, the University of Utah, and the University of North Carolina have also joined the project.) By 2003, forty-nine states (all but New York) had signed a memorandum of understanding that recognized the need for a national data set and that defined the data elements to be collected (New York has not signed as of 2012). Considerable progress has been made in creating a data dictionary and a technical assistance center has been established. A national EMS database has the potential to support the development of training curricula, the evaluation of care and outcomes, the facilitation of research, and the feasibility of cross-community comparisons. The main challenge to the adoption of NEMSIS by EMS systems around the country is its requirement that considerable resources be devoted to upgrading management systems and other kinds of change efforts, but without the support of federal dollars to underwrite these expenditures. Therefore, most localities view NEMSIS as an unfunded mandate. Many also see NEMSIS as having produced an unfocused encyclopedia of data, one into which the tiniest details of care have been collected without regard for their direct relevance either to improving outcomes or to furthering research. Despite these problems, however, a national database will draw attention to the issue of sudden cardiac arrest and allow new predictors of survival to be identified.

24 G. Nichol, J. Rumsfeld, B. Eigel, et al., "Essential Features of Designating Out-of-Hospital Cardiac Arrest as a Reportable Event," *Circulation* 117 (2008), 2299–2308.

25 R. W. Neuman, J. M. Barnhart, R. A Berg, P. S. Chan. R. G. Geocadin, R. V. Leupker, et al., "Implementation Strategies for Improving Survival after Out-of-Hospital Cardiac Arrest in the United States: Consensus Recommendations from the 2009 American Heart Association Cardiac Arrest Survival Summit." *Circulation* 123 (2011), 2898-2910.

26 In 2012, the ROC began two randomized clinical trials. One was designed to determine if antiarrhythmics are of value in shock resistant VF. The trial will have three interventions and will compare amiodarone, lidocaine and placebo for patients who are not defibrillated after one shock. The second trial will determine if continuous chest compression with one ventilation every 10 compressions results in higher survival than the traditional 30:2

sequence of 30 compressions and two ventilations.

27 Donald Berwick provides a useful commentary on traditional and nontraditional methods of assessing improvement. See D. M. Berwick, "The Science of Improvement," *Journal of the American Medical Association* 299 (2008), 1182–84.

ELEVEN A Vision of the Future

1 Survival from witnessed VF in Seattle and King County has hovered around 50 percent since 2008 and in 2011 both Seattle and King County surpassed 50 percent.

2 Defined by an ejection fraction of 35 percent or less, an ejection fraction being the proportion of blood expelled with each ventricular contraction; normally the ejection fraction is 50 to 60 percent.

3 Patients who have been shocked inappropriately liken the sensation to being kicked in the chest by a horse; inappropriate shocks occur in 15 percent of patients over the lifetime of the device. See P. J. Zimetbaum, "A 59-Year-Old Man Considering Implantation of a Cardiac Defibrillator," *Journal of the American Medical Association* 297 (2007), 1909–16.

4 L. A. Cobb, C. E. Fahrenbruch, M. Olsufka, and M. K. Copass, "Changing Incidence of Out-of-Hospital Ventricular Fibrillation, 1980–2000," *Journal of the American Medical Association* 288 (2002), 3008–13.

5 J. Herlitz, J. Engdahl, L. Svensson, M. Young, K. A. Angquist, and S. Holmberg, "Decrease in the Occurrence of Ventricular Fibrillation as the Initially Observed Arrhythmia after Out-of-Hospital Cardiac Arrest During 11 Years in Sweden," *Resuscitation* 60 (2004), 283–90; F. Kette, "Increased Survival Despite a Reduction in Out-of-Hospital Ventricular Fibrillation in North-East Italy," *Resuscitation* 72 (2006), 52–58.

6 T. D. Rea, M. S. Eisenberg, L. J. Becker, et al., "Emergency Medical Services and Mortality from Heart Disease: A Community Study," *Annals of Emergency Medicine* 41 (2003), 494–99.

7 W. D. Weaver, G. S. Lorch, H. A. Alvarez, and L. A. Cobb, "Angiographic Findings and Prognostic Indicators in Patients Resuscitated from Sudden Cardiac Death," *Circulation* 54 (1976), 895–900.

8 See chapter 4, note 16.

9 See chapter 10, note 15.

10 G. H. Bardy, K. L. Lee, J. E. Poole, et al., "Home Use of Automated External Defibrillators for Sudden Cardiac Arrest," *New England Journal of Medicine* 358 (2008), 1793–1804. The number of cardiac arrests among the 7,001 patients enrolled in the study was much lower than expected. There were 228 deaths in the control group and 222 deaths in the home AED group. There were only 160 sudden cardiac arrests considered to be the result of VF or VT and 117 occurred at home. Of the arrests at home, 58 were witnessed. AEDs were used in 32 patients, 14 received an appropriate shock, and 4 survived to hospital discharge.

11 C. W. Callaway and J. J. Menegazzi, "Waveform Analysis of Ventricular Fibrillation to Predict Defibrillation," *Current Opinion in Critical Care* 11 (2005), 192–99.

12 Y. Li, B. Bisera, F. Gehab, W. Tang, and M. H. Weil, "Identifying Potentially Shockable Rhythms without Interrupting Cardiopulmonary Resuscitation," *Critical Care Medicine* 36 (2008), 198–203.chapter 11, I think a survival rate of 60 percent is attainable.

13 M. S. Lloyd, B. Heeke, P. F. Walter, J. J. Langberg, "Hands-On Defibrillation: An Analysis of

Electrical Current Flow through Rescuers in Direct Contact with Patients During Biphasic External Defibrillation," *Circulation* 117 (2008), 2510–14.

14 I. Laurent, C. Adrie, C. Vinsonneau, et al., "High-Volume Hemofiltration after Out-of-Hospital Cardiac Arrest: A Randomized Study," *Journal of the American College of Cardiology* 46 (2005), 432–37.

15 I am indebted to Lewis Thomas, the medical essayist, who first pointed out the inverse relationship between level of technology and understanding of disease in his book *Lives of a Cell: Notes of a Biology Watcher*.

16 Brian Wansink, in *Mindless Eating: Why We Eat More Than We Think* (New York: Bantam, 2006), predicts that the twenty-first century will be the "century of behavior change." Behavioral changes and choices can add years and quality to our lives. Understanding how to motivate people to reduce risky behavior and embrace healthy behavior is the challenge of our century.

Index

Page numbers in italic refer to figures and tables; "n" and "nn" refer to endnotes.

A

academic medical centers, 190–91
accelerated (rapid) dispatch, 147, 152, 184
accessory pathways, 53
AC defibrillator, 34
acid buildup in bloodstream, 14
action plan: overview, 176; change agents, 173; citizen participation, 171; dispatcher-assisted telephone CPR, *176*, 177; guidelines for compassionate withholding of resuscitation, 203; implementation difficulty levels, *176*, 176; lead federal agency, *199*, 199; medical leadership, *170*, 170–71; National Institute of Resuscitation Research (proposed), 202–3; performance standards, national, 201, 202; political leadership, 173; prevention programs, 213; public access defibrillation (PAD), 191, 192; public expectations, 171–73; quality improvement, continuous, 170; rapid dispatch, *176*, 186-87; voice recordings, 189

acute coronary syndrome, 8
acute myocardial infarction (AMI): case examples, 46–47; as cause of sudden death, 46–48; description of, 47; heart disease with, 10; mobile coronary care units for, 36–37; symptoms, 10; treatment of, 10, 47
Adams, David, 31
administrative authority, *170*, 170–71
administrative control, on community report card, *157*
administrative support, level and nature of, 107–8
administrator perspectives, 147–49
advanced care, early, 153–54
advance directives, 165–67
advisory boards, 206
AEDs (automated external defibrillators): brands of, 240n38; clock synchronization, 236n21; defibrillator-guided therapy, 111; digital recording from, 58–59, 136; early prototype, 233n38; examples cases, 3; first EMT training program, 43; in homes, 255n10; long Q-T syndrome and, 52; paradox of, 177–78; placement of, 68–69; police AED model,

AEDs (*continued*)
133–34; public access defibrillation
(PAD), 109; survival rates and, 92, 109;
time stamp on, 71
African Americans, 84–85
age, 5, 61, 84
Aging with Dignity, 167
agonal respirations: CPR instructions and,
183; example case, 2; recognition of, 153;
survival rates and, 93–94
air pollution, 94–95
airway management, 114, 153
airway obstruction, 95
alternating current (AC), 34
ambulances: mobile coronary care units (MC-
CUs), 36–37, 38–39; private ambulance
model, 105–6, 130, 131–32
American Heart Association: on dispatcher-
assisted telephone CPR, 108–9, 253nn9–
10; four-link chain metaphor, 43; five-link
metaphor, *169*, 169, 251n1; on Hands-
Only CPR, 112, 229n69, 253n11; international guidelines, 100
American Medical Association, 27
AMI. *See* acute myocardial infarction
Amsterdam Society for Recovery of Drowned
Persons, 21–24, *22*, 232n25
anaphylaxis, 56–57
aneurysms, 19–20, 54–55
angina: case examples, 45–46; heart disease
with symptoms of, 9–10, 234n2; ischemia
and, 45–46
angina ("pre-infarction," "crescendo," or
"unstable"). *See* MI (myocardial
infarction)
Annals of Internal Medicine, 165
anti-arrhythmics, 110
aortic aneurysms, 54–55; ruptured, 12
aortic stenosis, 53
APCO (International Association of Public
Safety Communications Officials), 146
"arrest," defined, 12
arteriography (coronary arteriograms), 9
artificial circulation, 28. *See also* CPR (cardiopulmonary resuscitation)

Association of Physicians of Great Britain and
Ireland, 218n25
asystole (flatlining): in cardiac arrest, 15;
defined, 12–13; percent of cardiac arrests
associated with, *63*, 64, *64*; survival rate,
239n27; VF leading to, 12, 64
atherosclerotic heart disease (underlying
coronary artery disease or ischemic heart
disease), 45–46
athletes, 51
attitudes, 133, 142–43, 144–45
attrition rates in EMS agencies, 105
Aufderheide, T. P., 97
authority, sphere of, 103
automated external defibrillators. *See* AEDs
autonomic nervous system, 211
AutoPulse Assisted Prehospital International
Resuscitation (ASPIRE) trial, 138

B

back-pressure/arm-lift method, *23*, 24, 27
Baltimore City Hospital, 30–31
Bardy, G. H., 255n10
base-station hospitals, 246n7
Beck, Claude, 32–33, 161, 232n18
Becker, Lance, 86, 97
Belfast MCCU system, 36–37
Bellevue Hospital, New York City, 27–28
Berwick, Donald, 255n27
beta-blockers, 52, 87
biblical resuscitations, 19–21, *21*
blood chemistries, 217
brain and oxygen deprivation, 14–15
brain aneurysms, 19–20, 54–55
breathing. *See* agonal respirations; airway
management; airway obstruction
Brugada syndrome, 52–53
budgetary resources and survival, 107
bystanders: chain of survival and, 152–53;
chest-compression-only CPR and, 112–14;
CPR performed by, in King County,
65–66; CPR training for, 41–42; survival
rates and CPR initiated by, 91; witnessed
and unwitnessed arrests, 61–62. *See also*

CPR (cardiopulmonary resuscitation);
witnesses

C

call receivers, 235n5

cancer, 55–56

cardiac arrest. *See* sudden cardiac arrest
(sudden cardiac death)

cardiac arrest registries. *See* King County
registry of cardiac arrests; registries of
cardiac arrests

Cardiac Arrest Registry to Enhance Survival
(CARES) project, 178, 225

cardiac arrest tracking system, 225, *226*

Cardiac Arrhythmia Suppression Trial (CAST),
87

"cardiac," defined, 12

cardiac stimulants, 110

cardiomyopathy, 49–51

cardiopulmonary resuscitation. *See* CPR

CARES (Cardiac Arrest Registry to Enhance
Survival) project, 178, 225

Carville, James, 155

CAST (Cardiac Arrhythmia Suppression Trial),
87

catheter ablation, 53

causes of sudden cardiac arrest: overview,
44, *45*, *46*; acute myocardial infarction, 46–48; cardiomyopathy, 49–50;
congestive heart failure, 48–49; coronary
artery disease and ischemia, 45–46; non-
heart-related, 54–57; primary electrical
diseases, 51–53; primary ventricular
fibrillation, 48

causes of ventricular fibrillation, possible,
211–12

CCUs (coronary care units), 36

Center for Prehospital Emergency Care (University of Washington), 135

cerebral aneurysms, 19–20, 54–55

certification of EMTs and paramedics, 127–28

chain of command, medical, 141

chain of survival: overview, *151*, 151–54; case
example, 154–55; fifth link, 168-69m *169*,

250n3, 251n2 frame surrounding, *170*,
170–71

chest, placement of electrode pads on, 100

chest compression: defibrillation during, 217;
development of, 27–30; ratio of ventilations to, 139

chest-compression-only CPR, 112–14,
243nn68–69

chest pain, 18

CHF (congestive heart failure), 48–49

Chicago, 6, 86, 237n3

children: commotio cordis and, 53–54; long
Q-T syndrome and, 52; sudden infant
death syndrome (SIDS), 56

Chu, K., 85

circulation, 28

circulatory phase, 97

citizen participation, 171

citizens. *See* bystanders

Clark, J. J., 94

Clarke, S. O., 88

clock synchronization, 236n21

clots, 55

Cobb, Leonard, 41–42, 121–25, 134, 135, 245n2,
246n6

cold-related stress, 67

Columbus, Ohio, 138–39

commotio cordis, 53–54

community differences in survival rates, 6–8,
7, 80–81, 120–21, 135, 138–39

community report cards, 155–59, *157*

community support: and citizen participation, 171; on community report card, *157*;
public expectations, 171; Vickery on, 143

comorbidity, 85–86

compassionate withholding of resuscitation,
203–4

compressed-air piston devices, 111

compression straps, 112

computer-aided dispatch programs, 108–9,
191

computerized tomography (CT), 9

congestive heart failure (CHF), 48–49

continuous education, 145–46, 147

Copass, Michael, 121–23, 125, 134, 135, 250n7

coronary arteries, defined, 9

coronary arteriograms (arteriography), 9

coronary artery disease, 45–46

coronary care units (CCUs), 36

costs, 132, 233nn15–16

CPR (cardiopulmonary resuscitation): adjunct devices, 111–12; by bystanders, 65–66, 91; chain of survival and, 152–53, 154; chest-compression-only (hands-only), 112–14, 243nn68–69; during defibrillation, 174; defibrillation, interaction with, 100–101, 241n46; development of, 26–31, 30; examples cases, 2; high performance, 185–86; minimally interrupted, 202; in movies or television, 231n18; obesity and, 86; P-ROSC and, 173; quality of, 97–98, 139; ratio of ventilations to chest compressions, 139; telephone-assisted, 43, 65, 104–5, 108–9, 146, 147, 182–84, 240n37; time of initiation, 71, 72, 75; time to start of, 96, 96–97, 115, 127, 155, 250n4; training of public on, 41–43, 65, 108–9; victim position and, 153; vital role of, 15–16

crescendo angina. See myocardial infarction (MI)

critical mass of EMS responders, 103–4

CT (computerized tomography), 9

Culley, L. L., 242n62

culture, organizational, 107, 134, 147

culture of excellence, 107, 146, 149, 194–95

Cummins, Richard, 162

D

DART (Dispatcher Assisted Resuscitation Trial), 244n73

day of the week, 67, 67

DC defibrillator, 34

death, causes of. See causes of sudden cardiac arrest

death, declaration of, 251n7; rates, 5

death with dignity. See end-of-life decisions

decisions on resuscitation. See end-of-life decisions

The Deep End (movie), 17

defibrillation: aim of, 11; chain of survival and, 153–54; CPR, interaction with, 100–101, 241n46, 244n81; CPR during, 217; CPR quality assessment by, 98; development of, 31–34, 33; electrode pads, 100; example cases, 31–32; improvement of, 215–17; internal, 32–33, 33; quality of, 99–100; role of, 16; success, determinants of, 16; time of initiation, 71; time to start of, 98, 98–99, 99, 127, 155

defibrillators: development of, 31–34, 33; improvement of, 173; survival rates and defibrillator-guided therapy, 110–11; time stamp on, 71; voice recordings from, 136; wearable, 217. See also AEDs (automated external defibrillators)

defibrillatory wave forms, 217

Department of Health and Human Services, 200

Department of Transportation (DOT), 128, 200, 254n21

Diack, Arch, 233n38

dialysis, 56

diastolic heart failure, 49

diet, 86

digital recordings: from AEDs, 58–59; of dispatcher-assisted CPR, 146; voice recordings, 136, 189–90

dilated cardiomyopathy, 50–51

direct current (DC), 34

dispatcher-assisted CPR, 182–84

Dispatcher Assisted Resuscitation Trial (DART), 244n73

dispatchers: assertiveness and, 147; chain of survival and, 152; on community report card, 157; defined, 235n5; perspective of, 146–47; rapid (accelerated) dispatch, 147, 152, 186–87; review committee, 146–47; telephone-assisted CPR and, 43, 65, 104–5, 108–9, 146, 147, 182–84; training and continuing education, 147; training quality, 108; unwitnessed arrests and, 62 dispatch systems, *70*, 108–9, 187. *See also* 911 calls

diuretics, 87

DNR (do not resuscitate) orders, 164, 251n8

doctor's offices and clinics, 236n15

dogs, experimentation on, 28

do not resuscitate (DNR) orders, 164, 251n8

Dopplers, 140

down time, 71–72

drowning, sudden death by, 231n6

drug reactions, 56

E

ECGs (electrocardiograms), 9, 15, *33*, 174

economic cost of sudden death, 5

ejection fractions, 255n2

Elam, James, 26–27

electrical phase, 97

electrocardiograms (ECGs), 9, 15, *33*, 174

electrode pads, 100, 233n38

electrolytes, 234n6

Elijah (prophet), 20

Elisha (prophet), 20–21

"Emergency Medical Services at the Crossroads" (Institute of Medicine), 199

emergency medical technicians. *See* EMTs

emesis (vomiting), 92, 239n31

emotional cost of sudden death, 5

EMS Online, 145, *145*

EMS research centers, 203

EMS systems: attrition rates and salaries, 105–6; cardiac arrest management as surrogate for, 18; funding of, 132; organizational structure and culture, 107; quality of care, 105–6; size of, 103; types of, 101–2, 130–32, *131*

EMTs (emergency medical technicians): certification of, 127–28; chain of survival and, 153; collapse in presence of, 93; CPR quality and, 97–98; development of, 35–36; experience levels, 105; King County training programs, 43; perspectives of, 144–46; in tiered-response systems, 102; training quality, 108;

volunteer (examples case), 4–5; and withholding of resuscitation, 162–65. *See also* paramedics

end-of-life decisions: advance directives and *POLST*, 165–67, *166*; example case, 160; guidelines, need for, 203–4; hearts "too good to die" or "too sick to live," 160–63; withholding resuscitation for compelling reasons, 163–65, 251n7

endotracheal intubation: airway management systems and, 244n76; quality and speed of, 114; success rates of, 141; succinylcholine and, 141, 248n27

engine company, tiered response system with, *131*

Enlightenment, 21–22

environmental conditions and survival rates, 94–95

epinephrine, 110

estrogen, 61

European Resuscitation Council (ERC), 243n69

event factors in survival: overview, 88–89; activities and other possible triggers, 94; agonal breathing, 93–94; arrival of EMS personnel, arrest before or after, 93; bystander-initiated CPR, 91; cause of cardiac arrest, 91–92; circumstances surrounding decision to begin resuscitation, 95; emesis, 92; environmental conditions, 94–95; location of collapse, 90, *91*; on-scene AED, use of, 92; position of victim after collapse, 95; symptoms before collapse, 92–93; time of day, 90–91; type of heart rhythm, 89, *89*; witnesses, 89, *90*, *91*

exercise, 69

expectations, public, 171–72

F

fainting (syncope), 52

Feder, Sylvia, 163–65

federal performance standards, 144

fibrillation. *See* ventricular fibrillation (VF)

fine ventricular fibrillation, 15, 53–54

fire chiefs, 123–24, 141–44

fire-department based system. *See* Seattle–King County EMS system

fire departments, 35–36, 107

firefighters, 39. *See also* EMTs (emergency medical technicians); paramedics

fire-medic system, 130–31

fish oils, 86

Five Wishes, 167

flatlining. *See* asystole

foundation, 192

frame of survival, *170*, 170, 251n2

funding of EMS systems, 132, 246n10, 247n16

G

Geddes, John, 36–37, 39, 232n25

genetic abnormalities, 52

genetic factors in survival, 88

genetic predispositions for VF, 212

Gilmore, C. M., 240n39

glucose, 14

Gold Cross Ambulance Service, 133

Gordon, Archer, 31

Grace, William, 38–39

H

Hallstrom, Al P., 85, 87–88, 137–38, 151

hands-only CPR, 112–14, 243nn68–69

Harborview Hospital, Seattle, 41, 121, 124, 143, 148

hard and soft factors, 136

health-department model, 149

Hearne, Tom, 147–49, 249n33

heart: effects of cardiac arrest on, 15; filtration of, 218

"heart attack" as imprecise term, 8

heart disease: as cause of death, 5; continuum of, 8; magnitude of the problem, 5; modification of risk factors, 213–14; sudden cardiac death as first manifestation of, 213, 234n2; with symptoms of angina, 9–10; without symptoms, 9

heart failure. *See* congestive heart failure (CHF)

heart murmurs, 53

heart rhythms: associated with cardiac arrest, by percentage, *63*, 63–64, *64*; survival rates and, 89, *89*; and witnesses, presence or absence of, 64–65. *See also* asystole (flatlining); PEA (pulseless electrical activity); ventricular fibrillation (VF)

Helbock, Mike, 140–41

hemofiltration, 218

high-performance CPR, 185–86, 253n11

Hirschman, James, 39

histamine, 57

Hollywood heart attacks, 17–18

homes: AEDs in, 214; as location of cardiac arrest, 68, *68*

hospital-based model, 131, 132

hospital care, quality of, 115

hospital discharge, 7, 79, 242n63. *See also* survival

hypertrophic cardiomyopathy, 50, 51

hypothermia therapy, 114, 193–94

I

ICDs (implantable cardioverter defibrillators), 212, 218

impairment after resuscitation, 163

impedance threshold devices (ITDs), 111

implantable cardioverter defibrillators (ICDs), 212, 218

implantable defibrillators, 3–4, 52

implementation, 205–7

incident reports: medical control and, 157; NG911 and, 72; responder time and, 75; voice recordings and, 136. *See also* registries of cardiac arrests

Institute of Medicine, 199

internal defibrillation, 32–33, *33*

International Association of Public Safety Communications Officials (APCO), 146

International Liaison Committee on Resuscitation, 175

intubation. *See* endotracheal intubation

ischemia, 45–46

ischemic cardiomyopathy, 50

ischemic heart disease (underlying coronary artery disease or atherosclerotic heart disease), 45–46

ITDs (impedance threshold devices), 111

J

Japanese diet, 86

Journal of Emergency Medical Services (JEMS), 105, 131–32, 247n11

Journal of the American Medical Association (JAMA), 6, 26, 27, 28–29, *30*

Jude, James R., 28, *29*, 31

K

kidney failure, 56

Kim, C., 84

Kim, Francis, 194

King County, Washington: causes of cardiac arrest in, 44; pioneering programs in, 43; reporting requirements for cardiac arrest, 58–59. *See also* Seattle–King County EMS system

King County Medical Dispatch Training and QI, 147

King County Medic One, 125–26, 149, 163

King County registry of cardiac arrests: overview, 58–60; associated activities, 69–70; CPR-trained bystanders, 65–66; heart rhythms, 62–65, *63*, *64*; hour, day, and season, *66*, 66–67, *67*; location, 67–69, *68*; personnel, 235n3; response times and time intervals, 70–75, *73*, *74*; typical survivors, 75–76; victim characteristics, 60–61; witnessed and unwitnessed arrests, 61–62

Knickerbocker, G. Guy, 28, *29*, 31

Kouwenhoven, William, 28, *29*, 31

Kudenchuk, Peter, 136–37

L

leadership, administrative and medical, 170–71, 195

LEMAP (Loaned Executive Member Assistance Program), 146

Levesh, Tod, 139–40

living wills, 163, 165

Loaned Executive Member Assistance Program (LEMAP), 146

location of cardiac arrests, 67–69, *68*, 90, *91*

long Q-T syndrome, 52

Lown, Bernard, 34

M

MAAP (Member Advisory Assistance Program), 146

male-to-female ratio for cardiac arrests, 61

mantras, 221–25

manual defibrillators. *See* defibrillators

Maryland Medical Society, 31

Matheny, Roger, 164–65

Mayo Clinic College of Medicine, 134

MCCUs (mobile coronary care units), 36–37, 38–39

media attention, 172

medical control: on community report card, 157, *158*; as key factor, 137, 141; in Seattle–King County EMS system, 122–25, 143

medical directors: community report card and, 157; EMS system size and, 103; medical model and, 123–24; medical quality improvement (QI) and, 106; quality of medical direction, 106; in Seattle–King County EMS system, 245n5

MedicAlert, 60

medical leadership, 195

medical model, 122–25, 195

medical quality improvement (QI): as common denominator, 245n85; on community report card, *157*; continuous, 196–98; good data for, 136–37; in Seattle–King County EMS system, 128–30;

medical quality improvement (QI) (*continued*)
  survival and programs for, 106
medications, 86–87, 110, 169
Medic One Foundation, 192
Medic One program (Seattle), 41, 121–25,
  127, 128, 246n10. *See also* Seattle–King
  County EMS system
Medic Two program (Seattle), 41, 65–66, 108
medical model, 195–96
Mediterranean diet, 86
Member Advisory Assistance Program
  (MAAP), 146
men, 61, 84
metabolic phase, 97
MI (myocardial infarction), 10. *See also*
  acute myocardial infarction (AMI)
Miami paramedic program, 39–40
misperceptions by public, 17–18, 173
mitral valve prolapse, 53
mobile coronary care units (MCCUs), 36–37,
  38–39
mobile intensive care, 34–37
"A Mobile Intensive-Care Unit in the
  Management of Myocardial Infarction"
  (Pantridge and Geddes), 232n25
Morgan, Mark, 146–47
morning hours, *66*, 66–67
mouth-to-mouth ventilation: development
  of, 26–27, 231n4; hands-only CPR and,
  112–14; ratio to chest compressions, 139,
  229n1
movies and television, cardiac arrest in,
  17–18, 172, 231n18
multilayered systems. *See* tiered-response
  systems
murmurs, 53
Murray, Jack, 164
myocardial infarction (MI), 10. *See also*
  acute myocardial infarction (AMI)

N

NAEMSP (National Association of EMS
  Physicians), 254n23
Nagel, Eugene, 39–40

National Association of EMS Physicians
  (NAEMSP), 254n23
national action plan, 199
National EMS Information Systems (NEM-
  SIS), 201, 254n23
National EMS Research Agenda, 202, 253n20
National Fire Protection Association (NFPA),
  144, 201
National Heart, Lung, and Blood Institute,
  202
National Highway Safety and Traffic Act
  (1966), 35
National Highway Traffic and Safety Admin-
  istration (NHTSA), 200, 254n23
National Institute of Resuscitation Research
  (proposed), 202
National Institutes of Health, 202
national lead agency, need for, 199
National Registry of Emergency Medical
  Technicians (NREMT), 127
natural history of sudden cardiac arrest, 25
NEMSIS (National EMS Information Systems), 201, 254n23
NFPA (National Fire Protection Association),
  144, 202
NG911 network, 72
NHTSA (National Highway Traffic and Safety
  Administration), 200
Nichol, Graham, 135, 200
911 calls, *70*, 71–72
911 operators, 43. *See also* dispatchers
911 systems, 72
nitroglycerine, 10, 45
nonischemic cardiomyopathy, 50
NREMT (National Registry of Emergency
  Medical Technicians), 127
number of responders, 103–4, 135
nursing homes, 90

O

obesity, 86
omega-3 fatty acids, 86
Ontario Prehospital Advanced Life Support
  (OPALS) study, 102

Oregon Health & Sciences University, 166, 251n10

organizational culture, 107, 134, 147

overventiliation, 97

oxygenation, 26–27, 112–13

oxygen deprivation, 14–15

P

Pantridge, Frank, 36–37, 38, 39, 41, 232n25

paradox of technology, 218–19

paralytics, 141, 248n27

paramedic programs: development of, 37–41; example cases, 37–38; Medic One program (Seattle), 41, 121–25, 127, 128

paramedics: certification of, 127–28; chain of survival and, 154; culture and, 134–35; dual-training, 193; medical control and, 122–25; perspective of, 139–41; ratio to community population, 104, 135; skill levels, 139–40; skills improvement, 198–99; survival rates and addition of, 102; in tiered-response systems, 102; training quality, 108; and withholding of resuscitation, 162–65. *See also* EMTs (emergency medical technicians)

patient factors in survival: age, 84; comorbidity, 85–86; diet, 86; genetics, 88; medications, 86–87; obesity, 86; race, 84–85; sex, 84; socioeconomic status, 87–88

PEA (pulseless electrical activity): AMI and, 47; defined, 12–13; percent of cardiac arrests associated with, *63*, 64, *64*

perspectives on EMS systems: administrators, 147–49; dispatchers, 146–47; EMTs, 144–46; fire chiefs, 141–44; paramedics, 139–41; researchers, 134–39

pharmacotherapy at the scene, 110

physical activity and cardiac arrest, 69–70, 94. *See also* athletes

Physician Orders for Life-Sustaining Treatment (POLST) Paradigm to Improve End-of-Life Care, 166, 167, 251n10

physicians: medical control and, 122–25; in

mobile coronary care units (MCCUs), 36–37, 38–39; pushing resuscitation beyond the hands of, 39

pigs, experimentation on, 97

plan of action. *See* action plan

plunger devices, 111–12

police, tiered response system with, 130, *131*, 132–34, 190–91

police defibrillation, 191

political leadership, 170–71, 217–18

POLST (Physician Orders for Life-Sustaining Treatment) Paradigm to Improve End-of-Life Care, *166*, 167, 251n10

position of victim after collapse, 95, 153

post-resuscitation care, improving, 193–94

potassium depletion, 87

pre-infarction angina. *See* myocardial infarction (MI)

pressors, 110

prevention programs, 211–12

primary electrical diseases, 51–53

primary ventricular fibrillation, 48

private ambulance model, 105–6, 130, 131–32

probability of return of spontaneous circulation (P-ROSC), 216

probability thresholds, 111

P-ROSC (probability of return of spontaneous circulation), 216

protocols (standing orders) and standards: federal performance standards for EMS systems, 144, 201–2; medical model and minimization of, 124–25; regionalization, 148; survival rates and, 95

PSAPs (public safety answering points), *70*, 71, 72, 75

public access defibrillation (PAD), 109, 191–92. *See also* AEDs (automated external defibrillators)

public agency model, 130, 132

public expectations, 171

public misperceptions, 17–18, 172

public places: as locations of cardiac arrest, 68, *68*, 171; placement of AEDs in, 68–69; survival rates and, 90, *91*

public-private partnerships, 132

public safety answering points (PSAPs), *70*, 71, 72, 75
public utility model, 132
pulmonary embolus, 55
pulseless electrical activity. *See* PEA
The Pulse of Life (training film), 31

Q

qualitative factors, 148, 170–71
quality improvement (QI), continuous, 196–98 *See also* medical quality improvement (QI)
quantitative factors, 169–70

R

race, 84–85
rapid (accelerated) dispatch, 147, 152, 186–87
rate increasers, 110
Rea, Tom D., 88, 100, 105, 128–29, 134–35
recordings. *See* digital recordings
regionalization, 148
registries of cardiac arrests: developing, 178–81; personnel for, 246n9; quality of, 136, 252n2. *See also* King County registry of cardiac arrests
report cards, community, 155–59, *157*, 250n7
reporting requirements, 58–59, 157, 200
rescue societies in Enlightenment Europe, 21–24, *22*
research centers, EMS, 202
researcher perspectives, 134–39
residential facilities, 191–92
respiration. *See* agonal respirations; airway management
respiratory diseases, 54
response times and time intervals: community differences, 138; CPR, time to start of, *96*, 96–97, 115, 127; CPR initiation, time of, 71, 72, 75; defibrillation, time to start of, *98*, 98–99, *99*, 127; defibrillation initiation, time of, 71; in King County registry of cardiac arrests,

70–75, *73*, *74*; in Seattle–King County EMS system, 126–27, 246n8
restaurants, 236n18
restrictive cardiomyopathy, 50, 51
resuscitation, history of: ancient, 19–21, *20*; changing roles for EMTs, dispatchers, and bystanders, 43; citizen training, 41–42; before CPR, 24–25; CPR, development of, 26–31, *30*; defibrillation, development of, 31–34, *33*; eighteenth-century, 21–24, *22*; mobile intensive care, 34–37; paramedic programs, development of, 37–41
resuscitation, withholding of. *See* end-of-life decisions
Resuscitation Academy, vii, 221–28
Resuscitation Outcomes Consortium (ROC): about, 202; CPR-defibrillation interaction and, 101; ITDs and, 111; *JAMA* study and, 6; Nichol and, 135; registry quality and, 136; trials, 254n26
rhythms. *See* heart rhythms
risk factors for heart disease, modification of, 170–71
risk factors for VF, 211–12
ROC. *See* Resuscitation Outcomes Consortium
Rochester, Minnesota, 6, 120, 132–34, 191
Royal Human Society, London, *22*, 23
Royal Victoria Hospital, Belfast, Northern Ireland, 36–37, *37*–38
ruptured aortic aneurysm, 12
rural systems, *131*, 132

S

Safar Peter, 27, 31, 113, 161–62, 167
salaries, 105–6, 247n11
salvage, 175
San Francisco Fire Department, 142–43
Sayre, Michael, 138–39, 248n26
Schellenbaum, G. D., 88
score card, 188
seasonality of cardiac arrests, 67
Seattle Fire Department, 41, 143

Seattle–King County EMS system: overview, 120–21; administrator perspectives on, 147–49; AED program, 191; CPR training in, 41–42; design (one system, six programs), 125–26; dispatcher perspectives on, 146–47; EMT perspectives on, 144–46; fire chief perspectives on, 141–44; foundation of, 122–25; funding, 246n10, 247n16; history of, 121–22; medical directors, 245n5; other types of systems compared to, 130–34, *131*; paramedic perspectives on, 139–41; protocol on withholding resuscitation for compelling reasons, 163–65; researcher perspectives on, 134–39; response times, 126–27, 246n8; structure (response, training, and medical QI), 126–30. *See also* King County registry of cardiac arrests

seizure activity, 239n33

sex, 61, 84

sexual activity and cardiac arrest, 69–70

shocks, stacked, 100

"show" resuscitations, 163, 251n6

Shy, B. D., 114

Sinclair, Terry, 144–46

single-tier systems, 130, *131*

Siscovick, David, 86

Society for Recovery of Drowned Persons, Amsterdam, 21–24, *22*, 232n25

socioeconomic status, 87–88

soft and hard factors, 136

sphere of authority, 103

St. Vincent's Hospital, Greenwich Village, New York City, 38–39

stacked shocks, 100

standards. *See* protocols (standing orders) and standards

standing orders. *See* protocols (standing orders) and standards

stimulants, 110

strategic plans, 249n34

stress, 236n10

strokes, 55

subclinical heart disease, 9

Subido, Cleo, 147

succinylcholine, 141, 248n27

"sudden," defined, 11–12

sudden cardiac arrest (sudden cardiac death): as death before its time, 161; defined, 11–14; examples cases, 1–5; as first manifestation of heart disease, 171, 234n2; heart disease with, 11; history of, 16–17; incidence and prevalence of, 235n4; magnitude of the problem, 5; male-to-female ratio for, 61; moment of, 14–15; in movies, 17–18; natural history of, 25; and paramedic system, development of, 39; three-phase model of, 97; VF, PEA, and asystole, 12–13. *See also* causes of sudden cardiac arrest; end-of-life decisions; King County registry of cardiac arrests

sudden death by drowning, 231n6

sudden infant death syndrome (SIDS), 56

surveillance of cardiac arrests. *See* King County registry of cardiac arrests

survival: overview, 80–84, *82–83*; case examples, 77–79; chain of, *151*, 151–55; communities differences in rates of, 6–8, *7*, 80–81, 120–21, 135, 138–39; definitions of, 6, 80, 240n38; formula for, 115–19, *117*, *118*; limits of, 137; paramedic skill levels and, 139; patient factors, 84–88; for PEA and asystole, 239n27; post-resuscitation care and, 193–94; reporting on rates of, 79–80; typical survivor characteristics, 75–76; voice recordings and, 136. *See also* event factors in survival; system factors in survival; therapy factors in survival rates

Swor, R. A., 84

sympathetic stimulation of the heart, 169

synchronization of AED clocks, 236n21

syncope (fainting), 52

system factors in survival: overview, 96; administrative support, 107–8; community programs for CPR training, 108–9; community programs for public access defibrillation, 109; CPR, quality of, system factors in survival (*continued*) 97–98; CPR, time to start of, *96*, 96–97, 115, 127, 155; CPR and defibrillation, interaction between, 100–101; defibrillation, quality of, 99–100; defibrillation, time to start of, *98*, 98–99, *99*, 127, 155; dispatcher-assisted telephone CPR, 104–5; EMS care, quality of, 105–6; EMS culture and organizational structure, 107; EMS system size, 103; EMS system type, 101–2; EMS training, quality of, 108; formula based on, 115–19, *117*, *118*; medical direction quality, 106; medical quality improvement (QI) programs, 106; number of responders, 103–4; paramedic-to-population ratio, 104

systolic heart failure, 49

T

Take Heart American program, 248n26

TANGO study, 244n73

targeted community score card, 188

tax incentives, 202

technology, paradox of, 177–78

telecommunicators. *See* dispatchers

telemetry, 40. *See also* digital recordings

telephone-assisted CPR, 43, 65, 104–5, 108–9, 146, 147, 182–84

television and movies, cardiac arrests in, 17–18, 172

terminal illness, 164. *See also* end-of-life decisions

therapy factors in survival rates, 137; overview, 109–10; airway management, quality of, 114; chest-compression-only CPR, 112–14; CPR adjuncts, 111–12; defibrillator-guided therapy, 110–11; formula based on, 115–19, *117*, *118*; hospital care, quality of, 115; hypothermia, use of, 114; impedance threshold devices, 111; pharmacotherapy at the scene, 110

three-phase model of cardiac arrest, 97

tiered-response systems: order of action, 103; other types compared to, 130–32,

131; in Seattle–King County, 41, 126; structure of, 102

time. *See* response times and time intervals

timing of cardiac arrests, *66*, 66–67, *67*, 90–91

tobacco smoke, 24

toolkits, 227

training: on AEDs, 43; certification of EMTs and paramedics, 127–28; on community report card, *157*; continuous education, 145–46, 147; on CPR, 31, 41–43, 65; of dispatchers, 147; of EMTs, 43; quality of EMS training, 108; in Seattle–King County EMS system, 43, 127–28; telephone CPR instructions as, 43

treadmill exercise test, 9

Trevino, Mario, 141–43, 149

triple-response system, 132–34

Tyerman, Aaron, 139–40

U

underlying coronary artery disease (atherosclerotic heart disease or ischemic heart disease), 45–46

underlying heart disease as cause of death, 44

United States Military, 27

unstable angina. *See* myocardial infarction (MI)

unwitnessed arrests, 62, 70–71, 113. *See also* witnesses

U.S. Department of Transportation (DOT), 128, 200, 254n21

Utstein Criteria, 80, 109, *179*, 179

V

Valley Communications Center, King County, 146

valvular heart disease, 53

ventilation. *See* mouth-to-mouth ventilation

ventricular fibrillation (VF): causes of, 211; coarse, medium, and fine, 15, 53–54; CPR, vital role of, 15–16; description of,

12; ECGs during, *33*; heart disease with cardiac arrest, 11; percent of cardiac arrests associated with, *63*, 63–64, *64*; prediction of, 212; reducing incidence of, 213–14; risk factors for, 211–12; survival rates, 6–8, *7*. *See also* causes of sudden cardiac arrest

VF. *See* ventricular fibrillation

Vickery, Gordon, 41, 123–24

victim characteristics, typical, 60–61

video recording, 187–88

Vioxx, 87

voice recordings, 136, 189–90

volunteer firefighters and EMTs, 4–5

vomiting. *See* emesis

W

Washington Association of Sheriffs and Police Chiefs (WASPC), 146

wave forms, defibrillatory, 215–16

wearable defibrillators, 217

Weisfeldt, M. L., 97

White, R. D., 86

White, Roger, 133–34

withholding of resuscitation, 203, 204. *See* end-of-life decisions

witnesses: cardiac arrests, witnessed and unwitnessed, 61–62, 239n28, 240n38; chest-compression-only CPR and, 113; CPR, likelihood of, 66; heart rhythms and, 64–65; survival rates and, 89, *90*, *91*; time intervals and, 70–71. *See also* bystanders

Wolff-Parkinson-White syndrome (WPW), 52, 53

women, 61, 84

Z

Zoll, Paul, 33–34